A Textbook of
Clinical Research and Pharmacovigilance

A Textbook of Clinical Research and Pharmacovigilance

K. P. R. Chowdary

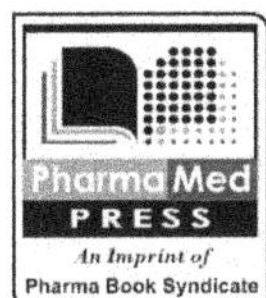

PharmaMed Press
An imprint of Pharma Book Syndicate
A unit of BSP Books Pvt. Ltd.
4-4-309/316, Giriraj Lane,
Sultan Bazar, Hyderabad - 500 095.

A Textbook of Clinical Research and Pharmacovigilance

by *K. P. R. Chowdary*

Published by

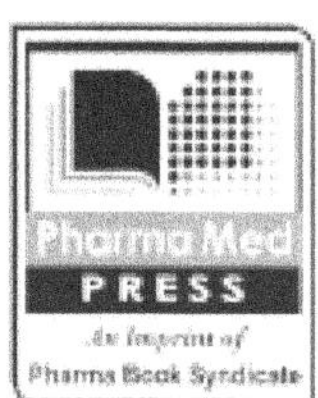

PharmaMed Press

An imprint of Pharma Book Syndicate

A unit of BSP Books Pvt. Ltd.

4-4-309/316, Giriraj Lane, Sultan Bazar, Hyderabad - 500 095.

Phone: 040-23445688; Fax: 91+40-23445611

e-mail: info@pharmamedpress.com

www.pharmamedpress.com/pharmamedpress.net

ISBN: 978-93-91910-51-8

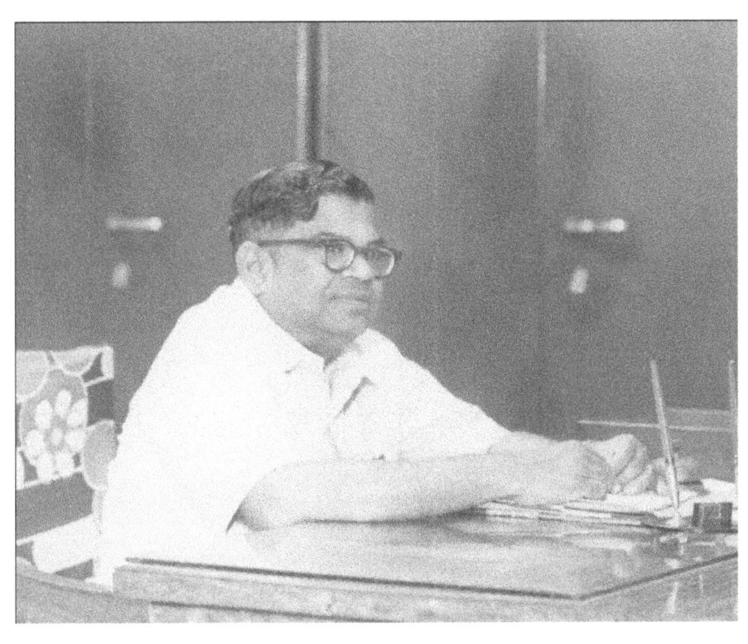

Dedicated to

My Teacher, Guide and Well Wisher

Prof. V. SUBBARAO

(1920-1990)

Preface

Clinical Research, Clinical Trials and Pharmacovigilance are essential and critical components of drug development research. Globally several regulations and guidelines are prescribed for Clinical Research and Clinical Trials by the Drug Regulatory Authorities and various governments to safeguard the health of patients and the human subjects participating in Clinical Trials. Voluminous literature has accumulated in this area making it difficult for pharmacy students and clinical research personnel to acquire good knowledge of the subject. The Pharmacy Council of India, New Delhi has also introduced courses on Clinical Research in the revised uniform syllabus prescribed for Pharm.D and M Pharm courses.

This book describes all concepts, practices, methods and regulatory guidelines related to clinical research, clinical trials and pharmacovigilance in a simple, lucid and easily understandable manner and covers the entire syllabus prescribed by Pharmacy Council of India (PCI) , New Delhi for Pharm.D and M. Pharm courses. The book provides a comprehensive knowledge of various aspects such as drug development and approval process, pharmacological and toxicological approaches and methods, pharmaceutical dosage form approaches for drug development, clinical approaches and clinical trials, phases, types, designs and statistical tests of clinical trials, regulatory aspects, GCP as per ICH, WHO, ICMR, Schedule Y and regulatory environment in US, Europe and India in 20 chapters. Special emphasis is given to Pharmacovigilance methods and Pharmacovigilance programme of India (PvPI). Latest practices and regulatory guidelines are included and hence the book provides updated knowledge.

This book is ideal for Pharm.D., M.Pharm, and Ph.D students of Pharmacy and also for research personnel involved in clinical research.

K. P. R. Chowdary

Author

Foreword

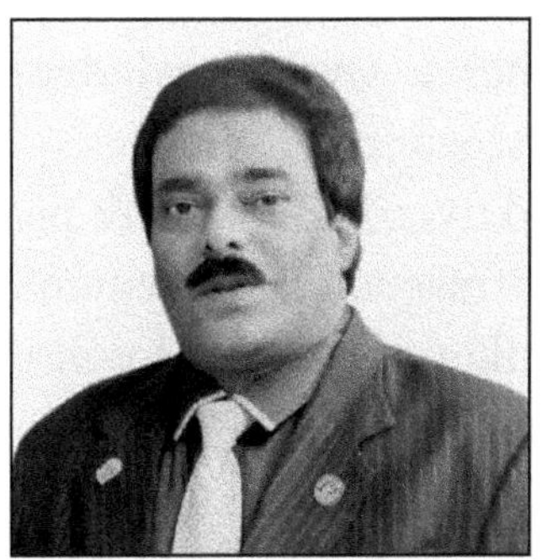

Dr. T. V. Narayana,
M.Pharm, PhD

National President
The Indian Pharmaceutical Association & President,
SEAR Pharm Forum & General Secretary, IPCA.

I am extremely happy and delighted to write the foreword to this textbook titled "Clinical Research and Pharmacovigilance" authored by Prof. K. P. R. Chowdary, one of the senior most teacher and researcher serving the pharmacy profession since five decades and associated in several professional activities. This textbook is a unique attempt by author, which fulfilled all the requirements of pharmacy students, teachers and clinical research personnel to acquire a comprehensive and updated knowledge of all aspects of clinical research, clinical trials and pharmacovigilance. The book was presented systematically and covers the entire syllabus prescribed by Pharmacy Council of India (PCI), New Delhi on clinical research with special emphasis on subjects of clinical trials, GCP, regulatory guidelines and pharmacovigilance of M.Pharm, Pharm.D and B.Pharm programmes. At present there is no comprehensive textbook available for this subject. I being the National President of Indian Pharmaceutical Association congratulate the author for his commendable efforts in bringing out this textbook on the most demanding and challenging area. I am sure that this textbook will be of immense use as ready reckoner and a great asset and I strongly recommend to all the students, teachers of pharmacy and as well as clinical research personnel.

With Best Wishes

(Dr. T. V. Narayana)

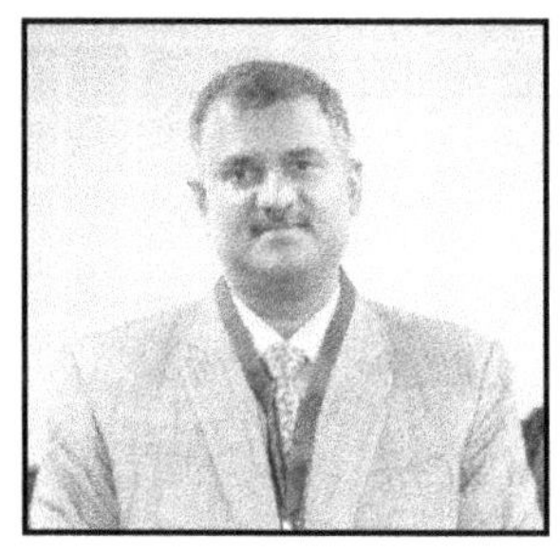

It gives me immense pleasure to write a foreword to this book "A Textbook of Clinical Research and Pharmacovigilance" authored by Prof. K. P. R. Chowdary, who has a vast knowledge & experience in the field of Pharmaceutical Sciences. The author has successfully guided over 100 PhD's & produced the pioneers in the field of Pharmaceutical Research & Practice. I am very glad that the author has done a lot of research in the areas of Clinical Research Methodology, Pharmacovigilance & Clinical Trials and put all of the information together meticulously in one book. I believe this is truly a distinctive book that would be extremely helpful to all PHARM.D, B.PHARM and M.PHARM students as well as Researchers in the field of Clinical Pharmacy & Practice. This book covers the entire syllabus for 4th & 5th Pharm.D Students for the Subjects Clinical Pharmacy, Research Methodology & Clinical Research as per the syllabus prescribed by Pharmacy Council of India, New Delhi. It also focuses on Comparison of Clinical Trial Regulations in India, Europe and USA which is very essential for budding Researchers working in our Pharmaceutical Companies as India is the world Capital for generic drugs. It also provides a lot of insight for carrying out project works in the hospitals by 5th Pharm.D students. I truly believe that this book will impart a lot of knowledge to its readers & I firmly recommend this book.

Hearty Greetings & Good Wishes!

Dr. Satheesh S. Gottipati, MS (USA), RPH (USA), CIP (USA)
Dean of Academics & Chief Preceptor
Department of Pharmacy Practice,
Vignan Pharmacy College, Vadlamudi, AP, India.

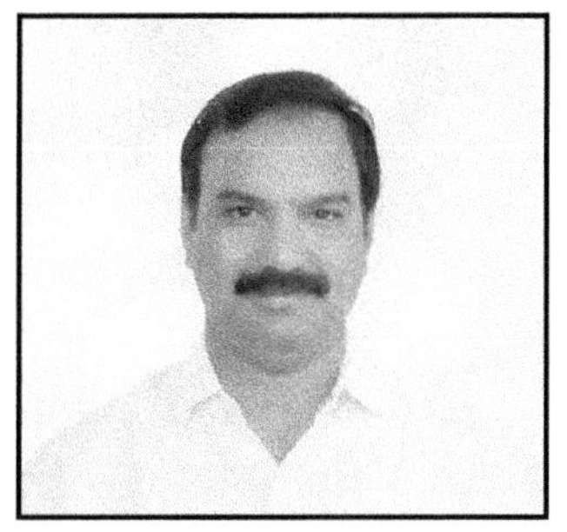

I feel very happy to write the Foreword to this textbook on Clinical Research and Pharmacovigilance authored by Prof. K. P. R. Chowdary who is having rich experience and expertise in teaching and research in pharmacy and clinical research. The book provides updated information on the principles, methods and regulatory guidelines of Clinical Research, Clinical Trials and Pharmacovigilance. The book is designed to aid the rapid and easy understanding of the subject by the students as well as industry persons involved in clinical research. The book covers all aspects and the entire syllabus prescribed by PCI, New Delhi for the subjects of clinical research, clinical trials and Pharmacovigilance for M. Pharm and Pharm. D programmes. I recommend this textbook to all pharmacy colleges and pharmacy students to acquire as it is a standard source of information. I congratulate the author for his efforts for bringing out this textbook on the most challenging and interesting subject of clinical research.

Dr. G. Vijaya Kumar
Professor & HOD of Pharmacy Practice
KVSR Siddhartha College of Pharmaceutical Sciences, Vijayawada

Contents

Dedication .... (v)

Preface .... (vii)

Foreword .... (ix)

Chapter 1

Drug Discovery, Development and Approval Process: An Overview 1

Chapter 2

Approaches to Drug Discovery (Pharmacological and Toxicological) 14

Chapter 3

Drug Characterization, Preformulation and Dosage Form Development 26

Chapter 4

The Investigational New Drug (IND) Application and New Drug Application (NDA) 46

Chapter 5

Clinical Development of Drugs – Introduction and Evolution of Clinical Research 58

Chapter 6

Clinical Research Methodology (Phases, Types, Designs and Statistical Concepts of Clinical Trials 66

Chapter 7

Clinical Trials Research in India (Clinical Trial Phases, Process, Documentation and Regulations) 85

Chapter 8

Methods of Post Marketing Surveillance (PMS) 100

Chapter 9

Abbreviated New Drug Application (ANDA) Submissions 113

Chapter 10

Guidelines and Principles of Good Clinical Practices (ICH & WHO) 133

Chapter 11

Comparison of Clinical Trial Regulations in India, Europe and USA 158

Chapter 12

Challenges in the Implementation of GCP Guidelines 175

Chapter 13

Ethical Guidelines in Clinical Research 179

Chapter 14

Composition, Role and Responsibilities of Institutional Ethics Committee (IEC) in Clinical Trials 191

Chapter 15

Regulatory Environment in US, India and Europe 195

Chapter 16

Role and Responsibilities of Clinical Trial Personnel as per GCP 210

Chapter 17

Designing of Clinical Study Documents and Informed Consent Process 219

Chapter 18

Data Management in Clinical Research 226

Chapter 19

Safety Monitoring in Clinical Trials 237

Chapter 20

Pharmacovigilance 251

Chapter 1

Drug Discovery, Development and Approval Process: An Overview

LEARNING OBJECTIVES

To understand

- Drug Discovery
- Methods for Drug Discovery
- Drug Development
- Steps Involved in Drug Development
- Preclinical Evaluation (Animal Studies)
- Clinical evaluation (Human Studies)
- Clinical Pharmacology
- Clinical Trials
- Drug Approval Process
- Drug Approval Process in United States
- Investigational New Drug (IND) Application
- New Drug Application (NDA)
- Abbreviated New Drug Application (ANDA)
- Drug Approval Process in Europe
- Drug Approval Process in India
- A Comparision of Drug Approval Process in US, Europe and India.

Introduction

In ancient time most of the drug used in the treatment of disease were derived from naturally occurring substances of plant origin, e.g. Opium from poppy, Quinine from cinchona, digitalis from foxglove. Presently, the majority of new therapeutics agent are synthetic in nature. Drug discovery and development is complex, time-consuming, costly process which carries commercial risk. Drug discovery and development is broadly divided into three main components:

i) drug discovery,

ii) preclinical evaluation,

iii) clinical trials.

Drug Discovery

Typically, researchers discover new drugs by the following methods:

i) Through new insights into a disease process that allow researchers to design a product to stop or reverse the effects of the disease.

ii) Through many tests of molecular compounds to find possible beneficial effects against a disease

iii) Through existing treatments that have unanticipated effects.

iv) Through new technologies that provide new ways to target products to specific diseases.

At this stage in the process, thousands of compounds may be potential candidates for development in to an effective and safe drug. After initial pharmacological and toxicity testing only a small number of compounds look promising and call for further studies.

Development: Once researchers identify a promising compound for development, they conduct experiments to gather information on: How it is absorbed, distributed, metabolized, and excreted. Its potential benefits and mechanisms of action. The best way to give the drug (such as by mouth or injection).

Side effects or adverse events that can often be referred to as toxicity. How it affects different groups of people (such as by gender, race or ethnicity) differently. How it interacts with other drugs and treatments. Its effectiveness as compared with similar drugs.

Methods for Drug Discovery

1. Random screening
2. Molecular manipulation
3. Molecular designing
4. Metabolites of drug
5. Serendipity

1. ***Random screening*:** In this procedure new chemical entities are subjected to battery of screening test designed to determine diff. types of biological activity. Such test include studies on animal behaviour. Isolated tissues, intact animal and sometimes even an animal models of disease. Such studies are time consuming, expensive and have a low yield. It is possible that the new drug thus found may be ultimately turn out to be similar in extraction to already existing drugs, with no added advantages.

2. ***Molecular manipulation***: In this procedure analogues of existing drugs are synthesized and tested for their biological activity. This is more logical approach and may yield new compounds with certain advantages like better absorption, greater potency, more selective action, fewer side effects.

3. ***Molecular designing***: This is the most rational form of drug R & D. It ends at designing of substances to fulfill of specific biological task. In its simplest form this may involve the synthesis of naturally occurring substance, a hormone, a vitamin o a precursor of a neurotransmitter. **e.g**. dopamine for cardiogenic shock, levodopa for parkinsonism.

4. ***Metabolites of Drug***: Sometimes active metabolites of drug are found to posses therapeutic advantages over parent compound. e.g. Paracetmol is metabolite of phenacetin and it is effective as an analgesic but does not cause renal damage.

5. ***Serendipity***: it means "happy observation by chance" and has led to introduction of many remedies in the past. *e.g.* use of organomercurials for cardiac oedema, penicillin as an antibacterial agent.

Drug Development

Once a new chemical entity is discovered it has to be subjected to the development process. Chemical synthetic activity is mostly carried out in R&D divisions of p'ceutical lab by synthetic chemistry. After synthesis the structure of new compound and its purity is determine and confirmed by analytical chemist.

Pharmacological evaluations can be divided into –

i) preclinical pharmacology and

ii) clinical pharmacology

Steps Involved in Drug Development

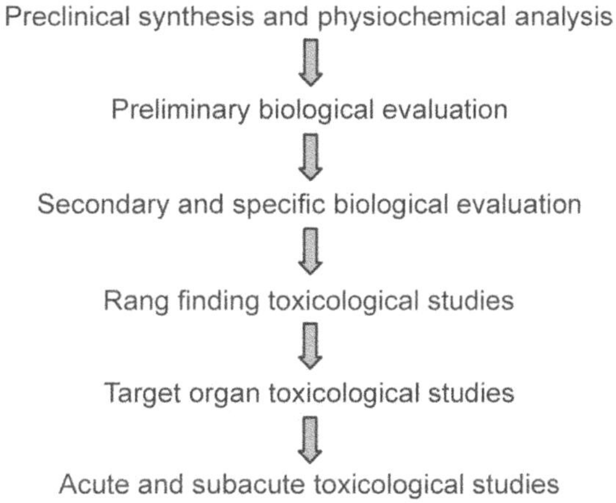

Preclinical synthesis and physiochemical analysis

⇩

Preliminary biological evaluation

⇩

Secondary and specific biological evaluation

⇩

Rang finding toxicological studies

⇩

Target organ toxicological studies

⇩

Acute and subacute toxicological studies

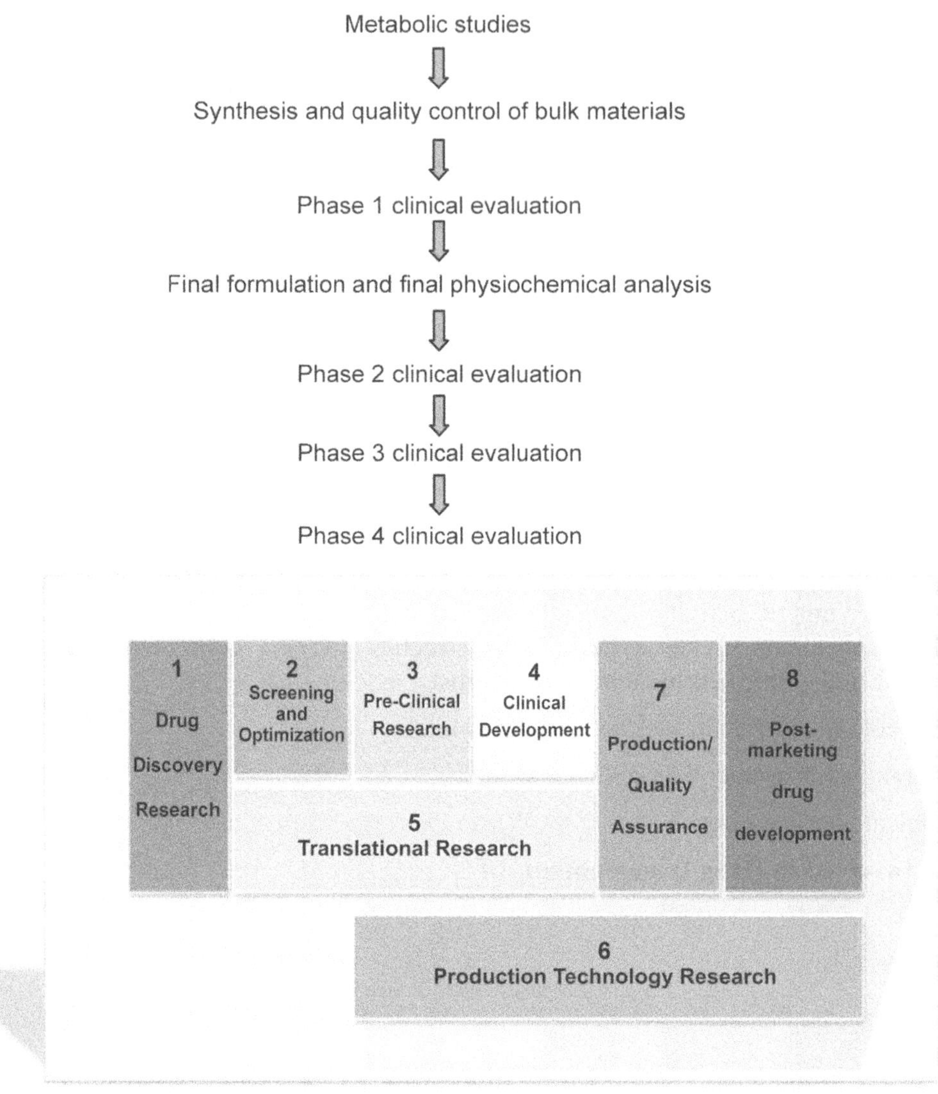

Fig.1.1 Various Stages in Drug Discovery Development and Approval Process.

Preclinical Evaluation (Animal Studies)

Before testing a drug in people, researchers must find out whether it has the potential to cause serious harm, also called toxicity. The two types of preclinical research are: -*In Vitro, In Vivo*. FDA requires researchers to use good laboratory practices (GLP), defined in medical product development regulations, for preclinical laboratory studies.

Usually, preclinical studies are not very large. However, these studies must provide detailed information on dosing and toxicity levels. After preclinical testing, researchers review their findings and decide whether the drug should be tested in people. The experimental animals used for preclinical testing include mice, rats, guinea pigs dogs, and sometimes monkeys.

The three major areas of preclinical evaluation are:

1. Acute, sub acute and chronic toxicity studies
2. Therapeutic index.
3. Absorption, distribution and elimination studies

Clinical Evaluation (Human Studies)

Preclinical data obtained from animal studies provide a general pharmacological, toxicological, and pharmacokinetic profile of a new drug. The New Drug application in the prescribed format, with all relevant literature and preclinical data must be submitted to Drug Control Authority for scrutiny, and sanction obtained before ***clinical evaluation*** studies are initiated.

Clinical Pharmacology

Clinical pharmacology deals with the effect of drugs on body and the effect of body on drugs in man, i.e. the *pharmacokinetic* and *pharmacodynamics studies in man.*

It has three distinct part:

1. Confirmatory pharmacology
2. Human biotransformation studies
3. Clinical trials.

Sir Bradford Hill (1966) defined a clinical trial as

"A carefull and ethnically designed human experiment with the aim of answering some precisely framed questions".

This definition is valid even today.

Clinical Trials

Here are some salient guidelines to design a perfect clinical trial:

1. **Ethics and patient selection:** Criteria for **selection of patient** should be well thought out and defined. Special care must be taken if more than one doctor is involved in the selection of patient in the trial specially in multicentric trials
2. **Response measurement:** The end point should be clearly defined. Side effect should be carefully observed and recorded.
3. **Experimental design:** For the design of an experimental design preferably a biostatistician should be consulted.

(a) In general, *controlled clinical trials* must include four safe guards against bias: double blind technique

(b) Randomization of treatment

(c) Matching of patient

(d) Cross over techniques.

Phases of Clinical Trials

- Phase I: Clinical pharmacologic Evaluation
- Phase II: Controlled clinical evaluation
- Phase III: Extended clinical Evaluation
- Phases IV: Surveillance during post marketing

Phase I:

Phase I are usually carried out on 20-50 healthy volunteers or patients, depending on class of drug and it's safety. This studies are mainly concerned with human toxicity, tolerated dosage range, pharmacological actions, and pharmacokinetics of drug.

Phase II:

These studies are carried out on 50-300 patients. These studies mainly aim to ascertain the safety and efficacy of the new drug, and are strictly controlled.

Phase III: Extended clinical Evaluation

These are formal therapeutic trials carried out in double blind Controlled manner in 250-100 patients. Efficacy and safety of the new drug is evaluated and even comparison with other drugs is undertaken.

Phase IV: Surveillance during Post marketing

After the drug release for general clinical use, certain unusual type of adverse reactions may be observed even after years of clinical usage. Thus, an adverse reaction monitoring is carried out in Phase IV evaluation.

For Further Reading

1. Pharmacology-I, Essential of pharmacotherapeutics, By F.S.K.Barar S.chand publication, 1st edition, 1985, Page no: 56-61 2
2. https://googleweblight.com/i?u=https://www.nature.com/subjects/drug discovery & grqid=DEji1MmA&hl=en-IN
3. https://googleweblight.com/i?u=https://www.slideshare.net/mobile/rahu l_pharma/drug discovery-and-development- 10698574&grqid=dRB10k76&hl=en-IN

DRUG APPROVAL PROCESS

Developing a new drug requires great amount of research work in chemistry, molecular biology, biochemistry, preformulation and formulation development, process development and manufacturing, quality control, preclinical and clinical studies. Drug regulatory agencies globally bear the responsibility of evaluating whether the research data support the safety, effectiveness and quality control of a new drug product to serve the public health. Every country has its own regulatory authority, which is responsible to enforce the rules and regulations and issue the guidelines to regulate the marketing of the drugs. Different countries have different regulatory requirements for approval of new drug. For IND, NDA or marketing authorization application (MAA) a single regulatory approach applicable to various countries is almost a difficult task, not available at present. Therefore it is necessary to have knowledge about regulatory requirements for drug approval process of each country.

The new drug approval process consists of two stages, the first stage is for IND and the second stage is for NDA and marketing authorization of drug. Firstly, non-clinical studies of drug are completed to ensure safety and efficacy. The next step is the submission of application for conduction of clinical trials to competent authority of respective country. In next step, clinical trials are carried out in four phases i.e. phase 1 to phase 4 study. These studies are carried out for the assurance of safety, efficacy and for optimization of dose of drug in human being. Then application for marketing of drug is verified by competent authorities. The competent authority review the application and approve the drug for marketing purpose, only if that drug is found to be safe and effective with desired therapeutic effect. The drug approval process in various countries is reviewed below.

Drug Approval Process in United States

The United States has the world's most stringent standards for approving new drugs. Drug approval standards in the United States are considered to be the most demanding in the world.[1-3]

Investigational New Drug (IND) Application

It's an application filed to the FDA in order to start clinical trials in humans if the drug was found to be safe from the reports of Preclinical trials. A firm or institution, called a Sponsor, is responsible for submitting the IND application.[4] A pre - IND meeting can be arranged with the FDA to discuss a number of issues like the design of animal research, which is required to lend support to the clinical studies, the intended protocol for conducting the clinical trial, the chemistry, manufacturing, and control of the investigational drug. Such a meeting will help the Sponsor to organize animal research, gather data, and design the clinical protocol based on suggestions by the FDA.

New Drug Application (NDA)

If clinical studies confirm that a new drug is relatively safe and effective, and will not pose unreasonable risks to patients, the manufacturer files a New Drug Application (NDA), the actual request to manufacture and sell the drug in the United States.[5-6]

Abbreviated New Drug Application (ANDA)

It's an application made for approval of Generic Drugs. The sponsor is not required to reproduce the clinical studies that were done for the original, brand name product. Instead, generic drug manufacturers must demonstrate that their product is the same as, and bioequivalent to, a previously approved brand name product.[7]For human testing in clinical trials Phase 1 studies (typically involve 20-80 people) Phase 2 studies (typically involve a few dozen to about 300 people). Phase 3 studies (typically involve several hundred to about 3,000 people). The pre-NDA period, just before a new drug application (NDA) is submitted, is a common time for the FDA and drug sponsors to meet Submission of an NDA is the formal step the FDA takes to consider a drug for marketing approval 8. After an NDA is received, the FDA has 60 days to decide whether to file it so it can be reviewed 9. If the FDA files the NDA, an FDA review team is assigned to evaluate the sponsor's research on the drug's safety and effectiveness. The FDA reviews information that goes on a drug's professional labeling (information on how to use the drug). The FDA inspects the facilities where the drug will be manufactured as part of the approval process. FDA reviewers will approve the application or find it either "approvable" or "not approvable"

Preclinical: Computer simulations, experimental animal studies, or *in vitro* studies are performed to identify a promising drug, test for promising biologic effects and test for adverse effects. A drug company may test many related compounds to identify 1 or 2 to take further in development. The FDA is not involved in this aspect of drug development but will review the study results for any compounds that are planned for clinical (human) testing.

New Drug Application (NDA): The IND is the formal process by which a sponsor requests approval for testing of a drug in humans and includes information developed during preclinical testing regarding safety and effectiveness. There are 3 phases in clinical testing of a new drug

Phase I studies are usually conducted in healthy volunteers. The emphasis in Phase I is on safety. The goal is to determine what the drug's most frequent side effects are often, to determine how the drug is absorbed, distributed, and excreted. The number of subjects typically ranges from 20 to 80.

The emphasis in Phase II is on effectiveness. The goal of a Phase II study is to obtain preliminary data on whether the drug works in people who have a specific disease or condition. For controlled trials, patients receiving the drug are compared with similar patients receiving a placebo or a different drug. Safety continues to be evaluated and short-term side effects are studied. Typically, the number of subjects in Phase II studies ranges from a few dozen to about 300 after Phase II.

At the end of Phase II, the FDA and sponsors negotiate about how the large-scale studies in Phase III should be done. The FDA usually meets with a sponsor several times, including prior to Phase III studies, and pre-NDA right before a new drug application is submitted.

All biologic agents or other products made using high-technology procedures. Products for HIV/AIDS, cancer, diabetes, neurodegenerative diseases, auto-immune and other immune dysfunctions and viral diseases. Products for orphan conditions.

Drug Approval Process in Europe

National authorization procedure: Each country within the EU has its own procedures for authorizing a marketing application for a new drug. A sponsor can consult the website of the regulatory agency in each country in which it is interested in obtaining marketing approval to obtain details of the approval process. A sponsor can also seek approval of several EU countries simultaneously using the decentralized or mutual recognition procedure.

Decentralized procedure: For products that fall outside the scope of the European Medicines Agency (EMA) with regard to centralized procedures, a sponsor can submit under the decentralized procedure. Using this process, a sponsor can apply for simultaneous authorization in more than one EU country for products that have not yet been authorized in any EU country. Mutual recognition procedure. With the mutual recognition procedure, a product is first authorized by one country in the EU in accordance with the national procedures of that country. Later, further marketing authorizations can be sought from other EU countries, who, rather than conducting their own review, agree to recognize the decision of the first country.

Centralized procedure: European drug approvals are overseen by the European Medicines Agency. The EMA is a decentralized body of the EU, with headquarters in London, England. It is responsible for the scientific evaluation of applications for authorization to market medicinal products in Europe (via the centralized procedure). Marketing applications for drugs for use in humans are evaluated by the Committee for Medicinal Products for Human Use (CHMP). Products that are eligible for review under the centralized procedure must meet the following criteria.

1. Biologic drugs developed by recombinant technology, controlled expression of genes coding for biologically active proteins in prokaryotes and eukaryotes including transformed mammalian cells, and hybridoma and monoclonal antibody methods medicinal products containing new active substances for the following indications: AIDS, cancer, neurodegenerative disorders, diabetes, autoimmune diseases and other immune dysfunctions, and viral diseases

2. Orphan medicinal products other new active substances may, at the request of the applicant, be accepted for consideration under the centralized procedure when it can be shown that the product constitutes a significant therapeutic, scientific or technical innovation, or the granting of a Community authorization is in the best interests of patients at the Community level.

Pre-submission process: At least seven months prior to submitting a marketing authorization application (MAA), a sponsor must notify the EMA of their intention to submit and the month of submission. This pre-submission involves a variety of information including a document outlining the reasons the sponsor believes the application should fall under the centralized procedure. The EMA will consider the pre-submission and notify the sponsor of its decision regarding acceptance of the MAA.

Selection of rapporteur/co-rapporteur: The rapporteur is a country-specific regulatory authority within the EU. The rapporteur (reviewer) and co-rapssporteur (if needed) are identified from the CHMP members. The selection of the rapporteur is based on objective criteria, to ensure objective scientific opinion and the best use of available expertise at the EMA. The role of the rapporteur is to perform the scientific evaluation and prepare an assessment report to the CHMP. If a co-rapporteur is involved, the co-rapporteur will prepare an independent assessment report, or provide a critique of the rapporteur's report, at the discretion of the CHMP. The process for assigning the rapporteur/co-rapporteur is usually initiated at the CHMP meeting following the receipt of a letter of an intention to submit. The sponsor is notified of the rapporteur/co-rapporteur once the EMA has deemed a submission admissible.

Product naming: A sponsor's name for the drug product should be the same in all countries within the EU, except where it violates trademark rules. The sponsor should submit the proposed name in advance (usually four to six months, and not more than 12 months) of the marketing authorization application.

Drug Approval Process in India

Passed by the India's parliament to regulate the import, manufacture, distribution and sale of drugs and cosmetics. The Central Drugs Standard Control Organization (CDSCO) and the office of its leader, the Drugs Controller General (India) [DCGI] was established. In 1988, the Indian government added Schedule Y to the Drug and Cosmetics Rules 1945. Schedule Y provides the guidelines and requirements for clinical trials, which was further revised in 2005 to bring it at par with internationally accepted procedure. The changes includes, establishing definitions for Phase I–IV trials and clear responsibilities for investigators and sponsors. The clinical trials were further divided into two categories in 2006. In one category (category A) clinical trials can be conducted in other markets with competent and mature regulatory systems whereas the remaining ones fall in to another category (category B) Other than A. Clinical trials of category A (approved in the U.S., Britain, Switzerland, Australia, Canada, Germany, South Africa, Japan and European Union) are eligible for fast tracking in India, and are likely to be approved within eight weeks. The clinical trials of category B are under more scrutiny, and approve within 16 to 18 weeks. An application to conduct clinical trials in India should be submitted along with the data of chemistry, manufacturing, control and animal studies to DCGI. The date regarding the trial protocol, investigator's brochures, and informed consent documents should also be attached. A copy of the application must be submitted to the ethical committee and the clinical trials are conducted only after approval of DCGI and ethical committee. To determine the maximum tolerated dose in humans, adverse reactions, etc. on healthy human volunteers, Phase I clinical trials are conducted. The therapeutic uses and effective dose ranges are determined in Phase II trials in 10-12 patients at each dose level. The confirmatory trials (Phase III) are conducted to generate data regarding the efficacy and safety of the drug in ~ 100 patients (in 3-4 centers) to confirm efficacy and safety claims. Phase III trials should be conducted on a minimum of 500 patients spread across 10-15 centers, If the new drug substance is not marketed in any other country. The new drug registration (using Form 44 along with full pre-clinical and clinical testing information) is applied after the completion of clinical trials. The comprehensive information on the marketing status of the drug in other countries is also required other than the information on safety and efficacy. The information regarding the prescription, samples and testing protocols, product monograph, labels, and cartons must also be submitted. The application can be reviewed in a range of about 12-18 months. Figure represents the new drug approval process of India. After the NDA approval, when a company is allowed to distribute and market the product, it is considered to be in Phase IV trials or pharmacovigilance.

A Comparision of Drug Approval Process Requirements in US, Europe and India

A comparision of Drug approval process requirements in US, Europe and India is shown in Tables 1-5.

Table 1.1 Comparison of Drug Approval Process Requirements in US, Europe and India (Administrative Requirements)

S.No.	REQUIREMENT	US FDA	EUROPEAN	INDIA
1.	Application	ND/NDA/ANDA	MAA	IND/MAA
2.	Number of copies	3	1	1
3.	Approval Timeline	18 months	12 months	12 months
4.	Fees	No Fees	10-20 Lakh	Rs 50,000
5.	Presentation	e CTD , Paper	e CTD, Paper	Paper

Table 1.2 Comparison of Drug Approval Process Requirements in US, Europe and India (Finished Product Control Requirements)

S.NO	REQUIREMENT	US FDA	EUROPEAN	INDIA
1.	Justification	ICH Q6A	ICH Q6A	-
2.	Assay	90-100%	95-105%	90-110%
3.	Disintegration	Not Required	Required	Required
4.	Color Identification	Not Required	Not Required	Required
5.	Water Content	Required	Not Required	Required

Table 1.3 Comparison of Drug Approval Process Requirements in US, Europe and India (Manufacturing and Control Requirements)

S.NO	REQUIREMENT	US FDA	EUROPEAN	INDIA
1.	Number of batches	1	3	3
2.	Packaging	A minimum of 1,00,000 units	Not Required	Not Adressed
3.	Process validation	Not required at the time of submission	Required	Required
4.	Batch size	Minimum of 1,00,000 units	Minimum of 1,00,000 units	3 pilot scale

Table 1.4 Comparison of Drug Approval Process Requirements in US, Europe and India (Stability Requirements)

S.NO	REQUIREMENT	US FDA	EUROPEAN	INDIA
1.	Number of batches	1	2	3
2.	Condition	25^0/60-40^0/75 RH	25^0/60-40^0/75 RH	30^0/35-30^0/75 RH
3.	Date & time of Submission	3 months accelerate &3 months long term	6 months accelerate& 6 months long term	6 months accelerate & 3 months long term
4.	Container Orientation	Inverted & upright	-------	Packing which simulate the final packaging for storage &distribution
5.	Clause	21 CFR part 210&211	Guidelines for medicinal products	ICH QF

Table 1.5 Comparison of Drug Approval Process Requirements in US, Europe and India (Bioequivalence Requirements)

S.NO	REQUIREMENT	USFDA	EUROPEAN	INDIA
1	CRO	Audited by FDA	Audited by MHRA	Audited by CDSCO
2	Reserve Sample	5 times the sample required for analysis	No such requirement	-----
3	Fasted/Fed	Must be as per OGD recommendation	No such requirement	As per CDSCO recommendation
4	Retention of samples	5 years from date of filling the application	No such requirement	3 years from the date of filling the application

For Further Reading

1. Rick NG, Drugs from discovery to approval. 2nd ed., John Wiley & Sons, Inc., (Hoboken, New Jersey). p.201.
2. Rick NG, Drugs from discovery to approval. 2nd ed., John Wiley & Sons, Inc., (Hoboken, New Jersey). p.202.
3. IRA R Berry, Robert P Martin, Editors, The Pharmaceutical Regulatory Process. 2nd ed., Informa Healthcare. p.45.
4. Rick NG, Drugs from discovery to approval. 2nd ed., John Wiley & Sons, Inc.,(Hoboken, New Jersey). p.203-4.
5. Rick NG, Drugs from discovery to approval. 2nd ed., John Wiley & Sons, Inc.,(Hoboken, New Jersey). p.205-7.
6. Rick NG, Drugs from discovery to approval. 2nd ed., John Wiley & Sons, Inc., (Hoboken, New Jersey). p. 208-10.
7. IRA R Berry, Robert P Martin, Editors, The Pharmaceutical Regulatory Process, 2nd ed., Informa Healthcare. p.46.

Chapter 2

Approaches to Drug Discovery (Pharmacological and Toxicological)

LEARNING OBJECTIVES

To understand

- Pharmacological Approaches to Drug Development
- Types of Pharmacological Studies

  (Research pharmacology studies, Primary pharmacology studies, secondary pharmacology studies, Safety pharmacology studies)
- Timing of Safety Pharmacology Studies in Relation to Clinical Development
- Toxicological Approach to Drug Development
- Outline of Typical Safety Program
- Systemic Toxicity Studies
- Doses for Carcinogenicity studies may be based one of the following;
- Duration of toxicity studies
- Factors in Designing Toxicity Studies
- Compound Libraries
- Systemic Toxicity Studies

  (Single dose study (Acute toxicity studies), Repeated-dose systemic toxicity studies, Male Fertility Studies, Female Reproduction and Developmental Toxicity Studies, Teratogenicity Study, Perinatal Study, Local Toxicity, Genotoxicity, Chronic toxicity studies, Carcinogenicity, special toxicity study)

Pharmacological Approaches

Pharmacology is a scientific discipline that specializes in the mechanism of action, uses and undesired effects of drugs. Pharmacological studies should be conducted to support use of therapeutics in humans. In the early stages of drug development enough information may not be available to rationally select study design for safety assessment. In such a situation, a general approach to safety pharmacology studies can be applied. Animal pharmacology testing provides the initial conformation that the molecular targets is involved in a metabolic pathway or integrated physiological process that is abnormal in the disease state. Animal pharmacology studies allow the effects of the lead compound on the disease process (Pharmacodynamic) to be correlated with the concentration of compound need to achieve these effects (Pharmacokinetics). If the results of the tests suggest potential beneficial activity, related compounds are tested to see which version of the molecule produces the highest level of pharmacological activity and demonstrates the most therapeutic promise, with the smallest number of potentially harmful biological properties.

Types of Pharmacological Studies

- ➢ Research pharmacology studies
- • Primary pharmacology studies
- • secondary pharmacology studies
- ➢ Safety pharmacology studies

Unlike primary and secondary pharmacology studies that explore the mode of action of the candidate drug and its effects related or unrelated to the therapeutic target, respectively, Safety Pharmacology identifies the "potential undesirable pharmacodynamic effects of a substance on physiological functions in relation to exposure in the therapeutic range and above" which are not identified by standard non-clinical toxicological studies.

Safety pharmacology studies are, therefore, performed to ensure the safety of clinical participants in first in human (FiH) trials through improved decision-making in the selection of lead candidate drugs.

1. Research pharmacological studies

- ➢ Research pharmacological studies are conducted at the starting of a drug development program. They need to be performed to GLP standards. There are two types:

a) Primary research pharmacology studies
b) Secondary research pharmacology studies

Primary Research Pharmacology Studies

Primary actions are related to proposed therapeutic use. These studies focus on the mechanism of action of drug and can be conducted *in vitro* and *in vivo.* Studies conducted *in vitro* include radiology and binding studies and focus on drugs action on specific receptor sites. Studies conducted *in vivo* investigate the pharmacological action of the drug in animal models.

Secondary Research Pharmacology Studies

Secondary actions focus on the overall pharmacological activity of the drug compound. And also relates to the actions that occur which is not directly related to the proposed therapeutic use. This can be conducted *in vitro* and *in vivo*. *In vitro* studies investigate the binding of the drug molecule with the non-target receptors. *In vivo* studies investigate the general pharmacological actions in animal models.

2. Safety pharmacology studies:

Safety pharmacology studies are studies that investigate potential undesirable pharmacodynamic effects of a substance on physiological functions in relation to exposure within the therapeutic range or above. Safety pharmacology studies investigate potentially undesirable effects of the drug compound. They are conducted in animal models, that are single dose studies using intended therapeutic dose.

In vitro studies should be designed to establish a concentration-effect relationship. The range of concentrations used should be selected to increase the likelihood of detecting an effect on the test system. The upper limit of this range may be influenced by physicochemical properties of the test substance and other assay specific factors.

In vivo safety pharmacology studies should be designed to define the dose- response relationship of the adverse effect observed. When feasible, the time course (e.g. onset and duration of response) of the adverse effect should be investigated.

The essential safety pharmacology is to study the effects of the test drug on vital functions. Vital organ systems such as cardiovascular, respiratory and central nervous systems should be studied.

Examples

CVS	blood pressure, heart rate, and the electrocardiogram.
CNS	motor activity, behavioural changes, coordination, sensory and motor reflex responses and body temperature
RS	tidal volume and haemoglobin oxygen saturation should be studied.

Supplemental Safety Pharmacology Studies

Required to investigate the possible adverse pharmacological effects that are not assessed in the essential safety pharmacological studies and are a cause for concern.

CVS	ventricular contractility, vascular resistance and the effects of chemical mediators, their agonists and antagonists on CVS
CNS	learning and memory, electrophysiology studies , neurochemistry and ligand binding studies.
RS	airway resistance, compliance, pulmonary arterial pressure, blood gases and blood pH.
Urinary system	urine volume, specific gravity, osmolality, pH, proteins, cytology and BUN, creatinine and plasma proteins estimation.
ANS	binding to receptors relevant for the autonomic nervous system, and functional response to agonist or antagonist responses *in vivo* or *in vitro,* and effects of direct stimulation of autonomic nerves and their effects on cardiovascular responses

GIS	gastric secretion, gastric pH measurement, gastric mucosal examination, bile secretion, gastric emptying time *in vivo* and ileocaecal contraction *in vitro.*
Others	Effects of the investigational drug on organ systems not investigated elsewhere should be assessed when there is a cause for concern. For example dependency potential, skeletal muscle, immune and endocrine functions may be investigated.

Safety Pharmacology Studies are usually not required when:

- Product is to be used for local application, e.g. dermal or ocular
- The pharmacology of the investigational drug is well known
- Systemic absorption from the site of application is low
- Safety pharmacology testing is also not necessary, in case of a new derivative having similar pharmacokinetics and pharmacodynamics.
- For biotechnology-derived products that achieve highly specific receptor targeting.

Timing of Safety Pharmacology Studies In Relation To Clinical Development

1. **Prior to First Administration in Humans**

   The effects of an investigational drug on the vital functions listed in the essential safety pharmacology should be studied prior to first administration in humans.

2. **During Clinical Development**

   Additional investigations may be warranted to clarify observed or suspected adverse effects in animals and humans during clinical development

3. **Before applying for marketing Approval**

   Follow-up and supplemental safety pharmacology studies should be assessed prior to approval unless not required, in which case this should be justified. Available information from toxicology studies addressing safety pharmacology endpoints or information from clinical studies can replace such studies.

4. **Application of Good Laboratory Practices (GLP)**

➢ The animal studies be conducted in an accredited laboratory. Where the safety pharmacology studies are part of toxicology studies, these studies should also be conducted in an accredited laboratory.

For Further Reading

1. Drug Discovery and Clinical Research - SK Guptha
2. https://www.fda.gov/ForPatients/Approvals/Drugs/ucm405382.htm
3. https://www.researchgate.net/profile/Dominic_Williams2/publication/23701632 5_Safety_pharmacology_-
4. _Current_and_emerging_concepts/links/59e07a4d45851537161225d5/Safety-pharmacology-Current-and-emerging-concepts.pdf
5. https://prezi.com/g95fbzxyu6fi/various-approaches-to-drug-discovery/
6. New drug development –design methodology & analysis by J. Rick Turner.

TOXICOLOGICAL APPROACH TO DRUG DEVELOPMENT

Toxicology is defined as the study of adverse effects of xenobiotic. Toxicology has evolved into three professional areas. Mechanistic toxicology deals with identifying and understanding mechanisms associated with toxic effects. Descriptive toxicology is toxicology testing to provide information for safety assessment & regulatory requirement. Regulatory toxicology deals with risk assessment based on the data generated by descriptive and mechanistic toxicity studies. Once a compound has evolved to lead status, its safety has to be evaluated in suitable in-vitro and in-vivo models. Toxicologists in pharmaceutical developments must properly design the toxicity studies to characterize the toxicity of a compound. It requires the highest possible dose be given for an adequate period of time to elicit a toxic response. The purpose of the toxicity studies in pharmaceutical development is to provide data in animals that can be used to assess the safety of a compound for human use. To accomplish this requires knowledge of toxic effects of a compound.

OUTLINE OF TYPICAL SAFETY PROGRAM

- A typical non-clinical safety program requires a 'staged approach'.
- With the staged approach, non clinical toxicity studies required to support the next clinical phase are conducted and the data made available prior to initiation of that clinical phase, the so-called "just in time" approach to clinical development.
- For the 1st dose in human study, the non clinical safety program generally consists of **single dose toxicity studies** (two species), **repeated-dose toxicity studies** (two species: one rodent &one non rodent), local tolerance (generally part of the repeated-dose toxicity studies), and Genotoxicity (Ames test: bacterial mutation assay and in vitro chromosomal damage with mammalian cells or in vitro mouse lymphoma assay) studies.
- These studies usually provide sufficient information to allow dose for 1st phase I study.

Systemic Toxicity Studies include

a) Single dose study (Acute toxicity studies)

b) Repeated-dose systemic toxicity studies

c) Male Fertility Studies

d) Female Reproduction and Developmental Toxicity Studies

e) Teratogenicity Study

f) Perinatal Study

g) Local Toxicity

h) Genotoxicity

i) Chronic toxicity studies

j) Carcinogenicity

k) special toxicity study

- As the data becomes available from the initial toxicity studies, the toxicologist assesses the findings, reassesses the clinical development plan, and prepares for the next toxicity studies.
- These studies involve the conduct of long term repeated-dose toxicity, reproductive toxicity, and in vivo Genotoxicity studies.
- The duration of the repeated-dose studies is dependent upon the duration of the clinical studies and the phase of clinical development.
- While the longer term repeated-dose toxicity studies are being conducted, reproduction and additional Genotoxicity studies are initiated.
- In all regions, male and female fertility studies, embryo-fetal development, and pre/postnatal development studies are required prior to marketing approval.
- Also concurrent with the conduct of long-term repeated-doses toxicity and reproduction toxicity studies, the remaining study in the standard battery of Genotoxicity studies, the in-vivo test for chromosomal damage using rodent hematopoietic cells, should be conducted.
- This is an in-vivo rodent micronucleus assay, which should be completed prior to initiation of phase 2 clinical studies.
- **Chronic toxicity studies** consist of 6-month studies in rodents and 9 or 12 month toxicity studies in non-rodents.
- This is required only when the duration of clinical use of drug is greater than 3 months.
- **Carcinogenicity studies** are required for drugs intended for continuous use for at least 6 months and /or there is a cause for concern.

Causes for concern include:

- Evidence of carcinogenicity in the compound class
- SAR suggesting carcinogenic risk
- Evidence of pre-neoplastic lesions in repeated-dose toxicity studies
- Long-term tissue retention of parent compound and/or metabolites resulting in local tissue reactions.

Doses for carcinogenicity studies may be based one of the following;

- Comparison of AUC in animals and man
- Saturation of absorption
- Pharmacodynamics
- Maximum feasible dose
- Maximum tolerated dose or
- Limit dose.
- The final type of toxicity is the **special toxicity study**.
- These studies are generally conducted when an issue arises and there is a need to better understand findings in other toxicity studies.

- A special toxicity study examining the toxicity of the metabolite alone may be conducted by administration of the metabolite to rats.

Duration of toxicity studies:

- For clinical studies of 2 weeks in duration, rodent toxicity studies of 2-4 weeks are required.
- For 2-4 week human trials, animal studies should be 1 month duration.
- For clinical trials of 1-3 months, 3 month toxicity studies is required
- The amount of planning, compound synthesis, and tissue assessment required for an in vivo toxicological evaluation can take from 3-6 months for sub acute toxicology.
- Chronic toxicity studies require 6-12 months of exposure.
- From these studies, a No Adverse Event Level (NOAL) can be determined.
- An NCE in clinical trials will also be evaluated over a 2 yr period for reproductive effects, teratogenicity and immunologic and behavioural toxicity both in adult mammal and their offspring.

Duration of Repeat Dose Toxicology Studies to Support Clinical Trials are summarized in the following tables:

Repeat-Dose Toxicology

Maximum duration of Clinical Trial	**Recommended minimum duration of repeat-dose toxicity studies to support clinical trials**	
	Rodent	Non-Rodent
Up to 2 weeks	2 weeks (a)	2 weeks (a)
Between 2 weeks to 6 months	Same as clinical trial duration (b)	Same as clinical trial duration (b)
Greater than 6 months	6 months (b, c)	9 months (b, c)

(a) In the US, an extended single dose design can support single dose human trials

(b) Longer trials can be initiated if equivalent duration toxicology studies are available before the duration of existing toxicity studies is exceeded in the trial

(c) Longer term juvenile toxicity studies may be required for pediatric drugs where there is evidence of developmental concerns.

Repeat-Dose Toxicology

Duration of indicated treatment	Recommended minimum duration of repeat-dose toxicity studies to support marketing	
	Rodent	Non-Rodent
Up to 2 weeks	1 month	1 month
> 2 weeks to 1 month	3 months	3 months
> 1 month to 3 months	6 months	6 months

(a) Longer term juvenile toxicity studies may be required for pediatric drugs where there is evidence of developmental concerns

FACTORS IN DESIGNING TOXICITY STUDIES

- Several factors must be considered when designing toxicity studies. These include the use of main study or satellite animals (In rodents, Toxicokinetics is commonly assessed in a so-called satellite group of animals which run in parallel to the main group devoted to toxicological evaluation.
- Satellite animals are extra animals dosed as per protocol but not subjected to toxicological and pathological observations and tests) for the collection of pharmacokinetic data, the total blood volume that can be extracted from animals during a given period of time, as well as the amount of blood that can be collected at each time point, route of exposure, sampling time points, number of animals per time point, number of sampling days and bio analytical support
- One of the 1st decisions is whether the matrix (generally plasma) will be obtained from animals being used for collection of toxicity data or from satellite animals.
- The next question is what matrix will be measured.
- Drug concentrations may be measured in a wide variety of matrices, but not limited to plasma, serum, tissue homogenates, urine and so on.
- For large animals (e.g., dogs) the samples are collected from main study animals, while for smaller animals (e.g., rodents) a satellite group is commonly used. Generally, 3 or more animals per time point are used.
- Sufficient sample times should be employed to allow calculation of an area under the curve and plasma concentrations should be determined on a sufficient number of days to establish the level of exposure achieved during the course of the study.
- In rodents, blood is not only required for the plasma concentration determination, but also for toxicity endpoints. Therefore, a spate satellite set of animals are used for the toxicity endpoint data.
- Blood volumes that will not alter physiological parameters vary depending upon the frequency of collection and the volume collected each time.
- Different route of exposure will require different study designs with respect to sampling for plasma concentration determination.

- Oral, intravenous, and subcutaneous administrations will all result in different plasma concentration vs. time curves. Therefore selection of time points for sampling will need to be adjusted accordingly.

Compound Libraries

- If the lead compound is found to be toxic it is kept in the compound library for future use.
- A compound library is a collection of compounds.
- Compound libraries from past projects are kept and may be screened for the biological activity you are looking for in a new project.
- New compounds may also be made "in-house" but nowadays specialist chemical companies are often contracted to simply make NCEs for big pharmaceutical companies.
- A disadvantage of synthetic libraries is that they are often limited.

Systemic Toxicity Studies

The following are the systemic toxicity studies needed

a) Single dose study (Acute toxicity studies)
b) Repeated-dose systemic toxicity studies
c) Male Fertility Studies
d) Female Reproduction and Developmental Toxicity Studies
e) Teratogenicity Study
f) Perinatal Study
g) Local Toxicity
h) Genotoxicity
i) Chronic toxicity studies
j) Carcinogenicity
k) special toxicity study

a) Single dose study (Acute toxicity studies)

Single dose studies in animals are essential for any pharmaceutical product intended for human use. The information obtained from these studies is useful in choosing doses for repeat dose studies, providing preliminary identification of target organs of toxicity and occasionally, revealing delayed toxicity. Acute toxicity studies may also aid in the selection of starting doses for phase I human studies, and provide information relevant to acute overdosing in humans. Acute toxicity studies should be carried out in at least two species, usually mice and rats using the same route as intended for humans. In addition, a least two more route should be used to ensuresystemic absorption of the drug, this route may depend on the nature of the drug.

Mortality should be looked for up to 72 hours after parenteral administration and up to 7 days after oral administration. Symptoms, signs and mode of death should be reported with appropriate macroscopic and microscopic findings where necessary.

b) Repeated-dose systemic toxicity studies

The primary goal of repeated dose toxicity studies is to characterize the toxicological profile of the test compound following repeated administration. This includes identification of potential target organs of toxicity and exposure/response relationships, and may include the potential reversibility of toxic effects. This information should be part of the safety assessment to support the conduct of human clinical trials and the approval of a marketing authorization. The decision whether a developmental toxicity study needs to be performed should be made on a case-by-case basis taking into consideration;

✓ Historical use,

✓ Product features,

✓ Intended target population

✓ Intended clinical use.

c) Male Fertility

Studies Male fertility studies are designed to provide general information concerning the effects of a test substance on male reproductive system such as gonadal function.

d) Female Reproduction and Developmental Toxicity Studies

Female fertility studies are designed to provide general information concerning the effects of a test substance on female reproductive system such as ovary function and lactation. These studies need to be carried out for all drugs proposed to be studied or used in women of childbearing age.

e) Teratogenicity Study

The drug should be administered throughout the period of organogenesis in animals if the test drug is intended for women of childbearing age and if women of childbearing age are to be included as subjects in the clinical trial stage, Using three dose levels. One of the doses should cause minimum maternal toxicity and one should be the proposed dose for clinical use in humans and other one will be multiple of it. The route of administration should be the same as for human therapeutic use.

f) Perinatal Study

This study is specially recommended if the drug is to be given to pregnant or nursing mothers for long periods or where there are indications of possible adverse effects on foetal development. The drug should be administered throughout the last third of pregnancy and then through lactation and weaning. The control of each treated group should have at least 12 pregnant females and the dose which causes low foetal loss should be continued throughout lactation weaning. Animals should be sacrificed and observations should include macroscopic autopsy and where necessary, histopathology

g) Local Toxicity

These studies are required when the new drug is proposed to be used by some special route (other than oral) in humans. The drug should be applied to an appropriate site (e.g. Skin, Ocular or Vaginal mucous membrane) to determine local effects in a suitable species. If the drug is absorbed from the site of application, appropriate systemic toxicity studies will also be required. *Examples:*-of local toxicity are Dermal Toxicity Study, Vaginal Toxicity Study, Photo allergy, Rectal Tolerance Test, Ocular Toxicity Studies, Inhalational Toxicity Studies, And Hypersensitivity. The control and the treated groups should consist of at least 20 pregnant females in case of non-rodents, on each dose used.

Observations should include the

a) number of implantation sites, restorations if any;

b) number foetuses with their Gender, weights and malformations if any.

h) Genotoxicity

➢ Genotoxicity refers to potentially harmful effects on genetic material (DNA) which may occur directly through the induction of permanent transmissible changes (mutations) in the amount or structure of the DNA within cells. *In vitro (artificial environment) and in vivo (in living organisms) genotoxicity tests* are conducted to detect compounds which induce genetic damage directly or indirectly. These tests should enable hazard identification with respect to damage to DNA and its fixation. Damage to DNA can occur at three levels:

  Point mutations (where a single nucleotide base is changed, inserted or deleted from a sequence of DNA or RNA inside the cell). Chromosomal mutations (changes involving whole chromosomes or parts of chromosomes). Genomic mutations (permanent alteration in the DNA sequence that makes up a gene, such that the sequence differs from what is found in most people).

The following *standard test battery is generally expected to be conducted*:

- A test for gene mutation in bacteria (Ames test)
- An *in vitro test with cytogenetic evaluation of chromosomal damage with*
- mammalian cells or an *in vitro mouse lymphoma assay*
- An *in vivo test for chromosomal damage using rodent hematopoietic* cells.

i) Chronic toxicity studies

Studies should be performed for all drugs that are expected to be clinically used for six months or more than six months as well as for drugs used frequently in an intermittent manner in the treatment of chronic or recurrent condition.

Fertility studies

➢ The drug should be administered to both males and females, beginning a sufficient number of days before mating.

➢ In females the medication should be continued after mating and the pregnant one should be treated throughout pregnancy.

- The highest dose used should not affect general health or growth of the animals.
- The route of administration should be the same as for therapeutic use in humans.
- The control and the treated group should be of similar size and large enough to give at least 20 pregnant animals in the control group of rodents and at least 8 pregnant animals in the control group of non-rodents.
- Observations should include total examination of the litters from both the groups, including spontaneous abortions, if any.

j) Carcinogenicity

- These studies are required to be carried out if the drug or its metabolite is related to a known carcinogen or when the nature and action of the drug is such as to suggest a carcinogenic/mutagenic potential. For carcinogenicity studies, at least two species should be used.
- These species should not have high incidence of spontaneous tumours and should preferably be known to metabolize the drug in the same manner as humans.
- At least three doses levels should be used;

a) The highest doses should be sub-lethal but cause observable toxicity;

b) The lowest doses should be comparable to the intended human therapeutic doses or a multiple of it, example 2.5x; to make allowance for the sensitivity of the species;

c) The intermediate doses to be placed logarithmically between the other two doses.

d) A control group should always be included.

e) The drug should be administered 7 days a week or a fraction of the life span comparable to the fraction of human life span over which the drug is likely to be used therapeutically.

f) Observations should include macroscopic changes observed at autopsy and detailed histopathology.

For Further Reading

1. Chapter 1- Drug Discovery and Clinical Research - SK Guptha
2. https://pdfs.semanticscholar.org/presentation/5c92/0271fc9f009c486ec3ab91d0 1e811bd58e60.pdf
3. Pharmacokinetics in drug development: Regulatory and developmental paradigms. By Peter Bonate, Danny Howard, Pg no: 87-94.
4. New drug development: Design methodology and analysis. By J. Rick Turner.

Chapter 3

Drug Characterization, Preformulation and Dosage Form Development

LEARNING OBJECTIVES

To understand

- Organoleptic Properties
- Purity of API and Excipients
- Analytical Method
- Solubility
- Hygroscopicity
- Dissociation/Ionization Constant (pK_a)
- Partition Coefficient (LOG P)
- Dissolution Behavior
- Crystallinity and Polymorphism
- Particle Size, Shape, and Surface Area
- Bulk Density
- Powder Flow Property
- Stability
- Drug-Excipient Compatibility Study
- Early Formulation Studies
- Preformulation Studies
- (Drug solubility, Partition coefficient, Dissolution rate, Physical form, Stability)
- Initial Product Formulation and Clinical Trial Materials
- Dosage Form Design
- Types of Dosage Forms
- Therapeutic Considerations

Introduction

It is expected for the pharmaceutical manufacturing industries to encounter product failure during routine production of commercial batch if it was not developed based on adequate biopharmaceutical knowledge. To identify the root causes of the failure and rectify them may incur huge loss in terms of money, man, power, and time. It is quite rational to sort out the problem from the very beginning during the stage of drug development and thus avoiding unnecessary losses especially in the case of new chemical entity (NCE).

Preformulation testing is considered as the first step before rational development of a dosage form with a drug molecule. It involves the exploitation of biopharmaceutical principles in selecting the right excipients, right composition, right processing steps, and right packaging materials. Obviously, the ultimate aim is to design an optimum drug product which is cost effective, safe, stable, patient-friendly and therapeutically effective. So, the preformulation testing is considered the fundamental aspect of developing robust formulations and can be considered as a learning process before actually developing the dosage forms. The overall objective of preformulation testing is to gather enough data in order to develop a chemically stable and therapeutically effective drug product that can be commercially produced at large scale. It also shortens the time of drug development process. The preformulation testing should start when the synthesized molecule passes the toxicity study and appears to show promising pharmacological response. Various preformulation tests are as follows.

Organoleptic Properties

Organoleptic properties of an API viz. colour, odour, flavour and taste need to be recorded at preformulation stage. Sometimes, these properties may vary from batch to batch depending on the specification of the API from a particular vendor. That is why those properties are recorded and compared against the reference. Once established, those specifications are compared for new batches of the drug to ensure batch to batch uniformity. If the API is coloured and with very low dose, it is very difficult to maintain colour uniformity in the finished uncoated tablets. To circumvent the problem with non-uniform colour, very often, uncoated tablets may need to be coated. Similarly, API with bad odour or unpalatable taste should not be considered as mouth-dissolving or chewable tablets, rather it should be considered for capsule or tablet (coated) dosage form.

Purity of API and Excipients

Drugs to be used in the various dosage forms are mainly available as solids, liquids and gases. Among these physical forms, solid drugs dominate the market, followed by the liquid form. Solid materials are preferred in formulation work because of their ease of preparation into solid oral dosage forms such as tablets and capsules. These solid drugs are pure organic compounds that exist as either crystalline or amorphous. The purity of the chemical substance is considered as its essential quality to comply with various pharmacopeial tests including therapeutic efficacy. API with impurities is not always necessary to be rejected, provided that the impurity is completely characterized. The major concern is that impurities can affect product stability. Impurity is often found to be carcinogenic in nature, e.g. aromatic amine (p- amino phenol).

Melting point of a chemical substance is considered its inherent property which can be used as an indicator of purity of that substance. As an example, a pure crystalline API can be identified by its unique and very sharp melting temperature determined by capillary method. Apart from that method, purity of an API can be determined by HPLC, TLC, DSC or GC. In chromatographic methods, reference standard of an API is considered 100% pure and unknown samples are compared against that reference standard. Impurity index, in those chromatographic analyses, is defined as the ratio of all responses (peak areas) due to components other than the main one to the total area response. Homogeneity index (HI) is defined as the ratio of the response (peak area) due to the main component, to the total response. According to ICH Q3A guidance, the allowable level of any given impurity or impurities that are permitted in API/drug product, without explicit non-clinical safety testing, (ICH, 2008).

Very often, the impurity originating from excipients needs to be considered at preformulation stage. Residue of organic solvents used in synthesis, extraction or purification of excipients may remain with them if the solvents are not removed completely. These solvent residues, apart from their toxicity, may destabilize the formulation. This is also true for excipients originating from natural source. So, impurity profiling of not only API but also excipients is important to avoid this unwanted consequence of drug degradation. Interestingly, this kind of problem is difficult to predict as it may not arise initially during product development, but at later stage of formulation development or even after commercial production; the product may undergo stability issue.

Analytical Method

It is very important to develop and validate appropriate analytical method at preformulation stage. It helps to quantify the API at various stages of product development, especially during optimization of in vitro drug release profile, product stability assessment, and drug-excipient compatibility study. Depending on response of chromophoric groups, UV spectrophotometric method is firstly attempted, provided that excipients present in the dosage form do not interfere with the detection at the particular wave-length (λ_{max}) of the drug. UV spectrophotometric method is quite rapid and easy to develop. Alternatively, suitable chromatographic methods such as High Performance Liquid Chromatography (HPLC), Thin Layer Chromatography (TLC) and Gas Chromatography (GC) may be used to avoid interference from excipients when API is present with other excipients. For all these analytical methods, initially, a standard curve is prepared within a working range with a reference sample at various concentrations. Unknown samples are then analyzed and their concentrations are estimated by applying calibration equation developed earlier by the reference calibration samples. Other useful analytical methods such TLC, GC, potentiometric titration, microbiological assay or atomic absorption spectroscopy (AAS) may be needed depending on the property of drug molecules and their sensitivity.

Solubility

The majority of existing drug candidates as well as emerging NCEs are lipophilic i.e. poorly soluble in water. This may be due to the high crystallinity/melting point and molecular weight of the drug or lack of ionisable groups present in the molecule (Lipinski, 2001). However, the drug has to be in solution in order to get absorbed through biological membrane, especially at the gastro-intestinal tract (GIT). Without proper solubilisation strategy, APIs with low solubility profile are very difficult to design into solid oral dosage forms due to their poor dissolution rate. The developed dosage forms also face potential food effect in achieving appropriate plasma-drug concentration. Also at pre- clinical toxicity study, they remain problematic in designing appropriate dosage form (even parenteral preparation) to deliver high dose. Most of the available drugs are weakly acidic and weekly basic in nature and their solubilities increase in basic and acidic pH respectively depending on their ionization state. However, neutral drugs remain unaffected. Hence, the estimation of aqueous solubility of any drug molecule within a pH range of 1 to 8 as well as its intrinsic solubility is important. Intrinsic solubility is the solubility of a drug at a particular temperature when the drug remains completely in the unionized state. Apart from water, at preformulation stage, solubility study of active drug is performed in various other solvents such as water, propylene glycol, polyethylene glycol, glycerine, ethyl alcohol, sorbitol, methanol, isopropyl alcohol, benzyl alcohol, polysorbate 20, polysorbate 80, castor oil, sesame oil, peanut oil, and buffers at various pH depending on the kind of dosage form to be developed.

For liquid oral formulation, solubility of the drug should be carried out in solubilisation agents/systems including co-solvents (e.g. propylene glycol, glycerine, and ethanol), surfactants (e.g. Span 20, Tween 80), and complexation agents (e.g. caffeine, cyclodextrin). On the other hand, if the drug is to be designed as a solid oral dosage form, solubility studies of the drug should be performed in simulated gastric fluid (SGF), simulated intestinal fluid (SIF) and pH 7.4 buffer. This would be helpful in developing suitable dissolution medium, granulating solvent, and coating fluid.

In order to get absorbed through the biological membrane, the solubility criteria of dosage form does not depend solely on aqueous solubility and log P value of the drug; rather, sometimes it depends on dose and permeability behaviour of the drug. Highly insoluble drug when administered in small dose may result in good absorption. In this regard, two important parameters namely dissolution time and maximum absorbable dose (MAD) need to be evaluated. Highly soluble drugs with rapid dissolution profile may result in poor bioavailability when passing through the acidic environment of the stomach where they are highly degraded.

According to Biopharmaceutical Classification System (BCS), based on solubility and permeability, drugs are classified into the following four groups:

Class I	High Permeability, High Solubility
Class II	High Permeability, Low Solubility
Class III	Low Permeability, High Solubility
Class IV	Low Permeability, Low Solubility

According to the above classification, a dosage form is termed as highly soluble if the highest dose is soluble in less than 250 mL water within a pH range of 1 to 7.5. Additionally, a dosage form is considered highly permeable if more than 90% dose is absorbed in human. On the other hand, the dosage form is termed rapidly dissolving if more than 85% of labelled amount of drug substance dissolves within 30 minutes. Compounds which show aqueous solubility of more than 1% w/v are not considered to exhibit dissolution-related absorption problems. In the case of drugs that show dissolution rate-limited absorption, the best way to increase the amount of drug absorbed is to increase their effective strength i.e. dose size. To assist it further, particle size of the drug can be reduced. If it does not help, then instead of the solid dosage form, liquid formulation may be tried, provided the drugs have sufficient solution stability. If the aqueous solubility of an API is below 1 to 10 mg/ml, it may be used as a salt of an appropriate acid or base depending on the dosage form requirement. As an example, non-steroidal anti-inflammatory drugs (NSAID) such as alclofenac, diclofenac, fenbufen, ibuprofen, and naproxen are weak acids with pK_a value approximately 4 and of low solubility. To overcome solubility and thereby bioavailability problems, most of the drugs are available as sodium salts. To be more specific, diclofenac (free acid) has solubility of only 0.8×10^{-5} M (25 °C). However, upon sodium salt formation, its solubility increases to around 24.5 mg/mL (37 °C). For drugs that are not acidic or basic, or not easy to modify their acidic or basic property to form a stable salt, other physical approaches such as the use of surfactant, particle size reduction (micronisation), solid dispersion and complexation, may be adopted to improve their solubility profile.

Hygroscopicity

Many drugs and excipients, essentially the water-soluble salts, have a high affinity to absorb environmental moisture. Changes in moisture level can greatly control many parameters such as chemical stability, flowability, and compatibility. When hygroscopic materials absorb adequate amount of water where they get dissolved completely, as observed with sodium chloride on a humid day; these are known as deliquescent materials. Equilibrium moisture content of any substance may depend on various parameters such as humidity, temperature, surface area, exposure time and the mechanism of moisture uptake.

As a test of hygroscopicity of any drug at preformulation stage, a weighed sample of that drug is placed in an open container and spread to form a thin bed to assure maximum atmospheric exposure. The drug sample is then exposed to a range of controlled relative humidity environments prepared with saturated aqueous salt solutions (e.g. ammonium sulphate at 25 °C gives 80% R.H. (relative humidity), potassium sulphate at 25 °C gives 97% R.H.). Moisture uptake by the sample is monitored over a period of time and analysed by methods e.g. gravimetric analysis (weight gained), Karl Fischer titration, or gas chromatography.

Depending on the hygroscopicity of the drug, suitable moisture-proof coating and storage in a low-humidity environment or in a special packaging with a desiccant can be adopted. It may also dictate the necessary action for smooth powder flow during processing of that drug in the manufacturing room. In general, hygroscopic compounds should be stored in a well-closed container preferably with a desiccant. If a granulation step is needed in tableting, non- aqueous granulating solvents should be recommended. If the drug is found to be moisture- sensitive, hygroscopic excipients should not be selected for development of solid oral dosage form.

Dissociation/Ionization Constant (pK_a)

Dissociation or ionisation constant (pK_a) is defined as the negative logarithm of the equilibrium coefficient of the neutral and charged forms of a compound. The pK_a allows us to estimate the effective charge present on a molecule at any particular pH. As mentioned earlier, majority of the drugs are weekly acidic or basic in nature. The unionized species are found to be highly lipid-soluble and they result in high absorption through biological membrane. That is why the GIT absorption of weakly acidic or basic drugs is dependent on the fraction of unionized drug present in the solution. If drug is strongly acidic or basic it will be ionized at all pH (pH 0 to 14), but the solubility of weakly acidic or basic drug will depend upon pH, which in turn will influence the extent to which drug enters the blood stream, its absorption and activity.

The degree of ionization of a drug molecule depends on pH and can be determined by the Henderson-Hasselbalch as per *Eq. 1 & 2.*

For acids:

$pH = pK_a + \log [\text{ionized form}]/[\text{unionized form}]$

For bases:

$pH = pK_a + \log [\text{unionized form}]/[\text{ionized form}]$

(Eq. 2)

pK_a values are temperature dependent in a non-linear fashion which are quite unpredictable. Thus pKa values are never reported without reporting the temperature which is traditionally measured at room temperature (25 ^{0}C). Determination of ionization constant can be done by various methods i.e. potentiometric pH-titration, pH-spectrophotometry method, or pH- solubility analysis. The measurements of pKa according to those methods are not straightforward. Appropriate method should be selected based on the solubility profile of the drug and experiments should be carried out carefully under specified conditions to assure that the results are valid. It may require a long time and good amount of expertise to interpret the data.

Partition Coefficient (LOG P)

Partition coefficient is the ratio in which a solute distributes itself between the two phases of two immiscible liquids (mostly n-octanol/water) when they are allowed to intimately mix with each other. As shown in *Eq. 3*, the value of Log P measures the affinity of a drug substance to partition between a lipid (oil) and water. It is a useful parameter in predicting the in vivo drug absorption through GIT or other biological membranes. Factors such as absorption, excretion and penetration of the drug through various biological membranes are found to be dependent on the Log P value of a drug. It also helps in determining the membrane permeability, plasma protein-binding, volume of distribution, renal and hepatic clearance. Log P value equal to 0 indicates that the compound is equally soluble in water and solvent. When the value is 5, the compound becomes more soluble in solvent (100,000 in solvent), whereas Log P value of 2 suggests that the compound is 100 times more soluble in water.

$$\text{Log}_{10}\text{P} = \text{Log}\frac{\text{Drug concentration in organic solvent}}{\text{Drug concentration in aqueous solvent}} \qquad .....3.3$$

Octanol/water is the preferred system to estimate Log P values. For a sufficient amount of any drug absorption, its Log P value should be in the range of 1 to 3. When Log P is greater than 6 or less than 3 it means they have poor transport characteristics (Log P and transport have a parabolic relationship). Increased Log P value indicates that compound is more soluble in the aqueous phase and hence will exhibit poor penetration into membrane barrier, while a compound with higher partitioning in organic solvent will be more confined to lipid phase of the membrane and may exhibit toxicity. Log P value of API at the preformulation stage can be measured by the Shake-Flask method, filter probe measurements and HPLC method. Dunn et al. (1986) reported a detail discussion on these methods.

Dissolution Behavior

Dissolution is a process which involves solubilization of a drug after its release from dosage form before being absorbed through the GIT membrane. It is a mass transfer phenomenon from a solid surface to a liquid phase. Dissolution rate may be defined as the amount of drug substance that goes in solution per unit time under standardized conditions of liquid/solid interface, temperature and solvent composition. It may be estimated by the Noyes-Whitney Equation given below:

$$-\frac{dW}{dt} = \frac{DAK(C_s - C)}{h} \qquad .....(3.4)$$

where

dW/dt	dissolution rate
A	surface area of the dissolving solid
D	diffusion coefficient
K	partition coefficient
h	aqueous diffusion layer
C_s	solubility of solute
C	solute concentration in the bulk medium

In vitro dissolution testing provides information regarding the behaviour of the drug product *in vivo*, especially how the drug is going to be released from the dosage form. In many circumstances, it may predict the bioavailability if the drug belongs to BCS Class I or Class

III. This may again lead to avoidance of very costly and time-consuming bioavailability/bioequivalence study which involves testing of drug in human volunteers or patient population before product registration with regulatory bodies. However, at preformulation stage, due to non-availability of proper dosage form, intrinsic dissolution rate is calculated instead of the conventional dissolution rate.

In order to find out the intrinsic dissolution rate of an API, study is conducted with constant surface area where dissolution rate is calculated as a function of intrinsic solubility. Dissolution parameters i.e. stirrer RPM, product surface area, bath temperature, pH and ionic strength of the dissolution medium are kept constant; dissolution is controlled solely by diffusion. The readers are advised to go through the details of their operation procedure mentioned in USP 29 (2006). As an example, ca. 500 mg drug is compressed to a 13-mm compact powder disc using 500 mPa compressional force. The disc is loaded onto a holder of the apparatus in such a way that only one surface of the disc is exposed to the dissolution medium. The apparatus is run for a certain period with specific operational parameters. Each drug candidate should be tested in 0.05 M HCl (gastric) and phosphate buffer pH 7 (intestinal), and distilled water as the dissolution medium. Finally intrinsic dissolution rate of the drug in water is compared with that obtained in acid and alkali. The results indicate the drug's ability to control its immediate microenvironment and give intrinsic dissolution rate in actual condition which the drug is going to encounter *in-vivo.*

The value of intrinsic dissolution rate ($mg/cm^2/min$) is considered unique for any drug molecule in a given hydrodynamic conditions. It helps in predicting in vivo dissolution behaviour in advance and if required, necessary strategy can be adopted to solve the same concern during product development. If the value is greater than 1 $mg/cm^2/min$, it implies that the drug is not likely to present dissolution rate-limited absorption problems. If the value is found to be less than 0.1 $mg/cm^2/min$, it usually exhibits dissolution rate-limited absorption.

However, if the value lies between 0.1 to 1.0 $mg/cm^2/min$, it indicates that more information is required before making any decision.

Crystallinity and Polymorphism

Solid drug substances may occur as amorphous and crystalline forms. Amorphous drug has atoms or molecules randomly placed (without definite structure) within it. Crystal is characterized by a highly ordered arrangement of the molecules, associated with a three-dimensional network. The repeating three-dimensional patterns are ideally depicted as lattice. Crystal habit is the description of the outer appearance of a crystal. Amorphous form is of a higher thermodynamic energy, of greater solubility as well as higher dissolution rate than the corresponding crystalline form. Many organic drug substances can exist in more than one crystalline form with different space-lattice arrangement; this property is called polymorphism. Solid crystal that contains entrapped solvent within its structure is called solvate, also known as a pseudo-polymorph. When the solvate is water, it is called a hydrate. Aqueous solubility of hydrate compounds can be significantly less than their anhydrous forms.

Different polymorphic forms may vary in biopharmaceutical properties such as solubility, hygroscopicity, diffusivity, dissolution rate, melting point, rates of reaction or stability. They also differ in various mechanical properties such as volume, density, crystal hardness and crystal shape. These properties may influence therapeutic efficacy, stability and manufacturing ability of a dosage form. In general, chemically, the most stable polymorph is found to have the highest melting point and the lowest solubility. However, sometimes a metastable form may need to be used in spite of its lower stability. Conversion from one polymorph to another or from metastable form to stable form can occur during processing or upon storage. Knowledge of polymorphism of active ingredient is very important at preformulation stage.

Polymorphism occurs due to variation in the conditions, temperature, solvent, and time under which crystallization is induced. The number of crystalline forms or polymorphs that can exist for a compound is proportional to the time and resources dedicated to the investigation of them. Polymorphs are unexpected and seems to be more common for compounds with low solubility in water, organic salts, larger molecules (hydrates), neutral compounds with larger molecular weights (organic solvates), and compounds with molecular weight below 350.

Chloramphenicol palmitate exists as three polymorphic forms (A, B, C) apart from its amorphous form, although only Form B and the amorphous form are found to be active. In one of the pharmacokinetic study, it was found that Form A produced sub-therapeutic level of plasma drug concentration when administered as oral suspension. It was demonstrated that polymorphic Form A was more hydrolyzed by pancreatin enzyme than Form B. Novobiocin, an aminocoumarin antibiotic, is available as crystalline and amorphous form. When its amorphous form is administered orally, it is well absorbed from GIT and produce good therapeutic response. However, its amorphous form is not very stable. On the other hand, its crystalline form is very stable, but suffers from solubility and thereby bioavailability. Under this circumstance, the FDA has asked its manufacturer to withdraw this drug from the market. On the same basis, the more stable crystalline form of penicillin G as potassium or sodium salt are preferred than the amorphous form.

Polymorphic disaster with ritonavir, a protease inhibitor, is a classic example that needs to be discussed in this regard. The drug was commercialized as capsule form (brand name Norvir®) in 1996 by Abbott Laboratories. However, during a routine quality control test for a commercial batch, the product failed the in vitro dissolution test which halted the marketing of the drug in early 1998. Later, in the summer of 1998, they discovered the most stable crystalline form (melting point 125 ^{0}C) with lower solubility profile. Till 2002, a total of five polymorphic forms were identified with different melting points. Various polymorphs and pseudo-polymorphs are characterized by several methods such as hot stage microscopy, Differential Scanning Calorimetry (DSC), X-ray Diffraction (XRD), Fourier Transform Infra-Red (FTIR), Scanning Electron Microscopy (SEM) and Thermal Gravimetric Analysis (TGA).

Particle Size, Shape, and Surface Area

Particle size, shape and surface area of an API play important roles for designing a solid oral dosage form. Necessary characterization of these particle properties is important at the preformulation stage. Certain physical properties (e.g. taste, texture, and colour), chemical reactivity, stability, bioavailability, content uniformity, sedimentation rate, flow and mixing homogeneity of powders and granules depend on particle size distribution and shape. Particle size significantly influences the oral absorption profiles of certain drugs such as griseofulvin, nitrofurantoin, spironolactone and procaine penicillin. Fine materials tend to require more amount of granulating liquid as compared to those with large particle size when they are processed for tablet formulation. Fine materials relatively are more open to attack from atmospheric oxygen, heat, light, humidity, and interacting excipients than coarse materials.

Very fine materials are difficult to handle as it produces lots of dust. They create problems in mixing and flow property. It is important to decide, maintain, and control a desired particle size range of the drugs before formulation development. However, if the particle size is too large, it is better to grind them; particle diameter more than 100 μm (mesh 140) down to approximately 10-40 μm (mesh 325). For particles with diameter less than 30 μm (mesh 400), grinding is unnecessary except for needle-like substances to improve flow property. Important drawbacks of grinding are material loss, static charge build-up, aggregation (increased hydrophobicity), lowering of dissolution rate, and polymorphic or chemical transformations. There are various techniques for particle size estimation: microscopy, sieving, sedimentation (Adreasen pipet), blockage of electrical conductivity path (Coulter counter), light blockage (HIAC/ROYCO®) and light diffraction or scattering techniques (Malvern®). Judicious selection of an appropriate method will depend on the availability or amount of drug sample, its shape and type of formulation.

Particle shape plays a major role in processing and formulation of solid dosage form. Unlike the regular or nearly spherical granules, irregular shape primary particle or granules do not flow properly and may lead to weight variation during capsule filling and tablet compression operation. Similarly, mixing non-uniformity may arise from irregular or needle shape particle. However, they are beneficial for drugs having poor compression property. Irregular shape powder or granules enhance particle to particle contact and lead strong bond formation during tablet compression.

Determination of surface area of powders has gained a lot of interest in recent years. Surface area reflects the particle size; the lower the particle size, the higher the total surface area. Brunauer-Emmett-Teller (BET) theory of adsorption is applied to estimate surface area of powder sample. As per BET theory, the powdered particle would adsorb gas molecules and form a monolayer at a specific temperature and pressure. The amount of the gas adsorbed on the powder will depend on the physical surface area available for that powder sample. This gives the measurement of powder surface area. Nitrogen is the gas that is usually used in combination with inert gas helium. Both gases are mixed in such a proportion that the mixture finally attains -195^0 C. It has been established then when nitrogen and helium are mixed at a ratio of 30:70 (v/v), the gas mixture attains -195^0 C and adsorbed on the powder sample forming a monolayer. It is hypothesized that the specified experimental condition helps the Van de Waals forces to act between adsorbed gas and powder sample. Under these circumstances, the kinetic energy of gas mixture is nullified by the intermolecular attraction between nitrogen atoms. At the same time, that kinetic energy is unable to exceed the bonding energy between nitrogen and atoms of the powder sample. This process involves physical adsorption in a nonspecific way instead of chemical interaction, thus truly serves the purpose of measuring the surface area of powder drug sample and especially important for characterising porous particles.

Bulk Density

Bulk density of powder drug is subjected to change during various manufacturing operation such as milling, precipitation, crystallization or dry granulation. Thus, knowing the bulk density is important when one considers the size of a high-dose capsule product or the homogeneity of a low-dose formulation in which there are large differences in drug and excipient densities (significant difference in the absolute densities of the components could lead to segregation). Thus, size of the finished product can be determined from such information. The design and the capacity of mixer are highly influenced by the bulk density of the powder. An example of calcium carbonate powder would be worthy to mention in this regard. Calcium carbonate is available with various powder specifications where bulk density varies from 0.1 to 1.3 g/mL. To accommodate the lightest (bulkiest) type calcium carbonate, it may require a mixer or storage container that is 13 times bigger than that required by the same calcium carbonate but with highest bulk density. Density problem may be corrected by milling, slugging, or formulation modification depending on the need. In order to measure bulk density (g/mL), a weighed powder sample is poured into a measuring cylinder with the help of a large funnel. The volume of the sample can be measured from the mark on the cylinder. On the other hand, for tapped density measurement, the same funnel filled with sample is fixed with mechanical tapper apparatus (tap densitometer). The apparatus is run for a fixed number of taps (approximately 500 or more) until the sample attains minimum fixed volume. Tapped density is measured from the tapped volume divided by the weight of the sample. In the absence of a tap densitometer, the same experiment can be executed by manual tapping of the measuring cylinder where the cylinder is allowed to fall repeatedly from a certain height.

Sometimes, it is required to know the true density of a powder to compute the void volume or porosity of packed powder bed. Void volume or porosity of packed powder bed is the ratio of void volume to bulk volume. Tapped density and bulk density can be used to determine % compressibility (Carr's index) as per *Equation 5*. Carr's index is the indirect measure of powder flow property although it deals with powder compressibility property. Table 2.1 enlists the powder flow property depending on the Carr's index results.

$$\text{Compressibility Index} = 100 \times \left(\frac{V_o - V_f}{V_o}\right) \qquad \text{.....3.5}$$

Where, V_0 = bulk density, V_f = tapped density.

Table 2.1 Relation between Carr's index and powder flow property

Carr's index	Flow description
5 to 15	Excellent (free-flowing granules)
12 to 16	Good (free flowing powdered granules)
18 to 21	Fair (powdered granules)
23 to 28	Poor (very fluid powders)
28 to 35	Poor (fluid cohesive powders)
35 to 38	Very poor (cohesive powders)
> 40	Extremely poor (cohesive powders)

Powder Flow Property

Investigation on powder flow property at preformulation stage is required to successfully manufacture tablet and capsule dosage form. Based on the prior knowledge of flow properties of API and excipients (either alone or in combination), a formulation recommendation such as granulation or densification via slugging may be adopted. One easy and quick method to estimate the powder flow property is to determine the angle of repose of that powder sample. Angle of repose, as represented by (Eq. 6), is defined as the maximum angle possible between the surface of a pile of powder sample and horizontal plane when the sample is poured from a fixed distance.

$$\tan \theta = h/r \qquad \text{.....(3.6)}$$

Where θ = angle of repose, h = height of the powder pile, r = radius of powder pile

Powder with rough and irregular surface produce higher angle of repose than regular or nearly spherical particles or granules. The relation between angle of repose and powder flow property is given in Table 2.2. Apart from the angle of repose method, based on the amount of sample available, various other techniques such as Jenike Shear Cell, bulk density method, powder flow tester etc can be adopted to characterize powder flow property. Presence of excessive moisture causes significant problem in powder flow. If required, moisture content of the powder material and granules should be optimum (2 to 4% w/w) to facilitate both powder flow and powder compression operation. To improve flow characteristics, glidants like colloidal silicone dioxide (Aerosil®), magnesium stearate, talcum powder, starch etc may be added to granular powders. However, concentration of glidant is critical to improve flow properties. Glidants are characterized by having a small particle size.

Table 2.2 Powder flow property depending on angle of repose value

Flow property	Angle of repose (θ)
Excellent	25-30
Good	31-35
Fair-aid not needed	36-40
Passable-may hang up	41-45
Poor-must agitate, vibrate	46-55
Very poor	56-65
Extremely poor	>66

Stability

Drug degradation occurs due to chemical interaction among drug and excipients or impurities present within the excipients in presence of favourable environmental conditions. However the structural features have lots of influence on its decomposition. There are some common pathways of degradation such as hydrolysis, oxidation, photolysis, isomerization and polymerization.

Hydrolysis and oxidation are the most common pathways for API degradation in the solid- state and in solution. Photolysis and trace metal catalysis are secondary processes of degradation. Temperature affects each of the above chemical degradation pathways; the rate of degradation increases with temperature. Extrapolation of accelerated temperature data to different temperatures, e.g. proposed storage conditions, is common practice (e.g. using Arrhenius plots) but we must be mindful of the pit-falls – the influence of the various degradation pathways and mechanisms might be changed with temperature. It is well understood that pH, particularly extremes, can encourage hydrolysis of API when ionised in aqueous solution. This necessitates buffer control if such a dosage form is required. Sometime microenvironment created inside the product in the presence of drug and excipients may influence the stability of the drug in the dosage form. This effect is more pronounced when the drug has pH-dependent stability profile. Even the drug with pH-dependent solubility may influence drug release on account of this microenvironment. Careful selection of excipients in compliance with drug property is necessary at preformulation stage.

Drug degradation may lead to substantial loss of its potency which fails to achieve required plasma level concentration to give therapeutic benefit of the drug. On the other hand, this degradation may convert the active drug to either totally inactive or toxic one. In both cases, the product may appear quite harmful to the patients. Even if the degradation occurs in the form of colour or odour alteration, the product loses its credibility to the patients as well as to the doctors. This explains why the stability profile of active drug when combined with other excipients is required to be submitted to regulatory agencies for pharmaceutical product registration.

Factors affecting solution state stability include pH of the solvent, temperature, light, oxygen, ionic strength, presence of surfactants, buffer salts and complexation agents. pH influences acid, base and water-catalysed hydrolysis. More complex shapes of kinetic profiles exist if the drug substance has (multiple) ionisable functionality. If the drug substance is found to be susceptible to degradation in solution (aqueous) state, strategies such as selection of a less soluble salt, co-solvent addition, micellar inclusion or complexation can be adopted to avoid that problem. Manufacturing conditions, storage conditions and packaging should be confirmed at the preformulation stage. If required, the micro-environment around the drug needs to be changed by adjusting the pH with acids, bases, or buffer salts. Complexation agents might be incorporated to inactivate trace metal ions. To prevent the drug from oxidation in liquid and parenteral preparation, if possible, the product should be supplied with nitrogen or argon. Alternatively, antioxidants can be incorporated within the formulation composition. At preformulation stage, parenteral dosage forms should be evaluated for injection site precipitation, pain upon injection, toxicity of new excipients, effect of excipients on crystallization or nucleation in suspensions, effect of processing and formulation parameters on both physical and chemical stability of the drug.

In solid-state stability, drug substance present on the surface is affected at first by environmental factors e.g. temperature, light and moisture including the reactive packaging materials in contact with the dosage form. Excipients, if not properly selected, may influence various chemical reactions with the drug. Bound or free moisture present in the excipients can initiate the drug degradation. This moisture also may change the microenvironment and pH inside the dosage form. So, excipients with low moisture content and low hygroscopicity in nature are preferable for the drugs that are sensitive to degradation by hydrolysis. Apart from environmental factors, various physical properties of the active drug such as particle size, shape, surface area, morphology and presence of impurities can play a major role in degradation of drug substances either alone or in the presence of excipients. If the drug substance is found to be sensitive to heat, processing condition can always be modified to expose the drug at reduced temperature environment. The reacting species should be separated to avoid intimate contact among the sensitive drugs and excipients. Coating with polymers or microencapsulation is another way to separate physical interaction with the reacting substance. Different novel formulation approaches e.g. multi-layer particles in capsule/tablet, tablets with moisture-proof coating, compression coating, tablet-in-a- tablet or tablet-in-a-capsule can be adopted. Solid-state stability of active drug can be evaluated by stressed conditions: high temperature studies, high humidity, exposure to high moisture and high intensity light environment. It gives an early indication of stability challenges for product development.

Drug-Excipient Compatibility Study

In addition to pharmacological inactivity, excipients are also supposed to be inactive chemically. However, this is not always true. Excipients may contain active functional groups which may initiate some kind of chemical reaction with the API. Even though this may not be visible at the beginning, after subsequent storage period this may cause havoc to the product. Moreover, impurities present in the excipient may initiate various catalytic reactions to destabilize drug products. Drug-excipient compatibility study at preformulation stage is very important.

In a typical drug-excipient compatibility testing program, binary (1:1 or any other ratio with proper justification) powder mixes are prepared by triturating API with the individual excipients. If the excipients are screened for solid oral dosage form, drug and excipients are fabricated into a compact mass, stored under an accelerated condition of temperature and humidity. The same sample is then analysed by some stability-indicating chromatographic method like HPLC, GC or TLC. The water slurry approach is preferred in case of liquid or suspension preparation to know the role of aqueous medium and pH in drug degradation when combined with excipient. Here water is added with drug-excipient mixture to prepare slurry and subjected to stressed condition. Alternatively, binary samples can be screened rapidly using thermal methods, such as DSC.

For a typical drug-excipient interaction study by DSC, active ingredient and suitable amount of an excipient are weighed in a DSC sample holder. Binary ratios between active drug and individual excipient followed for drug-excipient interaction study is about 1:5 for diluents, 3: l for binders or disintegrants, 5:1 for lubricants and 10: l for colorants. Around 5 to 10 mg sample is weighed, put in the DSC pan and set the instrument within a temperature range of 30-300 ^{0}C. Sample is heated at a rate of 5 to 10 K/min in the presence of an inert nitrogen atmosphere. The differences in the heat flow as a function of temperature between the sample and reference is recorded in the form of thermogram. When the sample is not going through any kind of physical or chemical change within it, the heat flow difference is negligible and that is represented by a flat base line on the DSC thermogram. The thermogram will record a peak when there is a difference of heat flow between the test and reference sample which indicates any exothermic or endothermic event occurring in the sample. If the characteristic melting point peak of individual drug and its physical mixture with excipient remains either the same or shows insignificant peak shifting, drug-excipient compatibility may be concluded. However, this kind of interpretation is not always straight forward and reliable, rather, it may be occasionally misleading with reports of false positive and negative. The reason could be due to the high temperature at which the drug is exposed. If the drug is thermolabile, it may show incompatibility with any excipient at elevated temperature, but in reality the drug may not undergo that stressed condition. Rather it is stored at room temperature only with some variation in temperature as a result of transport to different countries with different climates. To confirm, it is advisable to conduct further test by other methods such as TLC, stressed storage method, FTIR, powder-XRD, hot-stage microscopy, or SEM.

However, there is always criticism on the binary approach of drug-excipient compatibility study as it takes away a lot of time and is a financial constraint. The approach is not justified as it is unable to mimic the real composition of a prototype formulation. As an alternative, the prototype formulation can be tested. However, this approach is also not practical considering its complexity in data interpretation and insensitivity of the negligible reaction response. A complementary customised study could be justified if the need arises.

Chemical stability can be measured by chromatographic methods, whereas physical stability by microscopic, particle analysis and in vitro dissolution methods. Quantitative prediction of drug-excipient interaction is still difficult in spite of availability of vast literature on this topic. At preformulation stage, formulation scientists very often face lots of challenges for drug-excipient compatibility study which include low quantity and purity of drug substances, varieties of dosage form and time constraint. Formulation scientist should collect as many information as possible pertaining to the physicochemical parameters of the API and excipients, dosage form to be designed, proposed manufacturing steps and theirs process parameters prior to designing any dosage form.

Preformulation scientists act as mediators between synthetic chemists and formulation scientists. With a holistic aim of designing and developing a stable, cost-effective and therapeutically sound patient-friendly dosage form, they reduce the burden of formulation scientist and help the pharmaceutical industries to avoid unforeseen consequences. The right selection of API, excipients, dosage form, manufacturing processes, packaging materials, analytical methods and storage conditions among many others are important for the benefit of the product's life cycle and usage.

EARLY FORMULATION STUDIES

As a promising compound is characterized for biologic activity, it is also evaluated with regard to chemical and physical properties that have a bearing on its ultimate and successful formulation into a stable and effective pharmaceutical product. This is the area of responsibility of pharmaceutical scientists and formulation pharmacists. When sufficient information is gleaned on the compound's physical and chemical properties, initial formulations of the dosage form are developed for use in human clinical trials. During the course of the clinical trials, the proposed product is developed further, from initial formulation to final formulation and from pilot plant (or small-scale production) to scale-up, in preparation for large-scale manufacturing. To provide sufficient quantities of the bulk chemical (drug) compound for the sequence of preclinical studies, clinical trials, and small-scale and large-scale dosage form production, the careful planning, scheduling, and implementation of the bulk chemical's production must be undertaken by chemical engineers. Quality control and validation must be built into each step of the process. Full documentation of the CMCs is an essential part of all drug applications filed with the FDA.

Preformulation Studies

Each drug substance has intrinsic chemical and physical characteristics that must be considered before the development of a pharmaceutical formulation. Among these are the drug's solubility, partition coefficient, dissolution rate, physical form, and stability.

These and other factors are briefly noted here as an introduction to their importance in the preparation of dosage forms for drug evaluation in human clinical trials and in the development of a final product submitted to the FDA for marketing approval. The FDA's protocols seek to correlate in vitro drug product dissolution and in vivo bioavailability, since drug dissolution and gastrointestinal permeability are the fundamental parameters controlling the rate and extent of drug absorption.

Drug Solubility

A drug substance administered by any route must possess some aqueous solubility for systemic absorption and therapeutic response. Poorly soluble compounds (e.g., less than 10 mg/mL aqueous solubility) may exhibit incomplete, erratic, and/or slow absorption and thus produce a minimal response at desired dosage. Enhanced aqueous solubility may be achieved by preparing more soluble derivatives of the parent compound, such as salts or esters, by chemical complexation, or by reducing the drug's particle size.

Partition Coefficient

To produce a pharmacologic response, a drug molecule must first cross a biologic membrane of protein and lipid, which acts as a lipophilic barrier to many drugs. The ability of a drug molecule to penetrate this barrier is based in part on its preference for lipids (lipophilic) versus its preference for an aqueous phase (hydrophilic). A drug's partition coefficient is a measure of its distribution in a lipophilic– hydrophilic phase system and indicates its ability to penetrate biologic multiphase systems.

Dissolution Rate

The speed at which a drug substance dissolves in a medium is called its dissolution rate. Dissolution rate data, when considered along with data on a drug's solubility, dissolution constant, and partition coefficient, can provide an indication of the drug's absorption potential. For a chemical entity, its acid, base, or salt forms, as well as its physical form (e.g., particle size), may result in substantial differences in the dissolution rate.

Physical Form

The crystal or amorphous forms and/or the particle size of a powdered drug can affect the dissolution rate, and thus the rate and extent of absorption, for a number of drugs. For example, by reducing the particle size and increasing the powder fineness and therefore the surface area of a poorly soluble drug, its dissolution rate in the gut is enhanced (through greater exposure of the drug to gastrointestinal fluid) and its biologic absorption increased. Small and controlled particle size is also critical for drugs administered to the lung by inhalation. The smaller the particle, the deeper is the penetration into the alveoli. Thus, by selective control of the physical parameters of a drug, biologic response may be optimized.

Stability

The chemical and physical stability of a drug substance alone, and when combined with formulation components, is critical to preparing a successful pharmaceutical product. For a given drug, one type of crystal structure may provide greater stability than other structures and may therefore be preferred. For drugs susceptible to oxidative decomposition, the addition of antioxidant stabilizing agents to the formulation may be required to protect the potency. For drugs destroyed by hydrolysis, protection against moisture in formulation, processing, and packaging may be required to prevent decomposition. In every case, drug stability testing at various temperatures, conditions of relative humidity (RH) as 40°C 75% RH/30°C 60% RH durations, and environments of light, air, and packaging is essential in assessing drug and drug product stability. Such information is vital in developing label instructions for use and storage, assigning product expiration dating, and packaging and shipping.

Initial Product Formulation and Clinical Trial Materials

An initial product is formulated using the information gained during the preformulation studies and with the consideration of the dose or doses, dosage form, and route of administration desired for the clinical studies and for the proposed marketed product. Thus, depending upon the design of the clinical protocol and desired final product, formulation pharmacists are called upon to develop a specific dosage form (e.g., capsule, suppository, solution) of one or more dosage strengths for administration by the intended route of administration (e.g., oral, rectal, intravenous). Additional dosage forms for other than the initial route of administration may later be developed, depending on patients' requirements, therapeutic utility, and marketing assessments. This is especially important if the drug may be administered to children. The initial formulations prepared for Phase I and Phase II of the clinical trials, although not as sophisticated and elegant as the final formulation, should be of high pharmaceutical quality, meet analytical specifications for composition, manufacturing, and control, and be sufficiently stable for the period of use.

Often during Phase I studies, for orally administered drugs, capsules are employed containing the active ingredient alone, without pharmaceutical excipients. Excipients are included in the formulation for Phase II trials. During human trials, studies of the drug's ADME are undertaken to obtain a profile of the drug's human pharmacokinetics and biologic availability from the formulation administered. Different formulations may be prepared and examined to develop the one having the desired characteristics. During Phase II, the final dosage form is selected and developed for Phase III trials; this is the formulation that is submitted to the FDA for marketing approval.

Clinical supplies or clinical trial materials comprise all dosage formulations used in the clinical evaluation of a new drug. This includes the proposed new drug, placebos (inert substances), and drug products against which the new drug is to be compared (comparator drugs or drug products). They all must be prepared in indistinguishable dosage forms (look alike, taste alike, and so on) and packaged with coded labels to reduce possible bias when blinded studies are called for in the clinical protocol. Blinded studies are controlled studies in which at least one of the parties (e.g., patient, physician) does not know which product is being administered. At the conclusion of the clinical study, the codes for the products administered are broken and the clinical results statistically evaluated. Some studies are open label, in which case, all parties may know what products are administered.

Some pharmaceutical companies have special units for the preparation, analytical control, coding, packaging, labeling, shipping, and record maintenance of clinical supplies. Other companies integrate this activity within their existing drug product development and production operations. Still other companies employ contract firms specializing in this field to prepare and manage their clinical trial materials program.

In all clinical study programs, the package label of the investigational drug must bear the statement "Caution: new drug limited by federal [or United States] law to investigational use." Once received by the investigator, the clinical supplies may be administered only to subjects in the study. Blister packaging is commonly used in clinical studies, with immediate labels containing the clinical study or protocol number, patient identification number, sponsor number, directions for use, code number to distinguish between investigational drug, placebo, and/or comparator product, and other relevant information. Records of the disposition of the drug must be maintained by patient number, dates, and quantities administered. When there is a department of pharmacy at the site of the clinical study (e.g., university teaching hospital), pharmacists frequently assist in the control and management of clinical supplies. When an investigation is terminated, suspended, discontinued, or complete, all unused clinical supplies must be returned to the sponsor and an accounting made of used and unused products.

All formulations, from those developed initially through the final marketed version, must be prepared under the conditions and procedures set out by the FDA in its Current Good Manufacturing Practice guidelines.

DOSAGE FORMS

Dosage Form Design

At some stage, a decision needs to be made about the dosage form(s) for the delivery of the drug (e.g. a tablet, a capsule or an injection). The factors the determine which dosage form(s)is(are)to be used are many and involve marketing considerations apart from scientific considerations.

Types of Dosage Forms: Now a days there are many different dosage forms, including the three examples given above, and they all have their relative merits and demerits as given below

Dosage form	Relative merits & demerits
Tablets & capsules	Convenient and commonest dosage forms but likely to be no good if the drug cannot be absorbed in the alimentary tract or if the patient (e.g. A child cannot swallow them.)
Injections &infusion	Rapid action but impractical for treating chronic (long term) illnesses.
Pessaries & suppositories	Can deliver the drug to local area where required but have limited general use
Solution, Suspensions &Elixiris	Useful for children and the elderly but are bulky and less useful if the drug is unpalatable or unstable in the presence of water.
Ointments, Creams, &paints	Use is restricted to topical application.
Aerosols & Dry Powder inhalations	Good for drugs required in the but can be difficult to administer the dose correctly
Transdermal patches	Convenienent if the dose need to be released over a long period (eg. hormone replacement therapy) but can cause irritation.

Therapeutic Considerations

A therapeutic consideration plays an important role in deciding the dosage form to be formulated. Here are a few examples:

A tablet is not suitable dosage form if the drug cannot be absorbed in the alimentary tract - unless, of course, it Is required to treat an ailment in the tract itself (such as a gut infection). Instead of a tablet, an injection might be a Suitable alternative. •Even if the drug can be absorbed in the alimentary tract (saying the intestine), as the tablet will still be unsatisfactory if the drug is destroyed in the stomach acid. In such a case the tablet might be enteric coated to prevent drug destruction whilst the tablet is passing through the stomach. By the time the tablet reaches the intestine the coating has dissolved liberating the drug for absorption through the intestinal wall.

Drugs which need to act immediately (e.g. Bronchodilator drugs for treating asthmatic attacks where the airways suddenly become so constricted that the patient has difficulty in breathing) are best delivered by inhalation directly to the lungs where they can rapidly dilate the airways, rather than being swallowed in a tablet with the consequently delay in action whilst the drug is absorbed and delivered to the lungs.

To be effective, a drug must reach in desired concentration to the part of the body where it is required to act and, ideally, must be maintained at concentration for the appropriate period of time. This goal is influenced by the key interactions which takes place between the drug and the body after the drug has been administered. These are:

- Absorption (the way the drug enters the body and reaches the bloodstream).
- Distribution (where the drug goes in the body after it has been absorbed).
- Metabolism (how it is changed by the body - e.g. in the liver).
- Elimination (the route by which it, or its metabolites, leave the body - e.g. in the urine via the kidney).

These processes are referred to as ADME in short. The study of the pharmaceutical factors which affect the fate of the drug after administration is called biopharmaceutics and these factors will need to be evaluated in the development of a new drug.

Chapter 4

The Investigational New Drug (IND) Application and New Drug Application (NDA)

Learning Objectives

To understand

- Content of the IND
- The Clinical Protocol
- Pre-IND Meetings
- FDA Review of an IND Application
- The New Drug Application (NDA)
- General Content of the NDA Submission
- Drug Product Labeling
- FDA Review and Action Letters
- Phase IV Studies and Post Marketing Surveillance
- Supplemental, Abbreviated and Other Applications
- Supplemental New Drug Application (SNDA)
- Abbreviated New Drug Application (ANDA)
- Biologics License Application (BLA)
- Animal Drug Applications
- Medical Devices

Investigational New Drug (IND)

Under the Food, Drug, and Cosmetic Act as amended, the sponsor of a new drug is required to file with the FDA an IND before the drug may be given to human subjects (1). This is to protect the rights and safety of the subjects and to ensure that the investigational plan is sound and is designed to achieve the stated objectives. The sponsor of an IND takes responsibility for and initiates a clinical investigation. The sponsor may be an individual (a sponsor investigator), a pharmaceutical company, governmental agency, academic institution, or some other private or public organization. The sponsor may actually conduct the study or employ, designate, or contract other qualified persons to do so. Now-a-days, many contract research organizations conduct all or designated portions of clinical studies or clinical drug trials for others through contractual arrangements. After submission of the IND, the sponsor must delay the use of the drug in human subjects for not less than 30 days from the date the FDA acknowledges the receipt of the application. An IND automatically goes into effect following this period unless the FDA notifies the sponsor that as a result of its review of the submission, it is waiving the period and the sponsor may initiate the study early or the investigation is being placed on a clinical hold.

A clinical hold is an order issued by the FDA to delay the start of a clinical investigation or to suspend an ongoing study. During a clinical hold, the investigational drug may not be administered to human subjects (unless specifically permitted by the FDA for individual patients in an ongoing study). A clinical hold is issued when there is concern that human subjects will be exposed to unreasonable and significant risk of illness or injury, when there is a question of the qualifying credentials of the clinical investigators, or when the IND is considered incomplete, inaccurate, or misleading. If the concerns raised are addressed to the FDA's satisfaction, a clinical hold may be lifted and clinical investigations resumed; if not, an IND may be maintained in a clinical hold, declared inactive, withdrawn by the sponsor, or terminated by the FDA.

Content of the IND

The content of an IND is prescribed in the CFR and is submitted under a cover sheet (Form FDA-1571).

Among the items required

- Name, address, and telephone number of the sponsor of the drug
- Date of submission
- Name (s) of the drug, including all available names (generic, trade name, chemical, code)
- IND number (if one has been previously assigned)
- Indications for the proposed drug's use
- Indication of whether the application is a new submission, a response to a clinical hold, or an amendment to a previously submitted IND application
- Name and title of the person responsible for monitoring the conduct and progress of the investigation
- Name(s) and title(s) of the person(s) responsible for the review and evaluation of the information relevant to the safety of the drug
- Name and address of any contract research organization involved in the study
- Identification of the phase or phases of the clinical investigation to be conducted

- Introductory statement and general investigational plan: the name of the drug and all active ingredients, the drug's structural formula and pharmacologic class, the formulation of the dosage form and route of administration, and the broad objectives and planned duration of the study
- Description of the investigational plan: the rationale for the drug or research study, the indication or indications to be studied, the approach to evaluating the drug, the types of studies to be conducted, the estimated number of subjects to be given the drug, and any serious risks anticipated based on animal studies or other human experiences with the drug
- Brief summary of previous human experience with the drug (domestic or foreign), including the reasons if the drug has been withdrawn from any other investigation and/or marketing
- CMC information: a complete description of the drug substance, including its physical, chemical, and biologic characteristics; its method of preparation and analytical methods to ensure its identity, strength, quality, purity, and stability; a quantitative list of the active and inactive components of the dosage form to be administered; the methods, facilities, and controls employed in the manufacture, processing, packaging, and labeling of the new drug to ensure appropriate qualitative and quantitative standards; and product stability during the clinical investigation
- Pharmacology and toxicology information: the drug's mechanism of action if known; information on the drug's absorption, distribution, metabolism, and excretion; and acute, sub acute, chronic, and reproductive and developmental toxicity studies
- If the new drug is a combination of previously investigated components, a complete preclinical and clinical summary of these components when administered singly and any data or expectations relating to the effect when combined • Clinical protocol for each planned study
- Commitment that an Institutional Review Board (IRB) has approved the clinical study and will continue to review and monitor the investigation (discussed in the next section)
- Investigator brochure (discussed in the next section)
- Indication if any part of the study is to be conducted by a contract research organization, and, if so, the name and address of that organization
- Commitment not to begin clinical investigations until the IND is in effect, the signature of the sponsor or authorized representative, and the date of the signed application

The Clinical Protocol

As a part of the IND application, a clinical protocol must be submitted to ensure the appropriate design and conduct of the investigation. Clinical protocols include

- Statement of the purpose and objectives of the study

- Outline of the investigational plan and study design, including the kind of control group and methods to minimize bias on the part of the subjects, investigators, and analysts • Estimate of the number of patients to be involved
- Basis for subject selection, with inclusion and exclusion criteria
- Description of the dosing plan, including dose levels, route of administration, and duration of patient exposure
- Description of the patient observations, measurements, and tests to be used
- Clinical procedures, laboratory tests, and monitoring to be used in minimizing patient risk
- Names, addresses, and credentials of the principal investigators and co investigators
- Locations and descriptions of the clinical research facilities to be used
- Approval of the authorized Institutional Review Board

Once an IND is in effect, a sponsor must submit an amendment for approval of any proposed changes. This may involve changes of dosing levels, testing procedures, the addition of new investigators, additional sites for the study, and so on.

For many years, women and the elderly were included only rarely in clinical drug investigations. Women of childbearing age were excluded from early drug tests out of fear that the subject would become pregnant during the investigation with possible harm to the foetus. Exceptions were made only in cases of potentially lifesaving drugs. However, in recognition that the general exclusion of women from drug investigations results in inadequate data on any gender-based differences in a drug's effects, the FDA now calls for the inclusion of women in numbers adequate to allow detection of clinically significant differences in drug response.

The FDA "Guideline for the Study and Evaluation of Gender Differences in the Clinical Evaluation of Drugs" issued in 1993 states the agency's gender inclusion policy. Although the guideline does not require participation of women in any particular trial, it sets forth FDA's general expectations regarding the inclusion of both women and men in drug development, analysis of clinical data by gender, and assessment of potential pharmacokinetic differences between genders. In 1994, the National Institutes of Health (NIH) similarly issued its policy that women and minorities be included in all NIH-supported biomedical and behavioural research projects involving human subjects "unless there is a clear and compelling rationale and justification that their inclusion is inappropriate with respect to the health of the subjects or the purpose of the research".

Pregnancy is a concern in drug investigations because drugs are readily transported from the maternal to the foetal circulation. Because of undeveloped drug detoxication and excretion mechanisms in the foetus, concentrations of drugs may actually reach a higher level in the foetus than in the maternal circulation, with toxic levels resulting. To reduce the risk of foetal exposure to investigational drugs in women of childbearing age, the FDA guideline calls for pregnancy testing, use of contraception, and full information disclosure of potential foetal risks to prospective study subjects. The FDA has made a special effort to ensure that women who have a life-threatening disease (e.g., AIDS-related) are not automatically excluded from investigational trials of drug products for that disease because of a perceived risk of reproductive or developmental toxicity from use of the investigational drug. There are other instances in which drug studies or drug use during pregnancy is justified, for example, agents intended to prevent Rh immunization and haemolytic disease of the newborn.

When a proposed drug is likely to have significant use in the elderly, elderly patients are required to be included in clinical studies to yield age-related data of a drug's effectiveness and any adverse effects. Older people handle a drug differently because of altered body functions such as diminished liver and kidney function, reduced circulation, and changes in drug ADME. Furthermore, the elderly have a greater incidence of chronic illness and multiple disease states than younger adults, and as a result, take multiple medications daily, increasing the potential for drug–drug interactions. This potential is studied and defined.

Recognition of the need to examine in children new drugs intended for the pediatric patient has a similar requirement to ensure a drug's safe and effective use in this population. Also, differentiation in a drug's activity in minority groups and their subpopulations is important in the full assessment of a drug's potential. It is well known that there are interethnic variations both in disease incidence and in biologic response to some medications, and these factors must be considered in the clinical evaluation of drug substances.

Each IND submission must have the prior approval of the IRB with jurisdiction over the site of the proposed clinical investigation. An IRB is a body of professional and public members that has the responsibility for reviewing and approving any study involving human subjects in the institution they serve. The purpose of the IRB is to protect the safety of human subjects by assessing a proposed clinical protocol, evaluating the benefits against risks, and ensuring that the plan includes all needed measures for subject protection. By law, the IRB shall be constituted to include persons competent to review clinical research proposals and be diverse in membership, with consideration of race, gender, cultural background, and sensitivity to issues affecting the subjects and the community. Any substantive change or amendment to an originally approved clinical protocol must be submitted, reviewed, and approved by the IRB and the FDA before implementation.

Each clinical investigator must receive from the sponsor an investigator's brochure, which contains all of the pertinent information developed during the preclinical studies, including summary information on the drug's chemistry, pharmacology, toxicology, and pharmacokinetics; formulation of the clinical trial materials; any known information related to the drug's safety and effectiveness; a description of possible risks and side effects that may be anticipated and special monitoring required; the clinical protocol and study design; criteria for patient inclusion and exclusion; laboratory and clinical tests to be performed; and drug control and record-keeping information.

Each study has defined criteria for subject inclusion or exclusion. These criteria may relate to age, sex (as qualified earlier), smoking, health status (e.g., liver and/or renal function), and other factors deemed necessary in a given phase of investigation. Each subject in a clinical investigation must participate willingly and with full knowledge of the benefits and risks associated with the investigation.

The sponsor of the study must certify that each person who will receive the investigational drug has given informed consent that is, he or she has been informed of the following: participation in the study is voluntary; the purpose and nature of the study; the procedures involved; a description of any foreseeable risks or discomforts; the potential benefits for patients; disclosure of alternative procedures or courses of treatments, if any; the extent of confidentiality of records; conditions under which the subject's participation in the study may be terminated; consequences of a patient's decision to withdraw from the study; the approximate number of subjects to be enrolled; and whom to contact for answers to pertinent questions and/or in case of research-related illness or injury. These elements of informed consent, and additional protections that apply to prisoners in clinical investigations, must be in conformance with the Code of Federal Regulations. Individuals who agree to be subjects in an investigation indicate their consent by signing the form or document containing the above information.

Investigators selected by the sponsor to conduct a clinical investigation must be qualified as experts by training and experience to investigate a particular drug. Each investigator's qualifications are submitted to the FDA as a part of the IND application. To participate in an investigation, each investigator signs a form agreeing to comply with and to be responsible for ensuring that the study is conducted according to the IND's investigational plan and clinical protocol; protecting the rights, safety, and welfare of the human subjects; control of the investigational drug; written records of case histories and clinical observations; and the timely submission of progress reports, safety reports, and a final report. It is the responsibility of the sponsor to monitor the progress of all clinical investigations under its IND. If a sponsor discovers that an investigator is not in compliance with the investigational plan, it is the sponsor's responsibility to gain compliance or to terminate the investigator's participation in the study.

Any serious, unexpected, life-threatening, or fatal adverse experience that may be associated with the use of the drug during a clinical investigation must be reported promptly to the sponsor and subsequently to the FDA for investigation. Depending on the severity and assessment of the adverse experience, an alert notice may be sent to other investigators, a clinical hold may be placed on the study for further evaluation and assessment, or the IND may be withdrawn by the sponsor, placed on inactive status, or terminated by the FDA.

Pre-IND Meetings

On request, the FDA will advise a sponsor on scientific, technical, or formatting concerns relating to the preparation and submission of an IND. This may include advice on the adequacy of data to support an investigational plan, the design of a clinical trial, or whether the proposed investigation is likely to produce the data needed to meet the requirements of the next step, the filing of an NDA to gain approval for marketing.

FDA Review of an IND Application

The FDA's objectives in reviewing an IND are to protect the safety and rights of the human subjects and to help ensure that the study allows the evaluation of the drug's safety and effectiveness. These objectives are best met by the accuracy and completeness of the IND submission, the design and conduct of the investigational plan, and the expertise and diligence of the investigators. When received by the FDA, the IND submission is stamped with the date of receipt, assigned an application number, and forwarded to either the Center for Drug Evaluation and Research (CDER) or the Center for Biologics Evaluation and Research (CBER) for review. Applications for chemical agents are sent to CDER and applications for biologics to CBER.

Within CDER, applications are forwarded to the appropriate office of drug evaluation and then to one of its divisions for review.

After assignment to one of the divisions, the content of the application is thoroughly reviewed to determine whether the preclinical data indicate that the drug is sufficiently safe for administration to human subjects and that the proposed clinical studies are designed to provide the desired data on drug safety and efficacy while not exposing the human subjects to unnecessary risks.

The New Drug Application (NDA)

If the three phases of clinical testing during the IND period demonstrate sufficient drug safety and therapeutic effectiveness, the sponsor may file an NDA with the FDA. This filing may be preceded by a pre-NDA meeting between the sponsor and the FDA to discuss the content and format of the NDA. The purpose of the NDA is to gain permission to market the drug product in the United States.

General Content of the NDA Submission

An NDA contains a complete presentation of all of the preclinical and clinical results that the sponsor has obtained during the investigation of the drug. It is a highly organized document that may contain several hundred volumes of information. In recent years, a computer-assisted NDA process has been implemented whereby the sponsor may interact by computer with the FDA reviewers to facilitate the application review process.

The applicant submits three copies of the NDA: an archival copy, maintained by the FDA as the reference document; a review copy, used by the FDA review division; and a field copy, used by the FDA district office and field inspectors in an on-site preapproval inspection (1). The preapproval inspection is conducted in the facilities in which the approved product is to be produced. The inspectors assess the sponsor's capability to comply with all control and quality standards contained in the application, including the FDA's Current Good Manufacturing Practice standards. Final approval of an NDA can be contingent upon this inspection.

In part, an application for a new chemical entity contains the following components:

- Application form (form FDA 356 h) with the name, address, date, and signature of the applicant or the applicant's authorized representative
- Chemical, non-proprietary, code, and proprietary names of the drug, the dosage form its strength and route of administration
- Statement regarding the applicant's proposal to market the drug product as prescription only or as an OTC product
- Detailed summary of all aspects of the application, including the proposed text of the product's intended labelling, CMCs, nonclinical and clinical pharmacology and toxicology, human pharmacokinetics and bioavailability, statistical analysis, clinical trial data, benefit and risk considerations, and proposed additional or planned post marketing studies
- Detailed technical sections on the CMCs for the drug substance, including its physical and chemical characteristics, methods of identification, assay, and controls, and the drug product, including its composition, specifications, methods of manufacture and equipment used, in-process controls, batch and master production records, container and closure systems, stability, and expiration dating
- Detailed technical sections for nonclinical pharmacology and toxicology in relation to the proposed therapeutic indication, including acute, sub acute, and chronic toxicology, carcinogenicity, reproductive toxicology, and animal studies of absorption, distribution, metabolism, and excretion
- Detailed technical sections for human pharmacokinetics and bioavailability along with microbiology for antibiotic applications
- Detailed technical sections for clinical data for each controlled and uncontrolled study relating to the proposed indication, a copy of the study protocol, effectiveness and safety data including any updates on safety information, comparison of human and animal pharmacology and toxicology data, and support for the dosage and dose intervals and modifications for specific subgroups such as paediatric, geriatric, and renally impaired subjects
- Statement regarding compliance to IRB and informed consent requirements
- Statistical methods and analysis of the clinical data
- Samples of the drug substance, drug product proposed for marketing, reference standards, and finished market package, as requested
- Clinical case report forms for the archival copy of the application

The FDA accepts foreign clinical data if they are applicable to the U.S. population and domestic medical practice, if the studies were conducted by clinical investigators of recognized competence, and if the FDA considers the data to be valid without the need for an on-site inspection. The FDA has entered into bilateral agreements with some countries whereby inspections performed by the regulatory personnel of those countries are acceptable to the FDA.

Drug Product Labelling

The labelling of all drug products distributed in the United States must meet the specific labelling requirements set forth in the CFR and approved for each product by the FDA (56). Specific labelling requirements differ for prescription drugs, non-prescription drugs, and animal drugs. In each instance, however, the objective is the same to ensure the appropriate and safe use of the approved product.

According to federal regulations, drug labelling includes not only the labels placed on an immediate container but also the information on the packaging, in package inserts, and in company literature, advertising, and promotional materials.

For prescription drugs, labelling is a summary of all of the preclinical and clinical studies conducted over the period from drug discovery through product development to FDA approval. The essential prescribing information for a human prescription drug is provided in the package insert, which by law contains a balanced presentation of the usefulness and the risks associated with the product to enable safe and effective use. The package insert is required to contain the following summary information in the order listed.

1. Description of the product, including the proprietary and non-proprietary names, dosage form and route of administration, quantitative product composition, pharmacologic or therapeutic class of the drug, chemical name and structural formula of the drug compound, and important chemical and physical information (e.g., pH, sterility).
2. Clinical pharmacology, including a summary of actions of the drug in humans, relevant in vitro and animal studies essential to the biochemical and/or physiologic basis for action, pharmacokinetic information on rate and degree of absorption, biotransformation, and metabolite formation, degree of drug binding to plasma proteins, rate or half-time of elimination, uptake by a particular organ or foetus, and any toxic effects.
3. Indications and usage, including the FDA-approved indications in the treatment, prevention, or diagnosis of a disease or condition, evidence of effectiveness demonstrated by results of controlled clinical trials, and special conditions to the drug's use for short-term or long-term use.
4. Contraindications, situations in which the drug should not be used because the risk of use clearly outweighs any possible beneficial effect. Contraindications may be associated with drug hypersensitivity, concomitant therapy, disease state, pregnancy, and/or factors of age or gender.
5. Warnings, including descriptions of serious adverse reactions and potential safety hazards, limitations to use imposed by them, and steps to be taken if they occur.
6. Precautions, including special care to be exercised by prescriber and patient in the use of the drug; these include drug–drug, drug–food, and drug–laboratory test interactions, effects on fertility, use in pregnancy, and use in nursing mothers and children.

7. Adverse reactions, including predictable and potential unpredictable undesired (side) effects, categorized by organ system or severity of reaction and frequency of occurrence.
8. Drug abuse and dependence, including legal schedule if a controlled substance, types of abuse and resultant adverse reactions, psychologic and physical dependence potential, and treatment of withdrawal.
9. Overdosage, including signs, symptoms, and laboratory findings of acute over dosage, along with specifics or principles of treatment.
10. Dosage and administration, stating the recommended usual dose, the usual dosage range, the safe upper limit of dosage, duration of treatment, modification of dosage in special patient populations (children, elders, and patients with kidney and/or liver dysfunction), and special rates of administration (as with parenteral medications).
11. How supplied, including information on available dosage forms, strengths, and means of dosage form identification, as colour, coating, scoring, and National Drug Code.

FDA Review and Action Letters

The completed NDA is carefully reviewed by the FDA, which decides whether to allow the sponsor to market the drug, to disallow marketing, or to require additional data before rendering a judgment. By regulation, the FDA must respond within 180 days of receipt of an application. This 180-day period is called the review clock and is often extended by agreement between the applicant and the FDA, as additional information, studies, or clarifications are sought.

The NDA is reviewed by the same FDA division that reviewed the sponsor's original IND. However, for the NDA review, the FDA also obtains the recommendation of an outside advisory review committee composed of persons of recognized competence and stature in the clinical area of the proposed drug's use. Although not binding, this committee's recommendation has influence in the FDA's decision to issue an action letter after the entire review of the application is completed.

The FDA can respond to a sponsor of an NDA with one of the following types of letters:

1. Approval, meaning the drug has met agency standards for safety and efficacy and the drug can be marketed for sale in the United States.
2. Complete response, letting a company know that the review period for a drug is complete and that the application is not yet ready for approval. The letter will describe specific deficiencies and, when possible, will outline the recommended actions the applicant might take to get the application ready for approval.

After an NDA is approved and the product marketed, the FDA requires periodic safety and other reports, schedules plant inspections, and requires continued compliance with control and quality standards and current good manufacturing practices.

Phase IV Studies and Post Marketing Surveillance

The receipt of marketing status for a new drug product does not necessarily end a sponsor's investigation of the drug. Continued clinical investigations, often called Phase IV studies, may contribute to the understanding of the drug's mechanism or scope of action, mayindicate possible new therapeutic uses for the drug, and/or may demonstrate the need for additional dosage strengths, dosage forms, or routes of administration. Postmarketing studies may also reveal additional side effects, serious and unexpected adverse effects, and/ or drug interactions.

In applying for a new use, strength, dosage form, or route of administration for a previously approved drug, the sponsor must file a new IND, conduct all necessary additional nonclinical and clinical studies, and file a new NDA for FDA review.

Supplemental, Abbreviated and Other Applications

In addition to the IND and NDA, the following types of applications are filed with the FDA for the purposes described.

Supplemental New Drug Application (SNDA)

A sponsor of an approved NDA may make changes in that application through the filing of an SNDA. Depending on the changes proposed, some require FDA approval before implementing; others do not.

Among the changes requiring prior approval are the following:

- A change in the method of synthesis of the drug substance
- Use of a different facility to manufacture the drug substance where the facility has not been approved through inspection for Current Good Manufacturing Practice standards within the previous 2 years
- Change in the formulation, analytical standards, method of manufacture, or in-process controls of the drug product
- Use of a different facility or contractor to manufacture, process, or package the drug product
- Change in the container and closure system for a drug product
- Extension of the expiration date for a drug product based on new stability data
- Any labelling change that does not add to or strengthen a previously approved label statement

Examples of changes that may be made without prior approval are minor editorial or other changes in the labelling that add to or strengthen an approved label section, any analytical changes made to comply with the USP–NF, an extension of the product's expiration date based on full shelf-life data obtained from a protocol in the approved application, and a change in the size (not the type of system) of the container for a solid dosage form.

Abbreviated New Drug Application (ANDA)

An ANDA is one in which nonclinical laboratory studies and clinical investigations may be omitted, except those pertaining to the drug's bioavailability. These applications are usually filed for duplicates (generic copies) of drug products previously approved under a full NDA and for which the FDA has determined that information on the exempted nonclinical and clinical studies is already available at the agency. ANDAs commonly are filed by competing companies following the expiration of patent term protection of the innovator drug or drug product. Bioavailability and product bioequivalency are discussed in Chapter 5.

The Patient Protection and Affordable Care Act of 2010 created an abbreviated licensure pathway for biological products that are demonstrated to be "biosimilar" to or "interchangeable" with an FDA-licensed biological product. Under the Act, a biological product may be deemed to be "biosimilar" if data show that, among other things, the product is "highly similar" to an already-approved biological product.

Biologics License Application (BLA)

Biologics License Application (BLAs) are submitted to the FDA's Center for Biological Evaluation and Research (CBER) for the manufacture of biologics such as blood products, vaccines, and toxins. The applications for biologics approvals follow the regulatory requirements as stated specifically for these products in the relevant parts of the Code of Federal Regulations (CFR) (4).

Animal Drug Applications

The Federal Food, Drug, and Cosmetic Act, as amended, contains specific regulations pertaining to the approval for the marketing and labelling of drugs intended for animal use (6).

Included are NADAs, supplemental applications to an approved drug (SNADA), abbreviated new animal drug applications (ANADAs) for generic equivalents, and CNADAs, which are applications for conditional approval of new animal drugs which allow a drug sponsor to legally market a new animal drug intended for a minor use or a minor species after proving it is safe but before collecting all the necessary effectiveness data. The drug's sponsor can keep the product on the market for up to 5 years, while collecting the effectiveness data required for an NADA application.

Medical Devices

The Food and Drug Administration has regulatory authority over the manufacture and licensing of all medical devices, from surgical gloves and catheters to cardiac pacemakers and cardiopulmonary bypass blood gas monitors. Included in the regulations are standards and procedures for manufacturer registration, investigational studies, good manufacturing practices, and premarket approval.

Chapter 5

Clinical Development of Drugs – Introduction and Evolution of Clinical Research

LEARNING OBJECTIVES

To understand

- Clinical Research and Clinical Trials
- Introduction and Evolution of Clinical Research
- Arrival of Placebo (1800)
- The First Double blind Controlled Trial -Patulin for Common Cold (1943)
- First Randomized Curative Trial - The Randomized Controlled Trial of Streptomycin (1946)
- Evolution of Ethical and Regulatory Framework
- Evolution of Clinical Trials in India

Clinical Research and Clinical Trials

Clinical research is a branch of healthcare science that determines the safety and effectiveness (efficacy) of medications, devices, diagnostic products and treatment regimens intended for human use. These may be used for prevention, treatment, diagnosis or for relieving symptoms of a disease. Clinical research is different from clinical practice. In clinical practice established treatments are used, while in clinical research evidence is collected to establish a treatment.

Clinical research is a branch of medical science dealing with any research or study in living humans. 'Clinical trials' is the term interchangeably used with the terms 'clinical research' or 'clinical study'. Although there are many definitions of clinical trials, they are generally considered to be biomedical or health-related research studies in human beings that follow a pre-defined and –designed protocol. Clinical trial is defined as "a systematic study of new drug(s) in human subject(s) to generate data for discovering and/ or verifying the clinical, pharmacological (including pharmacodynamic and pharmacokinetic) and/ or adverse effects with the objective of determining safety and/ or efficacy of the new drug". Clinical trial is company-sponsored, meant for a new drug or device and carried out for a specific new use of an intervention; while clinical research is meant for academic and pharmacovigilance. Large number of literature describes on clinical trial and its phases. However, it has been now started to include a detailed description on clinical research or study.

Introduction and Evolution of Clinical Research

The world's first clinical trial is recorded in the "Book of Daniel" in The Bible.[1]This experiment resembling a clinical trial was not conducted by a medical, but by King Nebuchadnezzar a resourceful military leader. During his rule in Babylon, Nebuchadnezzar ordered his people to eat only meat and drink only wine, a diet he believed would keep them in sound physical condition. But several young men of royal blood, who preferred to eat vegetables, objected. The king allowed these rebels to follow a diet of legumes and water but only for 10 days. When Nebuchadnezzar's experiment ended, the vegetarians appeared better nourished than the meat-eaters, so the king permitted the legume lovers to continue their diet. This probably was the one of the first times in evolution of human species that an open uncontrolled human experiment guided a decision about public health.

Avicenna (1025 AD) in his encyclopedic 'Canon of Medicine' describes some interesting rules for the testing of drugs. He suggests that in the clinical trial a remedy should be used in its natural state in disease without complications. He recommends that two cases of contrary types be studied and that study be made of the time of action and of the reproducibility of the effects. These rules suggest a contemporary approach for clinical trials. However, there seems to be no record of the application of these principles in practice.

The first clinical trial of a novel therapy was conducted accidentally by the famous surgeon Ambroise Pare in 1537. In 1537 while serving with the Mareschal de Motegni he was responsible for the treatment of the battlefield wounded soldiers. As the number of wounded was high and the supply of conventional treatment – oil was not adequate to treat all the wounded, he had to resort to unconventional treatment. He describes, at length my oil lacked and I was constrained to apply in its place a digestive made of yolks of eggs, oil of roses and turpentine. That night I could not sleep at any ease, fearing that by lack of cauterization I would find the wounded upon which I had not used the said oil dead from the poison. I raised myself early to visit them, when beyond my hope I found those to whom I had applied the digestive medicament feeling but little pain, their wounds neither swollen nor inflamed, and having slept through the night. The others to whom I had applied the boiling oil were feverish with much pain and swelling about their wounds. Then I determined never again to burn thus so cruelly the poor wounded by arquebuses'.[2] However, it would take another 200 years before a planned controlled trial would be organized.

James Lind is considered as the first physician to have conducted a controlled clinical trial of the modern era. Dr Lind (1716-94), whilst working as a surgeon on a ship, was appalled by the high mortality of scurvy amongst the sailors. He planned a comparative trial of the most promising cure for scurvy. His vivid description of the trial covers the essential elements of a controlled trial.

Lind describe on the 20th of May 1747, I selected twelve patients in the scurvy, on board the Salisbury at sea. Their cases were as similar as I could have them. They all in general had putrid gums, the spots and lassitude, with weakness of the knees. They lay together in one place, being a proper apartment for the sick in the fore-hold; and had one diet common to all, viz. water gruel sweetened with sugar in the morning; fresh mutton-broth often times for dinner; at other times light puddings, boiled biscuit with sugar, etc., and for supper, barley and raisins, rice and currants, sago and wine or the like. Two were ordered each a quart of cyder a day. Two others took twenty-five drops of elixir vitriol three times a day. Two others took two spoonfuls of vinegar three times a day. Two of the worst patients were put on a course of sea-water. Two others had each two oranges and one lemon given them every day. The two remaining patients took an electary recommended by a hospital surgeon.

The consequence was, that the most sudden and visible good effects were perceived from the use of oranges and lemons; one of those who had taken them, being at the end of six days fit for duty. The other was the best recovered of any in his condition; and was appointed to attend the rest of the sick. Next to the oranges, I thought the cyder had the best effects" (Dr James Lind's "Treatise on Scurvy" published in Edinburgh in 1753). Although the results were clear, Lind hesitated to recommend the use of oranges and lemons because they were too expensive. It was nearly 50 years before the British Navy eventually made lemon juice a compulsory part of the seafarer's diet, and this was soon replaced by lime juice because it was cheaper.

Lind's Treatise of 1953, was written while he was resident in Edinburgh and a Fellow of the Royal College of Physicians, contains not only his well known description of a controlled trial showing that oranges and lemons were dramatically better than the other treatments for the disease, but also a systematic review of previous literature on scurvy.

In 2003, Royal College of Physicians established The James Lind Library to commemorate 250th anniversary of publication of Dr Lind's pioneering contribution "Treatise on Scurvy". The James Lind Library (www.jameslindlibrary.org) was created to improve public and professional general knowledge about fair tests of treatments in healthcare and their history. This library is a website (www.jameslindlibrary.org) that introduces visitors to the principles of fair tests of treatments, with a series of short, illustrated essays. In 2003, Scientific American awarded the Library a Sci/Tech web award. The publicity and popularity of the James Lind Library has made 20 May to be designated International Clinical Trials Day, because James Lind's celebrated controlled trial began on that day in1747.

Arrival of Placebo (1800)

It took another century before the emergence of another important mile stone in the history of modern clinical trial: the placebo. The word placebo first appeared in medical literature in the early 1800s. Hooper's Medical Dictionary of 1811 defined it as "an epithet given to any medicine more to please than benefit the patient." However, it was only in 1863 that United States physician Austin Flint planned the first clinical study comparing a dummy remedy to an active treatment. He treated 13 patients suffering from rheumatism with an herbal extract which was advised instead of an established remedy. In 1886, Flint described the study in his book A Treatise on the Principles and Practice of Medicine. "This was given regularly, and became well known in my wards as the 'placeboic remedy' for rheumatism. The favorable progress of the cases was such as to secure for the remedy generally the entire confidence of the patients."

The First Double blind Controlled Trial -Patulin for Common Cold (1943)

The Medical Research Council (MRC) UK carried out a trial in 1943-4 to investigate patulin treatment for (an extract of Penicillium patulinum) the common cold. This was the first double blind comparative trial with concurrent controls in the general population in recent times. It was one of the last trial with non-randomized or quasi-randomized allocation of subjects. The MRC Patulin Clinical Trials Committee (1943) was chaired by Sir Harold Himsworth, and its statisticians were M Greenwood and W J Martin. This nationwide study enrolled over a thousand British office and factory workers suffering from colds. This was quite a challenging endeavor in wartime,

The study was rigorously controlled by keeping the physician and the patient blinded to the treatment. The treatment allocation was done using an alternation procedure. A nurse allocated the treatment in strict rotation in a separate room. The nurse filed the record counterfoil separately, and detached the code label for the appropriate bottle before asking the patient to visit the doctor. The statisticians considered this an effective random concurrent allocation. .However, the outcome of the trial was disappointing as the analysis of trial data did not show any protective effect of patulin.

First Randomized Curative Trial - The Randomized Controlled Trial of Streptomycin (1946)

The idea of randomization was introduced in 1923. However, the first randomized control trial of streptomycin in pulmonary tuberculosis was carried out in 1946 by MRC of the UK. The MRC Streptomycin in Tuberculosis Trials Committee (1946) was chaired by Sir Geoffrey Marshall, and the statistician was Sir Austin Bradford Hill and Philip Hart, who later directed the MRC's tuberculosis research unit, served as secretary. Marc Daniels, as the "registrar" coordinated the clinicians at the participating hospitals. The trial began in 1947. As the amount of streptomycin available from US was limited, it was ethically acceptable for the control subjects to be untreated by the drug a statistician's dream. This trial was a model of meticulousness in design and implementation, with systematic enrolment criteria and data collection compared with the adhoc nature of other contemporary. A key advantage of Dr Hill's randomization scheme over alternation procedure was "allocation concealment" at the time patients were enrolled in the trial. Another significant feature of the trial was the use of objective measures such as interpretation of x-rays by experts who were blinded to the patient's treatment assignment.

Sir Bradford Hill had formed his allocation ideas over several years (with randomization replacing alternation in order to better conceal the allocation schedule), but had only tried them out in disease prevention. Dr Hill instituted randomization – a new statistical process which has been described in detail in the landmark BMJ paper of 1948.

"Determination of whether a patient would be treated by streptomycin and bed-rest (S case) or by bed-rest alone (C case) was made by reference to a statistical series based on random sampling numbers drawn up for each sex at each centre by Professor Bradford Hill; the details of the series were unknown to any of the investigators or to the co--coordinator and were contained in a set of sealed envelopes, each bearing on the outside only the name of the hospital and a number. After acceptance of a patient by the panel, and before admission to the streptomycin centre, the appropriate numbered envelope was opened at the central office; the card inside told if the patient was to be an S or a C case, and this information was then given to the medical officer of the centre. Patients were not told before admission that they were to get special treatment. C patients did not know throughout their stay in hospital that they were control patients in a special study; they were in fact treated as they would have been in the past, the sole difference being that they had been admitted to the centre more rapidly than was normal. Usually they were not in the same wards as S patients, but the same regime was maintained

Sir Bradford Hill had been anxious that physicians would be unwilling to give up the doctrine of anecdotal experience. However, the trial quickly became a model of design and implementation and gave a boost to Dr Hill's views and subsequent teaching, and resulted, after some years, in the present virtually universal use of randomized allocation in clinical trials. The greatest influence of this trial lay in its methods which have affected virtually every area of clinical medicine. Over the years, as the discipline of controlled trials grew in sophistication and influence, the streptomycin trial continues to be referred to as ground breaking.

Evolution of Ethical and Regulatory Framework

The ethical framework for human subject protection has its origins in the ancient Hippocratic Oath, which specified a prime duty of a physician – to avoid harming the patient. However, this oath was not much respected in human experimentation and most advances in protection for human subjects have been a response to human abuses e.g. World War II experiments.

The first International Guidance on the ethics of medical research involving subjects – the Nuremberg Code was formulated in 1947. Although informed consent for participation in research was described in 1900, the Nuremberg Code highlighted the essentiality of voluntariness of this consent. In 1948, Universal Declaration of Human Rights (adopted by the General Assembly of the United Nations) expressed concern about rights of human beings being subjected to involuntary maltreatment. The brush with thalidomide tragedy helped the U.S. pass the 1962 Kefauver-Harris amendments, which strengthened federal oversight of drug testing and included a requirement for informed consent.

In 1964 at Helsinki, the World Medical Association articulated general principles and specific guidelines on use of human subjects in medical research, known as the Helsinki Declaration. The Helsinki Declaration has been undergoing changes every few years the last one being in 2008. However, the use of placebo and post-trial access continue to be debatable issues.

In 1966, the International Covenant on Civil and Political Rights specifically stated, 'No one shall be subjected to torture or to cruel, inhuman or degrading treatment or punishment. In particular, no one shall be subjected without his consent to medical or scientific treatment. 'Dr. Henry Beecher's 1966 study of abuses and the discovery of human exploitation of Tuskegee study in the 1970s reinforced the call for tighter regulation of government funded human research. The US National Research Act of 1974 and Belmont Report of 1979 were major efforts in shaping ethics of human experimentation. In 1996, International Conference on Harmonization published Good Clinical Practice, which has become the universal standard for ethical conduct of clinical trials.

In parallel to ethical guidelines, clinical trials started to become embodied in regulation as government authorities began recognizing a need for controlling medical therapies in the early 20th century. The FDA was founded in 1862 as a scientific institution and became a law enforcement organization after the US Congress passed the Food and Drugs Act in 1906. After that, legislation progressively demanded greater accountability for marketing food and drugs and the need for testing drugs in clinical trials increased. The regulatory and ethical milieu will continue to evolve as new scientific disciplines and technologies become part of drug development.

Evolution of Clinical Trials in India

India has recently been recognized as an attractive country for clinical trials. But the country's journey in clinical research field has a long history. India has a rich heritage of traditional medicine – Ayurveda. The classic ayurvedic texts contain detailed observations on diseases and in-depth guidance on remedies. It is likely that these descriptions are based on direct observations made by the ancient ayurveda experts. However, there is no recorded documentation in the ancient texts of any clinical experiments. Hence, one has to fall back on current history of medical research in India.

The major historic milestones of the Indian Council of Medical Research reflect, in many ways, the growth and development of medical research in the country over the last nine decades. First meeting of the Governing Body of the Indian Research Fund Association (IRFA) was held on November 15, 1911 at the Plague Laboratory, Bombay, under the Chairmanship of Sir Harcourt Butler.[11] At the 2nd meeting of the Governing Body in 1912, a historic decision was taken to start a journal for Indian Medical research. Between 1918--20, several projects on beriberi, malaria, kalaazar and indigenous drugs were initiated. In 1945, a Clinical Research Unit – the first research unit of IRFA attached to a medical institution- was established at the Indian Cancer Research Centre, Bombay. In 1949, IRFA was redesignated as the Indian Council of Medical Research. Over next 60 years, ICMR established many national research centers in the fields of nutrition, tuberculosis, leprosy, viral disease, cholera, enteric disease, reproductive disorders, toxicology, cancer, traditional medicine, gas disaster, genetics, AIDS etc.

The Central Ethical Committee of ICMR on Human Research constituted under the Chairmanship of Hon'ble Justice (Retired) M.N. Venkatachaliah held its first meeting on September 10, 1996. Several subcommittees were constituted to consider ethical issues in specific areas e.g., Epidemiological Research; Clinical Evaluation of Products to be used on Humans; Organ Transplantation; Human Genetics, etc. The committee released Ethical Guidelines for Biomedical Research on Human Participants in 2000 which were revised in 2006.

Schedule Y of Drugs and Cosmetics Act came into force in 1988 and established the regulatory guidelines for clinical trial (CT) permission. The schedule did force the industry to conduct Phase III clinical trials for registration of a new drug and supported growth of a predominantly generic Indian pharmaceutical industry. However, this schedule only permitted clinical trials at a phase lower than its global status. This phase lag obstructed integration of India in global clinical development.

The next major step has been revision of Schedule Y in Jan 2005.As compared to Schedule Y 1988, which had narrow and restrictive definitions of clinical trial phases, the amended Schedule Y 2005 provided pragmatic definitions for Phase I to IV. The definitions and guidelines for clinical trial phases are broad and rational. The earlier restrictions on number patients and centers in early phases stipulated in Schedule Y 1988 were removed allowing the sponsor company freedom to decide these in relation to protocol requirements. The phase lag requirements gave way to acceptance of concurrent Phase II-III as part of global clinical trials.

Schedule Y 2005 legalized Indian GCP guidelines of 2001. This schedule stipulated GCP responsibilities of ethics committee (EC), investigator and sponsor and suggested formats for critical documents e.g. consent, report, EC approval, reporting of serious adverse event. These amendments in Schedule Y have been a major step forward in direction of GCP compliant trials and have provided the much-needed regulatory support to GCP guidelines.

Since the Scurvy trial, clinical trials have evolved into a standardized procedure, focusing on scientific assessment of efficacy and guarding the patient safety. As the discipline of drug development is enriched by novel therapies and technologies, there will always be a continuing need to balance medical progress and patient safety. As the scientific advances continue to occur, there will be new ethical and regulatory challenges requiring dynamic updates in ethical and legal framework of clinical trials.

For Further Reading

1. Collier R. Legumes, lemons and streptomycin: A short history of the clinical trial. CMAJ. 2009;180:23–24. [PMC free article] [PubMed] [Google Scholar]
2. Bull JP. MD Thesis: University of Cambridge; 1951. A study of the history and principles of clinical therapeutic trials. [Google Scholar]
3. Twyman R A. A brief history of clinical trials. The Human Genome. 2004. Sep, [Accessed 5 Oct 2009]. http://genome.wellcome.ac.uk/doc_WTD020948.html.
4. Dodgson S J. The evolution of clinical trials. The Journal of the European Medical Writers Association. 2006; 15:20–21. [Google Scholar]
5. Chalmers I, Milne I, Trohler U, Vandenbroucke J, Morabia A, Tait G, Dukan E The James Lind Library editorial team. The James Lind Library: explaining and illustrating the evolution of fair tests of medical treatments. J R Coll Physicians Edinb. 2008;38:259–64. [PubMed] [Google Scholar]
6. Hart PD. A change in scientific approach: from alternation to randomised allocation in clinical trials in the 1940s. BMJ. 1999 Aug 28;319(7209):572–573. [PMC free article] [PubMed] [Google Scholar]
7. MRC Streptomycin in Tuberculosis Trials Committee. Streptomycin treatment of pulmonary tuberculosis. BMJ. 1948;2:769–83. [PMC free article] [PubMed] [Google Scholar]
8. Yoshioka A. The Randomized Controlled Trial of Streptomycin in The Oxford Textbook of Clinical Research Ethics. In: Emanuel EJ, Grady C, Crouch RA, Lie RK, Miller FG, Wendler D, editors. Oxford: University Press Oxford; 2008. pp. 46–60. [Google Scholar]
9. Indian Council of Medical Research Ethical Guidelines for Biomedical Research on Human Participants. 2006 [Google Scholar]
10. Sparks J. Timeline of laws related to the protection of human subjects Office of History National Institutes of Health. html. [Accessed 20 Sep 09]. http://history.nih.gov/about/timelines_laws_human.html.

    [accessed on 8 Oct 2009]. http://www.icmr.nic.in/history.htm.
11. Bhatt A, Sewlikar S. India Steps towards Globalization-Reforms to Schedule Y Regulations. CR Focus. 2007; 18:21–26. [Google Scholar]

Chapter 6

Clinical Research Methodology (Phases, Types, Designs and Statistical Concepts of Clinical Trials)

LEARNING OBJECTIVES

To understand

- Ethics in Clinical Trial
- Phases of Clinical Trial

  (Phase I: Human/ Clinical Pharmacology trial, Phase II: Exploratory trial, Phase III: Confirmatory trial, Phase IV: Post-Marketing Surveillance)
- Types of Clinical studies

  (Descriptive studies, Explanatory studies, Observation studies, Aggregate observation studies, Individual observation studies)
- Case-control study
- Cohort
- Cross-sectional

  (Experimental studies, Non-randomized studies, Randomized controlled trials)
- Principles of Clinical Studies

  (Study design, Patient population, Control group, Randomization, Blinding, Treatment considerations, Outcome measures)
- Statistics in Clinical Research

  ('P' value and level of significance, Types of errors and power of study, Sample size formula for qualitative data, Confidence interval, Odds ratio and relative risk, Data analysis, Statistical tests)
- Status of Clinical Research in India

Introduction

Clinical research is a branch of medical science dealing with any research or study in living humans. 'Clinical trials' is the term interchangeably used with the terms 'clinical research' or 'clinical study'. Although there are many definitions of clinical trials, they are generally considered to be biomedical or health-related research studies in human beings that follow a pre-defined and –designed protocol. Clinical trial is defined as "a systematic study of new drug(s) in human subject(s) to generate data for discovering and/ or verifying the clinical, pharmacological (including pharmacodynamic and pharmacokinetic) and/ or adverse effects with the objective of determining safety and/ or efficacy of the new drug". Clinical trial is company-sponsored, meant for a new drug or device and carried out for a specific new use of an intervention; while clinical research is meant for academic and pharmacovigilance. Large number of literature describes on clinical trial and its phases. However, it has been now started to include a detailed description on clinical research or study.

Ethics in Clinical Trial

Depending upon the objective, clinical trial is conducted either on healthy volunteers or on volunteer patients. Healthy volunteers are generally included in such trial that determines pharmacokinetics, tolerability, safety and even efficacy of certain types of drugs (e.g. hypoglycemic, hypnotic, diuretic etc.). Otherwise, for majority of drugs (e.g. antiepileptic, antipsychotic, anti-inflammatory, antitubercular etc.), efficacy can only be assessed in patients.

The research entailing the use of human participants is considered to be absolutely essential after a due consideration of all alternatives in the light of the existing knowledge in the proposed area of research.

In other words, when a new drug is with clear significant benefit at human side, human as participants for trial experimentation becomes justified. International Conference on Harmonization has provided a guideline on Good Clinical Practice (ICH GCP) as an international ethical and scientific quality standard for designing, conducting, recording and reporting trials that involve the participation of human subjects.[3] World Health Organization Guidelines for good clinical practice for trials on pharmaceutical products also describe provisions and prerequisites for a clinical trial, protocol and protection of trial subjects, responsibilities of the investigator, responsibilities of the sponsor, responsibilities of the monitor, monitoring of safety, record-keeping and handling of data, statistics and calculations, handling of and accountability for pharmaceutical products, role of the drug regulatory authority, quality assurance for the conduct of a clinical trial and considerations for multicentre trials. United States Food and Drug Administration Guidelines for conduct of clinical trials provide guidance for institutional review boards and clinical investigators, information for health professionals on clinical trials and human subject protection, information for clinical investigators on drugs, devices and biologic as well as policies and regulatory matters regarding human subjects research. Several issues and principles have been discussed in various guidelines on conducting clinical trial (especially drug trial) which must be addressed while conducting a trial. These include the following:

1) Ethical justification and scientific validity of biomedical research involving humans
2) Ethics review board
3) Informed consent process
4) Choice of control in clinical trials
5) Research involving special group of research participants.

Moreover, clinical trial in India on a new drug or device or any surgical intervention shall be initiated only after the permission has been granted by the Licensing Authority under Rule 21 (b) and the approval obtained from the respective Ethics Committee(s).[7] Subjects who are relatively or absolutely incapable of protecting their own interests i.e. "vulnerable participants" include very poor, illiterate, terminally-ill, mentally-challenged, prisoners, students or employees are examples.[8] Clinical trial must preserve their rights while being conducted in such humans. Moreover, there must be equal distribution of burdens and benefits in terms of race (in case of genetic research), economic and social level, mental-healthiness and reduced autonomy, to avoid unintentional bias and to extend the benefit of trial to maximum of communities.

Phases of Clinical Trial

Clinical trial of a drug is conducted through various phases. The number of phases as trial varies from literature to literature and from author to author. Most literatures describe a clinical trial/ testing of a new molecule to comprise of four phases. These phases are as following:

1) Phase I : Human/ Clinical Pharmacology trial
2) Phase II : Exploratory trial
3) Phase III : Confirmatory trial
4) Phase IV : Post-Marketing Surveillance.

Some literatures describe the above-mentioned first three phases as actual phases of clinical trial while others consider phase II and III as the actual clinical trial. This may be because phase I is usually carried out on healthy volunteers except for diseases like cancer, acquired immuno-deficiency syndrome (AIDS) etc. Moreover, phase IV may not necessarily follow randomized, controlled trial (RCT) with blind fashion of the most commonly-employed type since the drug is available in market with known label-indication and it requires chronic drug administration and observation of patients.

1) Phase I: Human/ Clinical Pharmacology trial

This phase aims to obtain the precise information on a) initial safety in terms of safe dosage range and biological effects including adverse effects; b) metabolism and kinetics and c) drug interactions. The trial is carried out on healthy human volunteers (20-80 in number) except for life-saving drugs meant for treating life-threatening diseases such cancer, AIDS where actual patients only are included. The volunteers or patients are exposed to a single dose which is usually kept as $1/12^{th}$ of the effective dose found from animal studies especially from mice study.

2) Phase II: Exploratory trial

This phase is meant to find whether or not the drug possesses the actual therapeutic potential. It identifies the therapeutic efficacy of the drug with dose range, kinetics as well as metabolism. It follows RCT type with blinding of treatment. It is carried out at one or few clinical centers only on small but sufficient number of patients (100-300 in number) to reach clinical significance in outcomes. It also aims to find out therapeutic index of the drug being studied. It requires to be carried out in patients meeting selection criteria of age group, sex, presence of particular disease with pre-defined and –diagnosed severity etc. It also reports the adverse effects of the drug.

3) Phase III: Confirmatory trial

This phase applies the same study protocol designed for phase II to evaluate safety and efficacy at large. It is to confirm the effectiveness of the drug or treatment, to monitor side effects, to compare it to commonly used treatments and to collect information that will allow the drug or treatment to be used safely. It is simultaneously performed at a large number of clinical centers that include patients of various geographic origins with difference in responsiveness of the disease towards the drug treatment. Further, it covers large number of patients (1,000-3,000 in number) allowing the outcome to reach not only clinical significance but also statistical significance. Once the drug passes this phase successfully, it is licensed for commercial use. Thus, phase III of trial is a key study forming the primary basis for regulatory approval of an intervention and is often referred as pivotal trial. It general proceeds as randomized, placebo-controlled, double-blind clinical trial.

4) Phase IV: Post-Marketing Surveillance

This phase is so named because it is carried out after the drug is released in the market for therapeutic use. It is mainly to detect uncommon but significant adverse effects. Once the drug enters the market, it will be utilized by many more patients having other co-morbidity and co-existing diseases in addition to the disease for which the drug is indicated and licensed. This is also conducted to provide critical information on drug-drug interactions or iatrogenic diseases. The best example is of thiazolidinedione series of drugs, which were found to deteriorate heart failure (HF) if used as antidiabetic in HF-patients. Therefore, they are now contraindicated in diabetic patients with HF.

Clinical trials are conducted with the purpose of commercialization while clinical researches/ studies do not necessarily aim at commercialization. Clinical research can be based on any of the following four concepts:

1) treatment of a disease
2) diagnosis of a disease or disorder or dysfunction
3) systematic review of several clinical studies
4) prognosis of a particular disease.

Clinical research based on therapy/ treatment can be focused on any of the two areas; 1) pharmacology of a drug and 2) effects of a non-pharmacological intervention such as a surgery or a device. Clinical pharmacology is a branch of pharmacology dealing with study of a drug in humans (either healthy volunteers or patients). A large number of new drugs or molecules are synthesized in laboratories or are extracted from natural sources viz. plants or animal organs. However, only a small number enters pharmaceutical market as a successful drug for treatment of a disease. Many devices, as a disease-intervention or treatment, are also manufactured every year but only a few find a place in healthcare system. This is because of the stringent procedure for a drug or device to pass through the pre-clinical and clinical phases to prove its safety and efficacy as well. A drug cannot be marketed and hence not be used for treating a disease until and unless it passes all the phases and proves its effectiveness. Further, once a drug is registered and approved for general clinical use for one indication i.e. one therapeutic use, expansion of its therapeutic-use range requires additional clinical research and trial. Similarly, for any surgical intervention to be recommended by the healthcare system, it has to pass through various stages of pre-clinical and clinical studies.

Even though most of the new drugs are either structurally similar to or are the derivatives of already-existing drug molecule and are rarely with totally new basic structure, data from extensive pre-clinical i.e. animal studies are essential to conduct clinical trials of a new drug. When a drug molecule is a new chemical entity, detailed and extensive studies in animals become essential and more stringent. Biotechnology products, mainly all recombinant drugs are considered as new drugs (irrespective of international availability of the same formulation) and hence treated accordingly. Pre-clinical studies include those carried out in lower animals as well as higher primates with special emphasis on therapeutic and adverse effects. Further, it is also required to establish minimum dose producing the desired effect (i.e. therapeutic effect) and maximum dose causing adverse effects in specific animal species. The investigator should have data on acute, sub-acute and chronic toxicity studies. The investigator can initiate clinical experiment(s) only after he/ she gets all the following information and data about a new drug from animal studies:

1) The need of the new molecule over the existing drug range- the need can be either because of its different mechanism of action and hence additional benefit or due to less adverse effect or due to its greater efficacy and less cost at least.

2) Specific pharmacological actions i.e. those with therapeutic potential for humans and general pharmacological actions i.e. those on other organs and systems, especially cardiovascular, respiratory and central nervous system.
3) Pharmacokinetic data.[17]
4) Therapeutic index (i.e. ratio of dose lethal in 50% of the study population (LD_{50}) to dose effective in 50% of the study population (ED_{50}) which is denoted as $TI = LD_{50}/ED_{50}$) along with the minimum dose required to produce the desired therapeutic effect and the maximum dose producing the unwanted or lethal effect.
5) Toxicity data.
6) Nature of the adverse effects of the drug along with identified signs and symptoms in order to avail the possible treatment if the same occur in humans.

Clinical research based on clinical pharmacology includes exclusively the effect(s) of a drug in human and outweighs the other types of clinical studies in number.

Types of Clinical Studies

Descriptive studies

Descriptive studies report unusual or new events such as the occurrence of sudden infant death syndrome (SIDS) in several siblings within a single family, prevalence of albinism in a single family etc. The researcher simply records the observations and co-relates the events observed with possible reason. These are neither randomized nor pre-designed researches. They may be presented as case reports whereby certain individual patients with distinguished clinical characteristics are included in the study. All the baseline characteristics are recorded and the individual patient is treated as unique case with control over all the variables. The patient is observed and evaluated for the possible outcome. The results are compared with baseline values or are expressed as success or failure of the treatment given. If the treatment succeeded, a hypothesis is generated for an expanded and more rigorous study to find the relationship between the treatment and the outcome observed. In case-series, observations are documented at regular intervals from patients exposed to a particular drug or a group of drugs. They may also cover prior histories of patients with the same outcome, to find a possible cause-effect relationship if exists. These are useful in predicting the incidence of an adverse event of newly-marketed drug when reports on such events are limited.

Explanatory Studies

Observation studies

In an observational study, the subject to be observed chooses whether or not to take the drug or to have the surgery being studied.[20] Errors that are likely to occur include the differences in profile of the subjects since variables such as age, family history of disease, cause and severity of disease etc. may not be defined. For example, two patients have left ventricular (LV) dysfunction, in one it is because of ischemic heart disease (IHD) and in another it is because of severe mitral valve stenosis. Thus, the therapy of both the diseases differs due to different oetioes and hence both the patients cannot be compared in one study. Another example is of two patients suffering from headache, one because of migraine and the other because of common cold. These two patients cannot be compared for the analgesic activity of one drug since the cause and the severity of headache and hence the analgesic activity of the drug would vary greatly. Observational studies can never be blinded. Hence, biases from

Aggregate observation studies

Pandemic and epidemic studies on communicable diseases and their treatments are generally carried out as aggregate observation studies e.g. occurrence and effective treatment of malaria and its relapse in particular geographical area.

Individual observation studies

In individual observational study, the patients/ subjects are individually observed and they are assembled in groups on the basis of outcome or exposure or both. Depending upon the basis of the grouping, the individual observational study is sub-classified as 1) Case-control; 2) Cohort and 3) Cross-sectional.[19]

1) **Case-control study**

   Case-control study involves assembling of subjects in groups on the basis of the outcome found in those subjects. It compares the subjects with outcome in question (the group behaves as a case group) with the subjects without the outcome (the group acts as a control) e.g. occurrence or non-occurrence of myocardial infarction (MI) in patients with hypertension (HT). It generally follows the retrospective design and evaluates how the exposure is related to the well-defined outcome using control group.[19] However, grouping on the basis of outcome incorporates subjects with variety of distinguished characteristics. It is quick and inexpensive. Further, patients with rare outcome can be assembled in a group to study oetioes, pathophysioes and prognosis of a disease. Results are generally expressed in terms of odds ratio (OR) and risk ratio/ relative risk (RR). Although multiple exposure variables can be correlated with outcome, it does not allow the correlation of temporal sequence of cause and effect with the final outcome.

2) **Cohort**

   It includes groups assembled on the basis of exposure. Here the exposure is well-defined but the outcome is variable. Thus, it allows study of one exposure with many more outcomes.[19]

   Cohort study can be retrospective wherein the groups are defined in past or it can be prospective wherein the groups are defined in present. The retrospective cohort correlates the exposure occurred in past with the outcome resulted just in recent past. Here the patients have been followed forward and hence it associates the exposure with some temporal outcomes though not all. If the patients have been treated with different treatments to control outcome-related variables, it limits the correlation between exposure and one outcome only. Like case-control study, it is also quick and inexpensive. If carried out on the basis of well-defined, controlled exposure and followed with control over variables, retrospective cohort study suffices the requirements of prospective study with additional advantage of less time and money consumption. In prospective cohort study, the groups are observed for outcomes at particular, pre-decided time intervals. Thus, it finds firmly whether a particular exposure or sign or symptom is related with the outcomes. If the outcome is rare, the study requires inclusion of large number of patients and longer follow-up. Thus, it is expensive in terms of time and money. If the patients are not randomized and blinded, the outcomes may be influenced by bias and confounding.

3) Cross-sectional

Cross-sectional study assesses both the exposure and outcome concurrently. Generally it is survey or review based. Cross-sectional study is, therefore, good for prevalence research. However, it is not suitable for causal-outcome assessment.

Experimental studies

Non-randomized studies

Patients are selected on the basis of selection criteria. They are not randomized to the particular treatment(s) and are given a treatment depending upon course of disease. Generally, phase IV of clinical trial follows this way. Further, in many experimental studies in humans, randomization is not possible. Many of the surgical experiments have evolved with specific indication and application. They have a focused-patient group and therefore, randomization is not possible or is unethical. For example, patients with both the kidneys failed require undergoing kidney transplantation. Although, dialysis is an available option it is not comparable with renal transplantation and hence patients cannot be randomized to such options.

Randomized controlled trials

In the studies which are randomized controlled clinical trials (RCTs), human subjects (either healthy volunteers or patients) do not choose the therapy being studied or compared. Experimental clinical studies are generally RCTs. Randomized controlled trials are, as the name indicates, based on randomization. When a new drug successfully passes the pre-clinical studies, it is challenged to clinical experiments that follow random assignment of subjects to two or more groups one of which behaves as control group and therefore, such clinical experiments are called RCTs.

Principles of Clinical Studies

The principles to be considered include 1) Study design 2) Patient population 3) Control group 4) Randomization 5) Blinding or non-blinding/ open-labeling 6) Treatment considerations and 7) Outcome measures.

1) Study design

The common study designs employed in RCTs include parallel group design, matched pairs and cross-over designs. In parallel group design, the patients are enrolled, followed and observed for outcomes on parallel basis. Parallel group design requires large number of patients. In matched pairs, patients are matched for different variables and those matching the required variables are then randomized to various treatment groups. This type of study design overcomes the influence of variables on outcomes, although it is difficult to follow. Cross-over design is particularly used when the effect of a drug is reversible and transient. In cross-over design, the patients are given more than one treatment but in sequence i.e. one after another when the effect of previous treatment is washed out. Cross-over design, thus, requires less number of patients.

2) Patient population

As a common and required method, the RCTs are carried out on specific subject population selected on the basis of "selection criteria" which are derived in line with various fixed, independent and dependent variables. This is to overcome the misleading by variables. For example, if effects of angiotensin-converting enzyme inhibitor (ACEI) on cardiac function are to be studied in patients with LV systolic dysfunction, variables like family history of cardiac disease, presence of other cardiac diseases such as heart block or valve failure etc. should be avoided as patients with these variables are different from those not having the variables. Further, they may reveal different outcomes viz. the cardiac function and even survival. Depending upon the defined criteria, patients or healthy subjects are included in the study to randomize to various treatments for the comparison of outcomes and thus, to conclude. The criteria are namely (a) inclusion criteria; (b) exclusion criteria and (c) withdrawal criteria.

(a) Inclusion criteria: Specifications of subjects (patients or healthy volunteers) with regard to age, gender, ethnic groups, body mass index, prognostic factor, diagnostic admission criteria, should be clearly mentioned wherever relevant.

(b) Exclusion criteria: These specify the characteristics of the subjects on the basis of which they are excluded from the trial. For example, severity of the disease, concurrent medication etc.

(c) Withdrawal criteria: These specify the subjects on who the trial shall be terminated and mention when and how to withdraw the subjects from the study and to stop further follow-up in those.

To have comparison possible between or among various treatment groups, selection of patients must be done on the basis of inclusion and exclusion criteria. This allows enrollment of subjects with corresponding clinical characteristics.

3) Control group

Randomized controlled trial also includes control group (either placebo control or active control) to show the control and effect over dependent variables and to obtain clear effects of drug under consideration. Control group can be placebo control, no-treatment control, historical control or active control. The placebo means dummy to the drug under evaluation with regard to organoleptic properties but lacking any pharmacological actions. Thus, it is to overcome the psychological impact of drug administration manifested by an individual on disease progression. It allows the investigator to determine the true efficacy of the treatment being researched for a particular condition.

Some studies also include no-treatment control or historical control as types of controls. In no-treatment control group, the patients do not receive the placebo even. Therefore, they know that they do not receive any treatment and hence, individual bias due to psychic factors affects the study outcomes. In other words, it is least preferred type of control. Historical control is the control group of previous study that was a different with respect to treatment group. Here control group of one study is utilized for another study and both the studies differ with regard to treatment only. This is done for studies not allowing placebo control or no-treatment control and involving high mortality disease even after availability of effective treatment e.g. studies on treatment for cancer and human immune-deficiency virus (HIV) infection.

Inclusion of placebo in drug research and sham surgery has been debated. Moreover, when an effective established treatment is available, use of such placebo control group is unethical. For examples, a drug is to be assessed for its effects on cardiac function in patients with LV systolic dysfunction, as per American College of Cardiology/ American Heart Association (ACC/ AHA) guidelines all the patients would be necessarily receiving ACEI, if not contraindicated.[22] Therefore, in this type of study all the patients receive the recommended drug which has already proved its beneficial effect on cardiac function. Thus, one cannot have a placebo control group but will have an active control receiving the best current therapy. It provides information about relative efficacy of the investigational drug over existing one. In the present example, the patients would be randomly assigned to a group receiving ACEI or to a group receiving ACEI in addition to the drug being evaluated- the former behaving as an active control and the later as a treatment group.

4) Randomization

Randomization is an optimal method of distributing the variables between the treatment and control groups. Therefore, the bias of selecting specific treatment does not occur. Random assignment of subjects to various groups provides equal distribution of all variables in all the groups and does not let them influence the final outcomes. Randomization techniques mainly used in RCTs are simple randomization, cluster randomization and stratified randomization. In simple randomization, patients matching the selection criteria are randomized to various treatment groups. In cluster randomization various groups of patients matching the criteria are randomized to treatment under investigation. This kind of trial is especially used to find the geographical, genetic variations. In stratified randomization technique, subjects are classified in groups i.e. strata and then within a group they are randomized to various treatment groups. In RCTs, three main methods of randomization include 1) Tables of random numbers; 2) Mathematical algorithms for pseudorandom number generators and 3) Physical randomization devices such as coins, cards or sophisticated devices such as Electronic Random Number Indicator Equipment (ERNIE).

5) Blinding

To avoid bias, trial is carried out in blind fashion. Blinding means "concealing or masking of the patients-assignment to a study group (control or treatment) from those participating in the study i.e. patients, observer and experimenter". RCTs can be blinded or non-blinded. The non-blinded experiment is also called open-label study. In this type of study all three- the patient, the physician or the observer and the experimenter or the researcher, are aware of the treatment used. In many instances it is unethical to hide the treatment module from the patients especially those suffering from life-threatening disease such as cancer, AIDS, end-stage HF etc. Additionally, open-label study permits the patients to buy brand of the drug of his choice independently. However, it has the biggest disadvantage of introducing bias from any of the three components of the RCTs.

Blinding is carried out at the beginning of study. The blind RCT can be single-, double- or triple- blind. In a single-blind experiment, the participants either the patient or the healthy volunteer does not know whether he receives the test intervention or placebo. In double-blind trial, neither the patient/ subject nor the experimenter knows who belongs to the control group and who belongs to test group but the observer knows. In triple-blind RCT, none of the three components of study knows name or nature of the treatment given. Therefore, the triple-blind RCT is totally devoid of any kind of biases and allows the outcomes to be free from any such influence. In double- and triple-blind experiment the keys identifying the patients/ human subjects and the group they belonged to are preserved by a separate another party and given to the researcher only at the end of the study. Randomized controlled trial can also be conducted as PROBE. PROBE is an acronymus of Prospective, Randomized, Open-label, Blinded-End point as used earlier by Neutel and Smith (2003). This type of trial is easier to carry out than a double-blinded placebo controlled design (DBPC) because it does not require the "matched placebo group" and the "open-label" allows the enrolled patients to receive a marketed preparation of the drug. However, the PROBE studies have only the end-point blinded i.e. observer is unaware of the treatment being studied while investigator and patients are aware of it. Therefore, the investigator or the patient bias may be introduced and thus, the results obtained are less reliable than those with double- or triple-blind study.

6) Treatment considerations

While conducting RCTs, the treatment (either being studied or behaving as active-control) must be considered with regard to its dosages, dosing frequency and other concurrent medication. A drug is generally available in various dosage forms viz. tablet, capsule or injectable etc. and it varies in strength. Moreover, depending upon the dosage form, the route of administration differs and hence, the amount of administration and dosing frequency also. All these factors together affect the plasma concentration of drug and thereby the effects of the drug and hence the final outcome. Therefore, except dose and frequency of drug(s), all above-mentioned factors are kept unique and constant throughout the study. Whenever dose and frequency need to be changed, it is done gradually and stepwise. If two drugs are to be administered one of which is likely to interfere with the other either pharmacokinetically or pharmacodynamically, the dosage must be reconsidered to overcome the influence of such interference on study outcomes. Patient compliance is another important part of the treatment consideration. A treatment should not be non-compliant as the patient avoids or less prefers to take such medication resulting in erroneously less efficacious outcomes than those obtained with the other treatment group.

7) **Outcome measures**

The objective of the study determines the outcomes of interest to be measured. These measures are nothing but the points of checking and recording to accomplish the comparison. In experiments the outcomes are measured in terms of efficacy end-points i.e. primary end-points and surrogate end-points which are also called secondary end-points. For examples, in an experiment evaluating an antihypertensive agent, the clinical end-point of real interest is whether the treatment under investigation can reduce cardiovascular events; a surrogate is the ability of the treatment to reduce blood pressure. The primary end-points of the study are the main measures to support or refute the hypothesis of the study. They must be defined and specified by the investigator at the beginning of the study. Secondary measures, although pre-specified before the commencement of the study, can be further elaborated during the study. For example, when diuretics are used for treating hypertension, serum glucose level measurement can also be added though serum electrolytes are usually measured as main secondary end-point. Although various measures are determined as primary and secondary end-points, quality of life is now-a-days becoming main primary end-point.

STATISTICS IN CLINICAL RESEARCH

Statistics play a crucial role in concluding a clinical research. It is applied in clinical research to analyze data and to infer the results obtained. It is important to obtain a statistically significant difference between two or more groups being compared in a clinical research, in order to make the outcomes acceptable. Statistics is also required at the beginning of the trial to calculate the sample size required to reach a statistical significance in the findings.

'P' value and level of Significance

In a clinical research, a null hypothesis is stated and tested by finding the difference between/ among the results of groups involved in the research. The difference in the results obtained between/ among various groups should be of statistical significance in order to reject the null hypothesis and thus, to accept the alternative hypothesis i.e. "treatment being study as effective one". In many instances, clinical research finds the difference in the results of clinical significance but fails to attain a statistical significance and therefore, the null hypothesis is accepted. Rejection or acceptance of a null hypothesis is based on 'P' value. 'P' value is defined as "the smallest level of significance of the difference in the results that would reject the null hypothesis". It tells how likely it is that the difference between/ among groups occurred by chance rather than because of an effect of treatment.

Types of errors and power of study

The 'P' value is based on two types of errors that one may encounter during experiment. These two errors are designated as type I error and type II error. The former is also called alpha

(α) error and the later beta (β) error. A type I error occurs if a difference is found between A and B when none actually exists. Thus, α error indicates the chances of detecting a difference which does not actually exist i.e. the chances of having False Positive Difference. A type II error occurs if no difference is found though A and B do actually differ. Thus, β error indicates the chances of not detecting a difference which actually exists i.e. the chances of having False Negative Difference. Alpha error indicates the level of significance of the result difference among various treatment groups. The level of significance is usually set at the traditional value of 5%. Beta error gives an idea about power (1-β) of a clinical study. Beta error is often chosen to be between 5 and 20%.

Power is the ability of a statistical test to show significance if a specified difference truly exists. It is essential to minimize these errors at pre-decided levels or below to draw a conclusion in a clinical study. Furthermore, results of a statistical analysis are found conclusive only when the sample size is sufficiently large. However, because of time and cost factors, it may not be possible to enroll large sample size in a study. In that case, finding power of the study may disclose and support the inability of a test not to reach a statistically significant difference between the groups, even when the clinical difference is significant.

Sample size

Sample size depends upon the design of study, nature of variable and measurement scale.

Sample size formula for quantitative response

The number of patients required per group can be estimated using following formula:

$$\text{N per Group} = \frac{2(\text{SD})^2}{(\text{Diff})^2} \times \left(Z_\alpha + Z_\beta\right)^2$$

Where,

SD = estimated standard deviation – known or based on some other study

Diff. = expected difference between two treatment considered as clinically important

Z_α = Z value from statistical tables corresponding to level of significance (α)

Z_β = Z value from statistical tables corresponding to (β)

For 2 sided tests with $\alpha = 0.05$ and $\beta = 0.20$

Z_α = Corresponding to level of significance (0.05) = 1.96

Z_β = Corresponding to (β = 0.20) = 0.842

Sample size formula for qualitative data

The number of patients required per group can be calculated using following formula:

$$N = \frac{(2 \times \text{Joint Success rate} \times \text{Joint Failure rate})^2}{(\text{Diff})^2} \times \left(Z_\alpha + Z_\beta\right)$$

Confidence Interval

The confidence interval (CI) gives a range. It gives a measure of reproducibility of the results within the obtained range. Expression of 'P' value along with CI is clinically more useful and acceptable by many researchers. Generally, it is kept at level of 95%. A 95% CI indicates that if the study is repeated 100 times, the study results would fall within this interval 95 times. For example, if improvement in LV ejection fraction (LVEF) after revascularization in 95 patients is 6% on an average when compared with baseline with a 95% CI of 4.5 to 9% for the difference, it is concluded that the revascularization has the specificity of producing improvement in LVEF by 4.5 to 9% if this revascularization is performed in such 100 patient populations i.e. if it is repeated 100 times.

Odds Ratio and Relative Risk

Odds ratio (OR) and relative risk (RR) both are measures of the size of an association between an exposure and a disease or death. For example, association between smoking or HT and development of IHD; use of a medication and occurrence of a side effect; exposure to MI over global LV ischemia and mortality etc. are expressed in terms of OR or RR. Observational studies usually report their results as OR or RR, although experiments also include these types of measurements as safety and efficacy end-point. A RR of 1.0 indicates that the exposure does not change the risk of disease. A RR of 1.9 indicates that patients with the exposure are 1.9 times more likely to develop the disease or have a 90 percent higher risk of disease. For example, if the RR of hyperlipidemia is 1.4 for development of IHD indicates that patients with hyperlipidemia are 1.4 times more likely to develop IHD than those without hyperlipidemia or they have a 40% higher risk of developing IHD.

Odds ratio is a way to estimate relative risks in case-control studies, when the RR cannot be calculated specifically. Although it is accurate when the disease is rare, the approximation is not as good when the disease is common.

Data Analysis

Data analysis is carried out after compiling the observations and applying appropriate statistical test. The test to be applied depends on the type of data and their distribution in the study. At large, the data are categorized as parametric or non-parametric. However, in clinical study, the data collected for analysis can alternatively be classified in four classes.

1) Continuous e.g. blood pressure, blood sugar
2) Discrete, associated with numbers and ordered e.g. number of anginal episodes per week, number of MI attack in past etc.
3) Attributes: categorical, ordered e.g. degree of overweight, intensity of pain
4) Attributes: categorical, not ordered e.g. male or female, patients with diabetes mellitus or not

Data can also be typified alternatively as categorical or numerical. The categorical data can be nominal or ordinal in nature. Nominal data are expressed as proportion e.g. sex-male or female proportion in occurrence of a disease. Ordinal data are expressed as scores and ranks e.g. pain, categorized as mild, moderate and severe and can be scored as 1, 2 and 3 respectively. The numerical data are observed in form of interval measurements either continuous (e.g. blood sugar level, blood urea level) or discrete (e.g. number of patients admitted to a hospital, heart rate etc.).

Statistical tests

Application of most suitable statistical test allows analyzing the data and interpreting the results of the study. Different statistical tests are applied in a clinical research to analyze the data and to infer the results obtained depending upon the type of data and their distribution (Table 6.1)

Table 6.1 Statistical tests useful in Clinical Studies

		Type of Data		
Goal	**Numerical Measurement**	**Rank, Score**	**Binomial (Two Possible Outcomes)**	**Survival Time**
Describe one group	Mean, SD	Median, interquartile range	Proportion	Kaplan Meier Survival Curve
Compare one group to a hypothetical value	One-sample *t* test	Wilcoxon test	Chi-square or Binomial test	
Compare Two unpaired Group Compare Two paired Group	unpaired *t* test paired *t* test	Mann-Whitney Test Wilcoxon test	Fisher's test (chi-square for large samples) McNemar's test	Log-rank test or Mantel-Haenszel Conditional proportional hazards regression
Compare three or more unmatched group	One-way ANOVA	Kruskal-Wallis Test	Chi-square Test	Cox Proportional hazards regression
Compare three or more matched group	Repeated-measures ANOVA	Friedman Test	Cochrane Q	Conditional proportional hazards regression
Quantify association between two Variables	Pearson correlation	Spearman Correlation	Contingency coefficients	
Predict value from another measured variable	Simple linear regression or Nonlinear regression	Nonparametric Regression	Simple logistic Regression	Cox proportional hazards regression
Predict value from several measured or binomial variables	Multiple linear regression or Multiple nonlinear regression		Multiple logistic Regression	Cox proportional hazards regression

Status of Clinical Research in India

Clinical research in form of trial is conducted not only as unicenter but also as muticenter at various clinical research centers spread over various countries including India. In India, for international collaborative study, details about foreign collaborators and documents for review of Health Ministry's Screening Committee (HMSC) or appropriate Committees under other agencies/authority like Drug Controller General of India (DCGI) are implemented and followed in line with the guidelines by Indian Council of Medical

Research. The centers participating in the trial are taken care by clinical research organizations (CROs), which play a distinguished role of central facilities. With advancement and development of various guidelines to implement in such trials, more than 20 CROs have come up with many known to conduct trials at international level. Though developing at full swing, further expansion of field to include research on biologics and devices is needed.

For Further Reading

1. Part X-A Import or Manufacture of New Drug for Clinical Trials or Marketing. In: Malik V, editor. The Drugs and Cosmetics Act, 1940 and Drugs and Cosmetics Act, 1945 and their Allied Acts and Rules. Lucknow: Eastern Book Company; 2006. p.154-58.
2. Tripathi KD. Essentials of Medical Pharmacology. 6th ed. New Delhi: Jaypee Brothers Medical Publishers (P) Ltd.; 2009. p. 59-77.
3. International Conference on Harmonisation of Technical Requirements for Registration of Pharmaceuticals for Human Use. ICH Harmonised Tripartite Guideline: Guideline for Good Clinical Practice E6(R1) 10 JuneSD (standard Deviation), ANOVA (Analysis of Variance) 1996 [online. Available form: URL: http://www.ich.org/LOB/media/MEDIA482.pdf
4. World Health Organization Guidelines for good clinical practice (GCP) for trials on pharmaceutical products [online]. [cited 2010 Jul 29]. Available form: URL: http://apps.who.int/medicinedocs/pdf/whozip13e/whozi p13e.pdf
5. U. S. Food and Drug Administration (FDA) Guidelines for Conduct of Clinical trials (July 27, 2010) [online]. [cited 2010 Jul 29] Available form: URL: http://www.ninds.nih.gov/research/clinical_research/pol icies/fda.htm
6. Indian Council of Medical Research: Ethical Guidelines for Biomedical Research on Human Participants [online].2006 [cited 2007 Jul 21]. Available from: URL: http://www.icmr.nic.in/ethical.pdf
7. Gupta SK. Requirements and Guidelines to Undertake Clinical Trials in India-Schedule Y (Amended Version). In: Gupta SK, editor. Basic Principles of Clinical Research and Methodology. New Delhi: Jaypee Brothers; 2007. p. 233-52.
8. Thatte U. Ethical Issues in Clinical Research. In: Gupta SK, editor. Basic Principles of Clinical Research and Methodology. New Delhi: Jaypee Brothers; 2007. p. 58-72.
9. Oates JA. The Science of Drug Therapy. In: Brunton LL, Lazo JS and Parker KL, editors. Goodman & Gilman's The Pharmacological Basis of Therapeutics 11th ed. New York: McGraw-Hill Companies Inc.; 2006. p. 117-36.
10. Central Drugs Standard Control Organization, Directorate General of Health Services, Government of India: Good Clinical Practices for Clinical Research in India. Schedule

Y (Amended Version -2005) [online]. [cited 2007 Jul 21]. Available from: URL: http://www.cdsco.nic.in/html/GCP1.html

11. Rang HP, Dale MM, Ritter JM and Moore PK. Pharmacology 5th ed. New Delhi: Elsevier; 2003. p. 80-90.
12. Center Watch: Clinical Trials- Overview of Clinical Trials. [online] [cited 2010 Apr 28]. Available from: U R L : h t t p : / / w ww. c e n t e r w a t c h . c o m / c l i n i c a l-trials/overview.aspx
13. Reagan-Shaw S, Nihal M and Ahmad N. Dose translation from animal to human studies revisited. FASEB J. 2007;

    a. 659-61 [online]. [cited 2010 April 22]. Available from: URL: http://fasebj.org/cgi/reprint/22/3/659
14. Understanding Clinical Trials [online]. updated 2007 Sep20 [cited 2010 Apr 27]. Available from: URL: http://clinicaltrials.gov/ct2/info/understand
15. Vahle JL and TashjianJr AH. Clinical Drug Evaluation and Regulatory Approval. In: Golan DE, Tashjian Jr AH, Armstrong EJ and Armstrong AW, editors. Principles of Pharmacology- The Pathologic Basis of Drug Therapy 2nd ed. New Delhi: Wolter Kluwer (India) Pvt. Ltd.; 2008. p. 863-73.
16. POEMs and EBM Glossary: American Academy of Family Physicians- News and Publications [online]. [cited 2007 Jul 21]. Available from: URL: http://www.aafp.org/online/en/home/publications/journ als/afp/afppoems.html
17. The Drugs and Cosmetics Act, 1940 [online]. [cited 2010A p r 2 3] . A v a i l a b l e f r o m : U R L : http://cdsco.nic.in/html/Copy%20of%201.%20D&CAct 121.pdf
18. Abate MA and Hildebrand III JR. Clinical Drug Literature. In: Beringer P, Der Marderosian A, Felton L, Gelone S, Gennaro AR, Gupta PK, Hoover JE, Popovick NG, Reilly WJ and Hendrickson R, editors. Remington-The Science and Practice of Pharmacy 21st ed. New Delhi: Wolters Kluwer (India) Pvt. Ltd.; 2009. p. 74-86.
19. Grossi PM. Study Design and Validity. [online]. 2004 [cited 2007 Jul 21]. Available from: URL: http://dukehealth1.org/ surgery/documents /Clinical Studies. pdf
20. Rosenbaum PR. Observational Study. In: Everitt BS and Howell DC, editors. Encyclopedia of Statistics in Behavioral Science. Chichester: John Wiley & Sons Ltd; 2005(Vol. 3). p. 1451–62.
21. Bowalekar S. Biostatistics in Clinical Trials. In: Gupta SK, editor. Basic Principles of Clinical Research and Methodology. New Delhi: Jaypee Brothers; 2007. p. 233-52.
22. Hunt SA, Abraham WT, Mancini DM, Chin MH, Michl K, Feldman AM, Oates JA, Francis GS, Rahko PS, Ganiats TG, Silver MA, Jessup M, Stevenson LW, Konstam MA and Yancy CW. ACC/AHA 2005 Guideline Update for the Diagnosis and Management of Chronic Heart Failure in the Adult: a report of the American College of Cardiology/American Heart Association Task Force on Practice Guidelines (Writing Committee to Update the 2001 Guidelines for the Evaluation and Management of Heart

Failure) [online]. [cited 2007 Jul 23]. Available from: URL: http://circ.ahajournals.org/cgi/content/full/112/12/e154

23. Neutel JM and Smith DHG. Evaluation of angiotensin II receptor blockers for 24-hour blood pressure control: meta-analysis of a clinical database. J ClinHypertens. 2003; 5(1): 58-63.

24. D'Agostino RB Sr and Massaro JM. New developments in medical clinical trials. J Dent Res. 2004; 83(Spec Iss C): C18-C24.

25. Pais-Ribeiro JL. Quality of life is a primary end-point in clinical settings. Clinic Nutrit. 2004; 23(1): 121-30.

26. Montgomery DC. Introduction to statistical quality control 4th ed. John Wiley and Sons Inc.: 2003. p. 98.

27. Bolton S and Bon C. Pharmaceutical statistics: Practical and clinical applications 4th ed. New York: Marcel Dekker Inc.; 2004. p. 151-72.

28. Bolton S and Bon C. Pharmaceutical statistics: Practical and clinical applications 4th ed. New York: MarcelDekker Inc.: 2004. p. 1-30.

29. Motulsky H. Choosing a test. In: Intuitive Biostatistics.New York: GraphP ad Software, Oxford University Press:[online]. 1995 [cited 2007 Jul 21]. Available from: URL: http://www.graphpad.com/www/book/ Choose.htm

30. Patel BB, Tiwari S and Mishra B. Clinical research in India: An update. Ind J Pharm Pract. 2009; 2(2): 14-24 [online]. [cited 2010 Jul 29]. Available from: URL: http://ijopp.org/ijpp_3rd_issue/review_articles2.pdf

Chapter 7

Clinical Trials Research in India (Clinical Trial Phases, Process, Documentation and Regulations)

LEARNING OBJECTIVES

To understand

- Clinical Trials in India
- Phases of Clinical Trials
  (Phase 0, Phase I- Human/Clinical Pharmacology trials, Phase II - Exploratory trials, Phase III - Confirmatory trials, Phase IV - Post Marketing Trials)
- Clinical Trial Process
- Clinical Trial Application Filing
- Indian Clinical Trial Regulations
- Challenges in Indian Clinical Trials
  (Compensation Issue, Safety Reporting, Unethical Regulations, Ethics Committee Registration Informed Consent Form, Timelines, Documents, New Advisory Committee)
- Overcoming the Challenges

Introduction

"Clinical trial" is a systematic study of new drug(s) in human subject(s) to generate data for discovering and/or verifying the clinical, pharmacological (including pharmacodynamics and pharmacokinetics) and/or adverse effects with the objective of determining safety and / or efficacy of the new drug".

The perspective research in the area of drug discovery leads to newer, safer and more efficacious drugs being made available in the country. Before a new drug can be mass produced and distributed in the medical community, it must be thoroughly vetted. Clinical trials are the only way of establishing the safety and efficacy of any new drug before its introduction in the market for human use. Sulphanilamide and Thalidomide disasters, took place due to the deprived clinical trials. Hence, clinical trials are the most decisive part as a new molecule is administered into the humans to establish the safety and toxicity level.

The first recorded clinical trial reported is the biblical Daniel, who tested the effects of a diet of pulses rather than meat. The Edinburgh surgeon James Lind (1716-94) who investigated the best treatment for scurvy is considered as the first physician and father of clinical research.

Clinical trials are the key research tool for advancing medical knowledge and patient care.

Clinical trials are mainly done to confirm the following:

- whether a new approach works well with people and is safe
- which treatments or strategies work best for certain illnesses or groups of people

The global guidelines like Nuremberg Code, the Declaration of Helsinki, Belmont Report, Council for International Organizations of Medical Sciences' and World Health Organization's International Ethical Guidelines for Biomedical Research Involving Human Subjects and International Conference on Harmonization's Good Clinical Practice (GCP) provide the basis for fundamental ethical principles for conduct of clinical trial research.

In India, the legislative requirements of clinical trials are guided by the specifications of Schedule Y of the Drug & Cosmetics Act, 1940 and Drugs & Cosmetics Rules, 1945, which provides the guidelines and requirements for clinical trials. The Health authority in India is Central Drugs Standard Control Organization (CDSCO), Directorate General of Health Services, Ministry of Health and Family

Welfare, Government of India. The Drug Controller General of India (DCGI) is advised by the Drug Technical Advisory Board (DTAB) and the Drug Consultative Committee (DCC). India's Drugs and Cosmetics Act, 1940 (DCA) and Drugs and Cosmetics Rules, 1945 governs the registration, import, manufacture, testing, and sale of drugs and cosmetics.

Clinical Trials in India

The number of clinical trials conducted globally is increasing day by day for faster and better results of a drug to cure of disease/disorder. The Indian pharmaceutical industry is ranked fourth in terms of volume, globally, constituting 8% of total world's production. The number of approved trials hit a peak in 2010 with 529 approved trials by DCG (I).

According to National Institute of Health, United States of America, a total number of 1, 53, 773 clinical trials are registered globally by 2014 in which the number of clinical trials registered in India are 2,404.

Phases of Clinical Trials

There are four phases of clinical trials

Phase I – Human Pharmacology

Phase II – Therapeutic exploratory trials – II (a) & II (b)

Phase III – Therapeutic confirmatory trials – III (a) & III (b)

Phase IV – Post Marketing Trials

In addition there is a Phase 0 study also.

Phase 0

Phase 0 of a clinical trial is done with a very small number of people, usually fewer than 15. Investigators use a very small dose of medication to make sure it isn't harmful to humans before they start using it in higher doses for later phases. If the medication acts differently than expected, the investigators will likely to do some additional preclinical research before deciding whether to continue the trial.

Phase I - Human/Clinical Pharmacology Trials

The main objective of this phase study is to estimate the safety and tolerability of the investigational new drug with initial administration into human(s). The other objective of phase I trials is to determine the maximum tolerated dose in humans; pharmacodynamics effects, adverse reactions, if any, with their nature and intensity; and pharmacokinetic behaviours or the drug as far as possible. For the conduct of this phase study, an application in form 44 along with fee of Rs. 50,000/- and other required documents are submitted to CDSCO.

Phase II - Exploratory Trials

The primary objective of Phase II trials is to evaluate the effectiveness of a drug for a particular indication or indications in patients with the condition under study and to determine the common short-term side-effects and risks associated with the drug. For the conduct of a phase II study, an application in form 44 & form 12 for import license, along with fee of Rs. 25,000/- and other prerequisite documents are submitted to CDSCO.(10)

Phase II (a): Phase II (a) studies are pilot clinical trials designed primarily to evaluate safety in selected healthy population with main objectives, dose response, type of patient, frequency of dosing, or other characteristics related to the drug's safety.

Phase II (b): Phase II (b) studies are well- controlled clinical trials designed to evaluate both efficacy and safety in patients with a primary objective of determining a dose range to be studied in phase III. Phase II (b) studies are conducted in the patients suffering from the disease, for which trial drug is being tested.

Phase III - Confirmatory Trials

The primary objective of phase III trials is to demonstrate or confirm the therapeutic benefit(s). The studies in Phase III are designed to confirm the preliminary evidence accumulated in Phase II that the drug is safe and effective for using it in the intended indication and recipient population. For the conduct of this phase study, form 44 along with fee of Rs. 25,000/- and other required documents are submitted to CDSCO.

Phase III (a) trials: Phase III (a) trials are conducted after the drug's efficacy is demonstrated, but before regulatory submission of the New Drug Application (NDA). These trials are conducted in special patient populations, e.g., studies in children and in patients with renal dysfunction. (11)·

Phase III (b) trials: Phase III (b) trials are conducted after regulatory submission of the NDA, but prior to the drug's approval and launch. They may supplement or complete earlier trials. (11)

Phase IV - Post Marketing Trials

The post marketing trials are performed after drug approval and related to the approved indications. These trials go beyond the prior demonstration of the drug's safety, efficacy and dose definition. These trials may not be considered necessary at the time of new drug approval, but may be required by the Licensing Authority for optimizing the drug's use. They may be of any type, but should have valid scientific objectives. For new drug substances discovered in other countries, phase I trials are not usually allowed to be initiated in India unless, phase I data as required is available from other countries. However, such trials may be permitted even in the absence of phase I data from other countries if the drug is of special relevance to the health problem of India. For new drug substances discovered in India, clinical trials are required to be carried out in India right from phase I through phase III as required. The permission to carry out these trials is generally given in stages, considering the data emerging from the earlier phase studies.

Table 7.1 Phases of Clinical Trials

	Phases	Participants	Time period	Purpose
1	Phase I	20 – 80 Healthy volunteers	Several months	Safety and tolerability of medication
2	Phase II	100 - 300	Up to 2 years	Efficacy & short term side effects
3	Phase III	1,000 - 3,000	1- 4 years	Confirmation of therapeutic benefit
4	Phase IV	Thousands of participants	More than 1 year	Long term effectiveness, cost effectiveness

Clinical Trial Process

The Clinical trial process is mainly subdivided into 7 stages. The Complete clinical trial process in India involves following steps/stages:

1. **Planning:** Planning of the trial is based upon the persisting disease type and seeks to requirements for that trial.
2. **Compiling:** After planning of the trial, subsequent to the decided trial, the data required by the Health Authority is collected and compiled.
3. **Submission:** The complied clinical trial application is submitted to CDSCO, along with all specified documents.
4. **Questions & Answers:** After submission, soon there will be a meeting between the applicant and reviewers vis- à-vis on application.
5. **Approval:** After the meeting and complete review of the application, if application deems fit, No Objection Certificate (NOC) will be given by DCG

(I) to accomplish the trial.

6. **Amendments:** Any post approval changes persist, they need to be notified/ approved or status report on the clinical trial need to notify to the Licensing Authority at prescribed time.
7. **End of trial:** The trial tops with several risks & benefits. Notify clinical trial reports to DCG (I). The clinical trial reports are submitted annually based on annual progress and at the end the final report is submitted.

Clinical Trial Application Filing

The filing of the clinical trial application process involves several steps and departments. The Clinical trial application review involves several experts from different committees. The committees involved are

1. **New Drug Advisory Committee** – In the past, CDSCO alone used to review the applications for new drugs and clinical trials. In order to bring the transparency, consistency and accountability in the approval process of drugs & clinical trials, CDSCO introduced a Technical committee. For strengthening the scientific review and approval of new drugs/devices, the ministry has appointed 12 New Drug Advisory Committee's (NDAC) and 7 Medical Device Advisory Committee's (MDAC) to advise the CDSCO in making their decisions on approval of new drugs and global clinical trials, consisting of experts from government medical colleges and institutes, 6 experts & 2 pharmacologists. It is now renamed as Subject Expert Committee.
2. **Apex Committee & Technical Review Committee** – As there are more unethical clinical trials occurring in India and as the number of deaths of patients has been increased, the Supreme Court of India asked to make stricter regulations & stringent approvals of Clinical trials in India. In honour of it, the health ministry has constituted two - tier panel, an apex committee and a technical committee, consisting of senior ministry officials and experts. The Apex Committee meets every month to review new approvals, Secretary, will take the assistance of the technical committee to supervise and monitor the conduct of the clinical trials in the country.

3. **Ethics Committee** - Ethics Committee performs the responsibilities like verifying the protection of the rights, safety and well-being of human subjects involved in a clinical trial. An ethics committee is comprised of medical/scientific and non-medical/non-scientific members. It is also responsible for reviewing and approving the protocol, the suitability of the investigator's facilities, methods and adequacy of information to be used for obtaining and documenting "Informed Consent" of the study subjects and adequacy of confidentiality safeguards. It also performs other activities like, evaluation of possible risks to the subjects, expected benefits and adequacy of documentation for ensuring privacy, confidentiality & justice. In case of clinical trial related injury or death the ethics committee should review and make recommendations for compensation to be paid by the sponsor in stipulated manner & time period.

Clinical Trial Process

Clinical Trial process in India is divided into two stages. First stage gives the path of application from applicant to Health authority, i.e. CDSCO. The other stage gives the alleyway of documents from the applicant to the Ethics Committee. The timelines for the approval process vary from application to application, in some it may be more than 90 days.

Stage 1

The duly filled application (Form – 44) along with the prescribed fee (based on phase) is submitted by the applicant to CDSCO. The application is sent to DCG (I) for review, along with which extra 11 sets of documents are submitted to NDAC. The application and documents are reviewed by DCG (I) officers and NDAC simultaneously. The NDAC calls for a meeting with the applicant in the presence of CDSCO officials. The queries related to the subject of the application are asked by NDAC. Later, the Committee confers the perceptions on the application which are carried to technical review committee for further review. The technical review committee may support or may diverge on NDAC outlook. DCG (I) takes the final verdict and issues No Objection Certificate (NOC) for conducting the trial or Query letter for any clarifications or documents. By receiving NOC the applicant can set out to Stage 2 path for Ethics Committee approval.

Stage 2

After the approval from DCG (I), the applicant seeks for the Principal Investigator and takes the undertaking from investigator to conduct trial. The investigator, who conducts the trial, should be a qualified and registered person. The applicant gives the NOC, issued by DCG (I) and set of documents, which are submitted to the Ethics Committee for the approval by the Investigator. Clinical trials are conducted only in sites which are approved by Ethics committee and are registered in DCG (I). The documents are reviewed by Ethics Committee members and the approval is given, after clarifying any questionnaires on application. After the approval, the clinical trial is commenced at the respective sites. The investigator is responsible to update the sponsor regarding the trial and should also report the Health authority along with the sponsor about serious adverse events.

Documents Required / Information Required

1. Name of the Applicant
2. Name of the Sponsor
3. Authorization Letter from Sponsor
4. Treasury Challan along with Form 44 (amount)
5. Name of the Study Drug
6. Dosage form
7. Therapeutic class
8. Study Protocol & Phase of Study
9. Undertaking by the Investigators as per Appendix VII of Schedule 'Y'
10. Patient Information Sheet (PIS) /Informed consent form (ICF) as per Appendix V of Schedule 'Y'
11. Justification for conducting the study in India
12. Name of the Participating Countries
13. Total Number of patients to be enrolled globally
14. Total Number of patients to be enrolled in India
15. Status of Drug in India & other countries
16. Status of the proposed study in other participating countries
17. Approvals of the proposed protocol from other participating countries
18. Ethics Committee approvals if available
19. Investigator Brochure
20. Investigational Medicinal Products Dossier(IMPD)
21. Technical Documents
    - Package Insert
    - Preclinical Data
        - Animal Pharmacological Data
        - Animal toxicology data as per Schedule Y
    - Clinical Data
        - Human / Clinical pharmacology (Phase I)
        - Therapeutic exploratory trials (Phase II)
        - Therapeutic confirmatory trials (Phase III)
    - Post Marketing Surveillance / Periodic Safety Update Report data (Phase IV)
    - Treasury Challan along with Form 12 (amount)

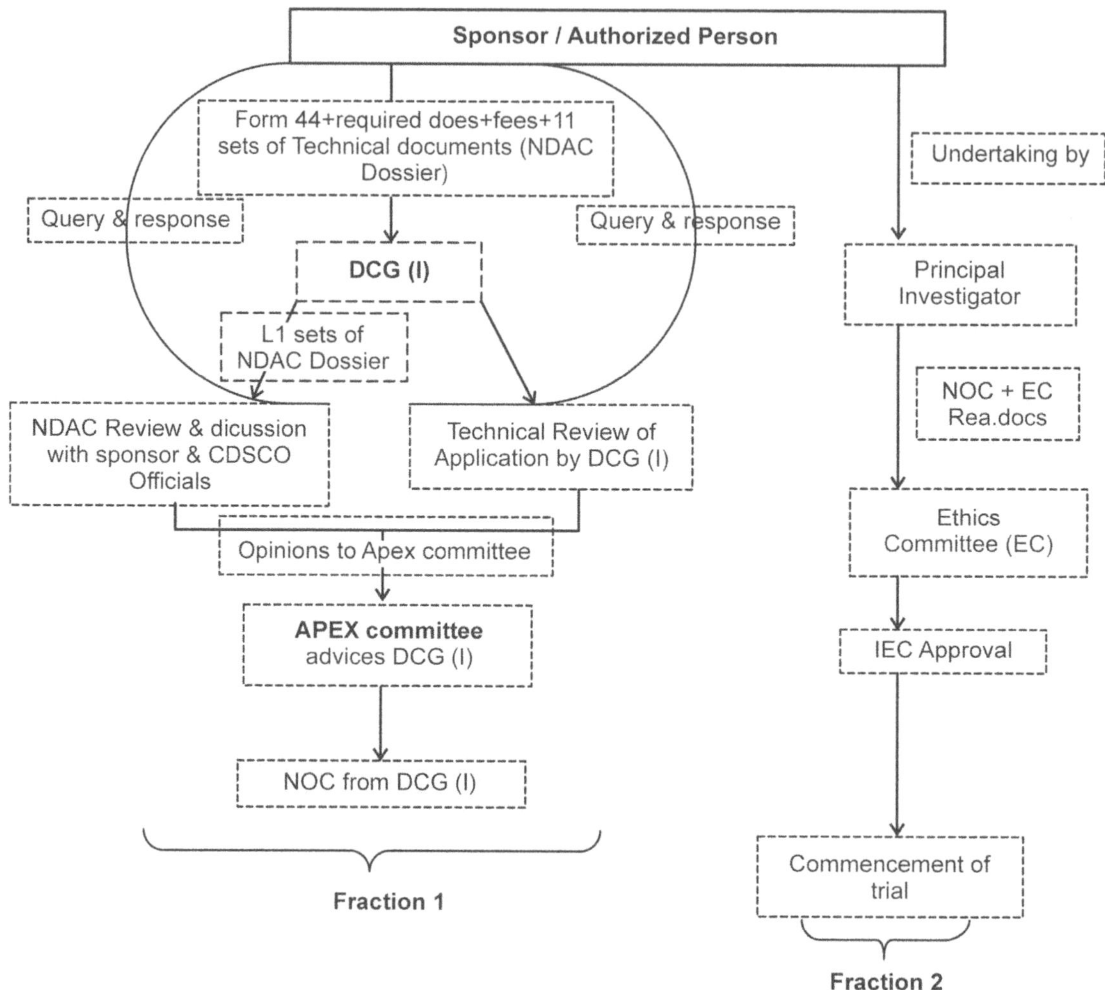

Fig.7.2 Clinical Trial Approval Process.

Indian Clinical Trial Regulations

1988: The local clinical trials were made mandatory in the year 1988, with a Phase lag, such that, the clinical trial in India will be one phase behind when compared to rest of the world.

2000: Many incidents due to the violations of ethical issues related to informed consent were reported. Based on these incidents Central Ethics Committee on Human Research (CECHR) and Indian Council of Medical Research (ICMR) took a regulatory initiative & conceptualized and issued Ethical Guidelines for Biomedical Research on Human Subjects in 2000. Trials were allowed to conduct only after approval from Ethics Committees, apart from DCG (I) and the informed consent of the subject participating in the trial was made mandatory.

2001: Good Clinical Practice (GCP) guidelines were developed in line with ICH and GCP.

2005: DTAB made Good Laboratory Practices (GLP) mandatory for all the laboratories. (16)

CDSCO made elaborate revisions to Schedule Y to bring it on at par with internationally accepted definitions and procedures. The changes which took place were

1. Definitions for Phase I-IV trials, which eliminated the Phase lag.
2. Clear responsibilities of investigators; and sponsors.
3. Requirements for notifying changes in protocol.(17)

2006: CDSCO issued draft regulations which included

- Checklist for filing Global Clinical Trial Applications
- Categorization of approval of protocol amendments(18)

2007: Schedule Y revisions in 2007 permitted Phase I trials to be carried out concurrently in India along with the rest of the world. This removed the phase lag and clinical trial registry was launched.

2008: CDSCO started inspection of clinical trial centers in India. A full fledge onsite inspection by US-FDA trained Indian Inspectors & regulatory experts started. (16)

2011- 2012: Several steps have been taken by the Government, to strengthen the clinical trial approval procedures and their monitoring mechanism to ensure that the safety, rights and well-being of clinical trial subjects are protected:

1. Registration of clinical trials in the ICMR's registry at www.ctri.in has been made mandatory.
2. Guidelines for conducting inspection of clinical trial sites and sponsor / Clinical Research Organizations (CROs) have been prepared.
3. Applications of Investigational New Drugs (IND) i.e., New Drug Substances which have never earlier been used in human beings are evaluated by an IND Committee, chaired by the Director General, Indian Council of Medical Research (ICMR).
4. 12 NDAC's and 7 MDAC's consisting of leading experts mostly from the Government medical colleges and institutes from all over the country have been constituted to advise the CDSCO on matters related to approval of clinical trials and new drugs.
5. Proposals to amend the toxicity study data requirements for approval of clinical trial / new drugs to make it harmonized with the international guidelines have been approved by DTAB.(19)

2013: For further strengthening of the regulatory provisions for approval of the conduct of clinical trials and safety and well-being of trial participants, there have been several new amendments made in schedule Y,

Drugs and Cosmetics Act, 1940 and Drugs & Cosmetics Rules, 1945. The amendments include in the Drugs and Cosmetics rules, 1945:

- Rule 122-DAB is inserted related to Appendix XII-Compensation in case of injury or deat during Clinical Trial.
- In Part X-A, after rule 122 DAB, a new rule 122 DAC inserted-related to Permission of Clinical Trials.
- After rule 122 DC, a new rule 122 DD inserted related to Registration of Ethics Committee.(7)

The Ministry of Health has appointed a two tier panel, an apex committee and a technical committee. Apex committee will take the assistance of the technical committee to supervise and monitor the conduct of the clinical trials in the country.

DCG (I) constituted three Independent Expert Committees in pursuance of sub-clause (6) of appendix XII of the Schedule Y to the Drug & Cosmetics Rules 1945 on 14thMarch, 2013 to examine the Serious Adverse Events of deaths occurring during clinical trials and to recommend the cause of death, and to determine the quantum of compensation, if any, to be paid by the Sponsor or his representative, whosoever had obtained permission from the DCG (I). The Committee after deliberation prepared formula to be followed in the determination of Quantum of Compensation in case of Clinical Trial related death.

$$\text{Compensation} = B \times F \times R$$

Where,

B = Base amount (i.e. 8 lacs)

F = Factor depending on the age of the subject as per Annexure 1 (based on Workmen Compensation Act)

R = Risk Factor depending on the seriousness and severity of the disease.

In 2013, a new office order has been passed by DCG (I) regarding the financial support, fees, honorarium, payments, etc. to be paid to investigator by the sponsor for each contract.

The GCP guideline states that the sponsor should have a legal agreement / contract with the investigator before the start of the trial. Now DCG (I) has recommended the sponsor to submit the details of the financial support, fees, honorarium, payments, etc. given to his investigator, while making a clinical trial application to DCG (I).

CDSCO has granted certain recommendations on Ranjit Roy's report, which insists that all clinical trials should be carried only in accredited sites by an accredited Investigator with the oversight of accredited Ethics Committees, renaming NDAC as Subject Expert Committee. The Technical Review Committee should examine the application concisely and should decide whether the approval should be given for the protocols which have a definitive need in the country, which is done on a case by case basis. The time period for the approvals of the clinical trial applications and for new drugs has been fixed as six months. The audio visual recording of the informed consent process is to be submitted along with written informed consent for all the participants enrolled in clinical trials including global trials.

Compensation should be paid to the patient or their legal heirs in case of death or injury/disability, which is related to the trial drug, in case of any injury or death occurring during clinical trial due to adverse effect of the investigational product or any clinical trial procedures involved in the study, and also if any drug-related anomaly is discerned at a later stage and accepted to be drug related by a competent authority whether in India or abroad.

Challenges in Indian Clinical Trials

There are many challenges in Indian clinical trials, which tumbled India to last option for global clinical trials. Some of the major challenges are

1. Compensation Issue

   - In Jan 2013, CDSCO released a gazette notification (1st amendment in the Drugs and Cosmetics Rules, 1945:122-DAB) describing the Compensation to be paid in case of injury or death during CT. After this amendment, many US companies withdraw or stopped conducting Global Clinical trials in India. The compensation and medical coverage for an injury/ death to the subject, whether it is related to the trial drug or not, for an uncertain period, has turned as a major challenge for Indian Clinical trials
   - In term of compensation issues, there is no clarity on the time period, i.e., for how long the compensation has to be paid, which will be decided by the regulatory authorities and EC's on case by case basis. If the compensation is not provided as per the authorities, it leads to suspension/losing of their license to conduct Clinical trials which stand as a check for many companies

2. Safety Reporting

   - In Drugs and Cosmetics rules, 1945, the time period for reporting the serious adverse event by the investigator to the sponsor, licensing authority, EC is given as 24 hours. But in some cases it will be practically impossible as the investigator may not get the full and correct information about the SAE within such a short period
   - Timelines for reporting any SAE of death by the sponsor to the EC and expert committee is within as 10 days of occurrence. But internationally, the timelines required for reporting such cases is 14 days
   - The timelines given to the Ethics Committee to examine the SAE of death and to send its opinion on compensation to be given is 21 days and for expert committee it is 30 days and for DCG (I) to give its compensation report is 90 days look arbitrary

3. Unethical Regulations

   - Between 2005 and 2012; 2,644 people died during the clinical trials of 475 new drugs out of which 80 deaths were found to be attributable to the trials
   - In January 2013, the Supreme Court observed that unregulated clinical trials had caused chaos to the human life, and the Court denounces the central government for failing to take proper note on the legal and ethical bifurcations of clinical trials. The Court said: "the subjects of the country are being used as guinea pigs by the

companies". It also criticized the state government for failing to penalize and punish the criminal medical practitioners.

- The government immediately announced for a proper regulatory structure for monitoring clinical trials. For an efficient and ethical clinical trial environment, the presence of a strong centralized regulatory regime is needed. Regulatory bodies are working towards new challenges and government is bringing in more changes in the regulations for reducing the time limits for approvals and making more accessible and approachable for global communities.
- The court also pointed out that the CDSCO had approved 33 drugs, out of a randomly selected sample of 42, without clinical trials on Indian patients. The reports of unethical trials conducted on children and mentally challenged patients in Madhya Pradesh have also surfaced recently. Numerous unethical regulations taking away the lives of many innocent subjects were also reported.

4. Ethics Committee Registration

- The latest amendment to schedule Y stating "Registration of Ethics Committee" have raised challenges for the pharmaceutical/device/biotech industry/academic investigators and regulators who have to realign themselves with these requirements, which are now becoming mandatory
- The unregistered ECs cannot review and accord their approval for CT protocols legally which has led to the delays in study initiation at those sites and slowed down the recruitments for such approved CTs from the licensing authority(LA)
- For this reason, the sponsor is advised to select the sites, which have got to register ECs, rather than risking unregistered sites. The approvals being issued for CT protocols have to see that the study is conducted by abiding to the new rules by the applicant. The registration will be valid up to 3 years, after which it should be reviewed and renewed. The rules also require that the ethics committee maintains records and documents that can be reviewed by the licensing authority at any time. The ethics committee should allow the CDSCO investigators to enter their trial sites to inspect records, data and other documents.

5. Informed Consent Form

- There were many unethical issues noticed regarding incomplete and inappropriate Informed consent forms
- The trial, including human papilloma virus (HPV) vaccine was suspended since March 2010, but was carried out by the Program for Appropriate Technology and Health (PATH), an NGO, in collaboration with the Andhra Pradesh and Gujarat governments and the ICMR. It was conducted on nearly 23,500 girls in the 10-14 years age group in Khammam district (Andhra Pradesh) and Vadodra (Gujarat) and has led to many deaths. When the informed consent forms are seen, they were being filled very carelessly with incomplete and probably inaccurate information. In Andhra Pradesh, nearly 2,800 consent forms were signed by a hostel warden or headmaster, as the 'guardian'. Not only has this case, there were many other cases regarding

informed consents which are drawing India back from conducting ethical clinical trials.

6. Timelines

- In the viewpoint of global pharmaceutical industries, a country is mostly attracted for conducting the clinical trials depends on its speed and quality of data. The speed is affected by the factors like regulatory permission time, Ethics Committee (EC) approval, patient recruitment and retention.
- There were no specific timelines given for the approval of clinical trials. Previously the timelines were about 45 days. But after the amendments i.e., adding NDAC, it is raised to 90 days approximately. CDSCO again failed to address the variable timelines for CT approval leading to significant delays and lost trust of the sponsor companies.

7. Documents

- As mentioned above, the global pharmaceutical industries look for the complete quality data. The quality of data is largely influenced by GCP culture, ethics, documentation and record keeping. But in India, the documentation of the data, informed consent forms, patient records were not on their track, which as returned out as a hurdle for global industries.
- The clinical trial application is submitted as per the health authority requirements. But there are some problems in compiling all the necessary documents as some of them are very confidential, like a certificate of analysis, documents regarding drug substance, etc.,

8. New Advisory Committee

- The CDSCO set up a new process for referring all the clinical trials to NDAC. Instead of improving the decision making, it has become as a hurdle for global pharmaceutical industries resulting in delays and uncertainties in the Clinical trial approval.
- The NDAC process should be made more transparent & time bound.
- There is no clarity on scheduling of NDACs. The roles of NDACs need to be reviewed.
- The Committee should be reviewed on 6 months basis to ensure that no member is retired or moved out of their role.
- Distinction should be made for the type of application to be referred to NDAC

  Early phase studies (I/II/IIIA) should be referred to NDAC

Phase IV studies need not to be referred to NDAC

- Phase II/III studies with a molecule, where the study is already approved, unless if it had any safety /ethical concerns should not be referred to NDAC.
- Planning of the meetings should be revised. The applicant should get the prior notice of at least 2 weeks & the meeting calendar should be displayed in CDSCO website in 4 weeks advance.

Overcoming the Challenges

To overcome the challenges, the experts along with government should revise the new amendments and should bring more transparency among them. The main issues which are drawing India back are related to the committee functions, compensation, timelines & safety of patients.

- The compensation to be given, should be limited to an injury or death of the subject, which is directly or justifiably related to the clinical trial in which the subject has participated and it should not be for unrelated events or any injury
- There should be clarity on the compensation amount to be reimbursed and the sponsors are responsible for contributing the amount required for the medical treatment, related to trial injury
- However, there should be more clarity on the amount of compensation to be given, for how long the medical treatment should be given, and industry also should be able to participate in this calculation along with DCGI and ECs
- On May 16th, 2013, DTAB proposed a few changes to the compensation amendments. For example: "In the case of CT related injury" the compensation clause clearly mentions that only trial related death/injury needs to be compensated for. The DTAB has also recommended the removal of the compensation for the failure of the investigational drug for intended therapeutic effect as well
- It is also crucial to increase the technical staff with advanced industry training at the DCGI office, the further training by international regulator exchange programs as well as advanced training in clinical trial design, implementation, monitoring, data management, and quality assurance might help to improve the consistency of approvals and reduce the time taken
- Empowering DCGI's office to make the decisions might be useful to reduce the time required for approval of clinical trials. Further, the support from technical and regulatory expert committee for CT application filing, review and related activities will also decline the approval timelines
- The functions of NDAC and the apex committee should be more transparent and strict in reviewing the applications. The communication and cooperation between the other agencies involved in the CT process approvals will also be useful
- Ethics committees should have appropriate representatives and should be monitored centrally. Through constant monitoring and accountability of the ECs, the quality & ethics operation can be ensured. They should also monitor trials, including the consent aspects, ensuring the diversity of trial populations so as to avoid misuse of vulnerable population including recruitment of poor homogeneous rural communities
- There should be transparency among all the participants like the sponsors, investigators, regulators and ECs. The sponsors should also communicate the risks & status of the trials to the authorities at specified time. Investigators should be

transparent about the treatment given, adverse events, relatedness to the trial activities etc. with the public and regulators

- The transparency by the regulators in the entire review process of the CT application along with the appropriate reasons for the approval or rejection of the application and the approval criteria for the applications will be very useful
- It is also crucial to increase the technical staff with advanced industry training at the DCGI office, the further training by international regulator exchange programs as well as advanced training in clinical trial design, implementation, monitoring, data management, and quality assurance might help to improve the consistency of approvals and reduce the time taken
- The Informed consent process needs to be highly transparent and it should be voluntary and documented properly. There should be audit conducted on Clinical Trials, which will be useful to build confidence in the integrity of the data coming out of India
- People should owe their own responsibilities and the casual attitude towards consenting, ethical/quality trials process including documentation need to be vanished
- It is very important for the regulators, the industry and the Government to come together and plan the regulations that protect the interest of the public at all times and also to have the regulations that are supportive to the industry leading to the economic growth of the country.

The stringent upcoming clinical trial regulations menace the investigators of unethical clinical trials. These stringent rules are preparing India with more ethical trials by philanthropic safer drugs, assembling Indian Clinical trials again as a flipside into Global Clinical trials. As they are in edifice stage, they cause annoyance of clinical trials over a period of time.

A Clinical trial is obligatory for a drug/device to ensure its safety & efficacy in humans before their usage. The filing process of the clinical trial application in India is a lengthy process; it involves many committees like NDAC, Technical review committee, Apex Committee, Ethics Committee. The clinical trial in India had undergone many changes from 2008 to till date, still altering. These changes made India to be a global hub for clinical trials for many years. Recent amendments collapsed India as a last predilection for clinical trials due to some gaps. By plugging these gaps suitably, and by addressing the needs of stakeholders, India can definitely bounce back as the preferred destination for clinical trials, benefiting the Indian population.

Chapter 8

Methods of Post Marketing Surveillance (PMS)

LEARNING OBJECTIVES

To understand

- Post marketing surveillance: (By MHRA in UK)
- History of the Yellow Card scheme
- PMS in the UK: Features and Aspects
- Reporting an ADR
- Communication between Healthcare Professionals and Patients
- Minimizing the Risk: A Regulatory Perspective
- Safety Assessment Marketed Medicines
- PMS in Canada
- Current Post Marketing Surveillance System
- ADR Reporting Requirements
- Data Assessment and Management
- Risk Minimization
- Risk Communication

Introduction

In the field of pharmaceutical sciences, drug innovation is a continual process that more often than not culminates in the discovery of potential new medicines. The development of a drug, right from conceptual stages to the finished product, is considered to be a highly complex process that scrutinizes every little aspect of the drug, thereby providing adequate assurance of its safety at the time of approval. However, to further ascertain the safety of new drugs for human consumption, investigative studies tend to continue after approval. These studies are commonly called 'post marketing studies' or 'phase IV trials'.

Post marketing surveillance (PMS), in simple terms, refers to the process of monitoring the safety of drugs once they reach the market after the successful completion of clinical trials.[1] The primary purpose for the conduct of PMS is to identify previously unrecognized adverse effects as well as positive effects. Other essential components can include off-label drug use, issues with orphan drugs and problems associated with the conduct of international clinical trials in the pediatric population.

While premarketing trials are conducted with the intention of establishing the toxicity profile of a drug, they are frequently found to be lacking in capacity when it comes down to the detection of important adverse drug reactions (ADRs). This can be attributed to limitations in the number of participants in the trials, as some ADRs may be observed at rates of 1 in 10,000 or fewer drug exposures. ADRs are defined by the World Health Organization (WHO) as 'a response to a drug that is noxious and unintended and occurs at doses normally used in man for the prophylaxis, diagnosis or therapy of disease, or for modification of physiological function'. They have different categories such as dose-related, non-dose related, time-related and unexpected failure of therapy. Follow ups are integral to the detection of adverse reactions associated with the long-term use of drugs or the intake of drugs at widely separated intervals. Taken as a whole, the shortcomings posed by premarketing trials necessitate the conduct of continual investigative studies after drug approval.

PMS is an essential tool that helps to correlate the strength of the exposed drug with that of the adverse events, thereby painting a clearer picture with regard to the types of positive or negative effects that a drug may threaten to pose, over a prolonged period of administration.

Over the years, PMS practices have undergone considerable evolution, with regulatory authorities realizing the importance of applying appropriate measures to stifle the increasing incidences of adverse reactions. This has ushered in an era of 'proactive approaches' rather than 'reactive approaches' with a focus on risk prevention and necessary communication measures. Examples of this can be seen in the United Kingdom (UK) and Canada, two of the most regulated pharmaceutical markets in the world.

In 2013, an average of 176 out of 100,000 people reported an adverse event in the UK. Similarly, around 200,000 ADRs are reported in Canada every year, of which up to 22,000 resultant deaths are reported. These statistics were accountable for reported ADRs only, and it is widely believed that around 90% of ADRs go unreported. However, in the years to come, these stats are expected to reflect more accurate numbers with the implementation of a more robust PMS and pharmacovigilance (PV) system.

Post Marketing Surveillance: (By MHRA in UK)

PMS or pharmacovigilance in the UK is practiced in the form of the Yellow Card scheme that is jointly operated by the MHRA and the Committee of Human Medicines (CHM). The Yellow Card scheme is credited as being one of the first PV schemes aimed at mitigating ADRs. PV encompasses the following objectives:

- Monitoring the use of medicines in everyday practice with the aim to identify erstwhile unrecognized ADRs and also changes in the patterns of adverse effects.

- Carrying out risk benefit analysis for medicines and suggesting suitable actions, if and when necessitated.
- Providing regular updates to healthcare professionals and patients with regard to the safe and efficacious use of medicines.

In addition to the Yellow Card scheme, the MHRA brought into effect an updated black triangle scheme in 2009 that was aimed at increasing the awareness of healthcare professionals and the public in general towards drugs and vaccines that required intensive monitoring. Any suspected adverse effects caused by such drugs and vaccines were to be immediately brought to the attention of the MHRA and the CHM. The symbol, which is denoted by an inverted black triangle, is found imprinted beside the name of the relevant drug product.

History of the Yellow Card scheme The scheme, established in 1964, was an outcome of the thalidomide tragedy that occurred in the early 1960s. This Yellow Card reporting system, based on the concept of voluntary reporting of suspected adverse reactions, is considered to be one of the first ADR reporting systems in the world. From the inception of the scheme until 1997, the reporting system was open only to doctors and dentists and therefore was restrictive in nature. However, from early 1997 onwards, the scope of the scheme was considerably widened to include hospital pharmacists. This move was widely recognized and appreciated by the healthcare community at the time as pharmacists were better placed to report and counter the adverse reactions caused by a rampant increase in the use of nonprescription medicines as well as complementary medicines.[9] Further, in 1999, community pharmacists were added into the system, and since then, a substantial increase has been witnessed in the proportion of ADRs being reported. Since 2003, the scheme was amended to include nurses and coroners, following which a pilot scheme was implemented which persuaded patients and guardians to directly report ADRs to the MHRA through the Yellow Card scheme. The insight gained through this pilot project encouraged the MHRA to develop the scheme on a nationwide basis, which was rolled out in February 2008.

Through the years, the emergence of information technology has had a significant impact on the Yellow Card scheme. When initiated in 1964, the system was entirely paper-based. Over the years, the authorities realized that paper forms do not make the most convenient and accessible method for reporting ADRs. As a result, the MHRA launched the Yellow Card scheme website in 2002 which provided the reporting population with access to the electronic Yellow Card reporting form. This website has been updated by the MHRA on a regular basis to keep up with advances in technology. In 2008, the website was redeveloped and launched, coinciding with the launch of the Patient Reporting scheme.

PMS in the UK: Features and Aspects: Spontaneous reporting of ADRs is an integral mechanism of PV, and the Yellow Card scheme in the UK fulfills this requirement. Yellow Card reports can be submitted directly to the MHRA *via* post, telephone or the internet. The essential reason to establish spontaneous reporting schemes is to detect adverse reactions to new drugs as well as established drugs, as clinical trials cannot define rare but important ADRs. Although clinical trials are funded by large sums of money running into millions, companies usually fail to detect rare ADRs, as drugs will be administered to a relatively smaller population base of 2,500 volunteers, out of which only about a 100 or so will have taken the drug for a duration lasting more than 1 year. Therefore, it is prudent that the MHRA functions efficiently in operating the Yellow Card scheme in order to discern previously known ADRs and convey information about the same to the health care community.

The following are the features of the Yellow Card scheme employed by the MHRA in the UK.

Reporting an ADR: The ADR should be reported using a Yellow Card. All ADRs associated with prescription as well as non-prescription drugs should be reported. The MHRA and the CHM do not specify the need for causality to report an ADR. On the contrary, patients and healthcare professionals are encouraged to submit reports, even in the event of doubt with regards to the ADR having occurred. Some instances where reporting a suspected ADR is considered mandatory are described below.

- **Black triangle drugs**: In the UK, newly introduced pharmaceutical products including biologicals, are labelled with an inverted black triangle when they are first marketed. This black triangle indicates that all suspected ADRs occurring with respect to the marked drug product needs to be brought to the notice of the authorities, regardless of the severity of the adverse reaction. This intensive monitoring of the drug continues for a minimum of 2 years from the launch of the product and can be extended further if necessitated. In addition, a black triangle can be indicated on any medication that requires extensive monitoring. This can be observed in the case of a proven product being marketed as a combination product with another market-proven API.
- **Serious reactions:** In the event of serious suspected reactions taking place, it is recommended that they are reported through the Yellow Card scheme, irrespective of whether the pharmaceutical product belongs to the category of a black triangle product or not. Such reactions can include fatal and life-threatening reactions, disabling or incapacitating reactions, congenital abnormalities and also medically significant reactions. The reporting of such ADRs is highly encouraged as increasingly specific advice on side-effects which are likely to occur and corresponding comprehensive data obtained can be employed to compare the safety standards of drug products belonging to the same therapeutic class. When a Yellow Card is intended to be submitted to the agency, it should include all possible information of the drug that is responsible for the adverse reaction and also document the characteristics of the reaction that occurred. Apart from this, essential information with regard to the patient and information of the healthcare professional should also be provided. The age, sex and weight of the patient should be included, as well as the patient's initials and a number to identify the patient to the reporter, known as the local identification number. While submitting the report, it is not prudent for the reporter to inform the patient; however, the MHRA advises the reporter to inform the patient of the report and also to keep a copy of the Yellow Card on the patient's chart. Once a Yellow Card is completed, it is forwarded to the MHRA. Alternatively, the Yellow Card can also be provided to any of the five regional

monitoring centres, who forward it to the MHRA. Upon successful acceptance of the report, an acknowledgement is provided to the reporter containing a UIN (unique identification number). Further, the UIN will be affixed to the Yellow Card and all patient-identifying information, except the contact information of the reporter is removed by the MHRA. The report is then entered into the MHRA database to enable rapid analysis of the ADR report. The reporter can be contacted by the MHRA at any point of this entire operation, to provide further data or to provide clarifications about the adverse reaction observed. The scientists and concerned officials at the MHRA will use data provided on the Yellow Card to check for signs of suspected drug safety issues. These signs are then used to develop the overall ADR profile of the drug product, where alternatives to the drug can be used to carry out a comparison on the probable benefits, both on the basis of indication and efficacy. The CHM and the Pharmacovigilance Expert Advisory Group advise the MHRA on drug safety issues, and based on this advice, a decision will be taken on whether the drug should be withdrawn from the market or whether any changes are necessitated in the use of the drug.

Communication between Healthcare Professionals and Patients: The MHRA realizes that frequent communication with professionals from the healthcare sector as well as the general population is crucial in ensuring that awareness is created about the prevalence of new ADRs and also to impart valuable feedback. The MHRA achieves this in the following ways:

- An independent review carried out on the Yellow Card scheme in 2004 suggested possible ideas that can be implemented to further streamline the system that included the introduction of drug analysis prints (DAPs). A DAP provides information on the reactions reported for all drugs and this database can be accessed from the MHRA database.
- Updating patient information leaflets and summaries of product characteristics for drug products when new safety concerns are identified. Also, the MHRA publishes safety concerns regarding drug products on its website.
- Doctors and other healthcare professionals are immediately informed of any urgent drug hazard warnings. The MHRA publishes a monthly bulletin *Drug Safety Update* that provides the latest advice to enable safer use of medicines. At the same time, the CHM publishes *Current Problems in Pharmacovigilance*, a drug safety bulletin which is circulated among all doctors as well as professionals from the pharmaceutical field, a copy of which is also provided on the MHRA website.
- The MHRA uses the Public Health Link, which is an electronic cascade system, to propagate urgent information about ADRs to all concerned individuals, particularly from the healthcare sector. This system helps disseminate information when sufficient time is not available to do the same through hard copies.

Minimizing the Risk: A Regulatory Perspective: When warranted, the MHRA may adopt approaches that will ensure that a drug can be used in a way to minimize its risks, thereby delivering optimum benefits to patients. These approaches are as follows:

- Changes to warnings provided on product packaging and labels.
- The regulatory authorities will restrict the indications for the use of a drug.
- In certain instances, if the use of a drug is deemed to be subject to adverse reactions or is considered to be harmful when taken in higher doses, the regulatory authorities will change the legal status of the drug, for example, an over-the-counter medicine to a prescription medicine.
- In rare situations, if the MHRA deems that the adverse effects associated with the use of a marketed product are far too severe compared with the relative benefits, and then it will take the decision to withdraw the product from the market.

Safety Assessment Marketed Medicines: The launch of the Safety Assessment Marketed Medicines (SAMM) guidelines in 1994 was an attempt at providing post-approval safety assessment studies of greater scientific credibility. The SAMM guidelines were formalized by a working group containing the MHRA (formerly known as the Medicines Control Agency), Committee on Safety of Medicines, the Association of the British Pharmaceutical Industry, the British Medical Association (BMA) and the Royal College of General Practitioners. These guidelines were also made available in other European countries including Germany and the Netherlands in order to create an easier passage for the conduct of multinational multicentre studies. This enabled researchers to incorporate thousands of patients in the clinical studies and safety surveillance. In the UK, an SAMM study is 'a formal investigation conducted for the purpose of assessing clinical safety of marketed medicines in clinical practice.' This definition of SAMM guidelines encompasses all studies sponsored by the marketing company that are aimed at evaluating the safety of marketed medicinal products. These studies are designed on an objective-based approach but can include observational cohort studies, case-by-case surveillance and clinical trials. The highlights of the guidance were asfollows:[18]

(1) Study patients should be selected from a pool that is representative of the general population of users.
(2) The comparator groups (i.e. patients with similar parameters but on an alternate drug therapy) should ideally be included.
(3) For a patient to be incorporated in a study, the drug should have been prescribed under normal clinical practice circumstances. The subsequent recruitment of the patient into the study shall be as per the study protocol.

For all studies the general advice is also clear:

(1) The draft study plan shall be discussed by the companies with the MCA (now MHRA) prior to submitting a finalized plan.
(2) An adequate ethics committee approval is mandatory.
(3) The company is held responsible for ensuring the conduct of the study as per the approved study protocol under the supervision of aUK-registered medical practitioner.

(4) In the instance that an appointed agent conducts the study on behalf of the company, the agent will be held responsible for the conduct of the study as per the protocol and should liaise with the company.

(5) The entire study should be overseen by an independent advisory board.

(6) Studies should not be instituted with the any ill intent, such as a promotional exercise. The study payment to doctors should be in accordance with BMA guidelines.

PMS in Canada

Drug approvals in Canada are based on the presentation of substantive documentation of a drug's quality and safety, by the manufacturer to the regulatory authority, Health Canada. The conduct of clinical trials is subject to the submission of a clinical trial application. After this, Health Canada can authorize the manufacturer to conduct developmental phase clinical trials, involving drugs where the suggested trial is outside the parameters of the marketing authorization of the drug. If the drug manufacturer is able to provide substantial evidence of the fulfilment of all applicable requirements, Health Canada will grant an no objection certificate and a drug identification number that authorizes the manufacturer to sell the drug in the pharmaceutical market.

In accordance with the Good Pharmacovigilance Practices guidelines, drug manufacturers have a binding obligation to monitor the safety and efficacy of their medicines post-approval. Section C.01.016 to C.01.019 of the guidelines[21] strictly forbid a drug manufacturer from engaging in the active sale of a drug unless all necessary information regarding any serious unexpected adverse effect has been reported to Health Canada within 15 days of the occurrence. According to Health Canada, a serious unexpected adverse reaction is "a noxious and unintended response to a drug which may occur at any dose and which will require the hospitalization of the patient or prolonging of existing hospitalization, causes malformation, results in persistent or significant disability or is fatal and life-threatening in nature". Hence, Health Canada employs a three-pronged approach to assure decreased incidences of serious unexpected adverse reactions of marketed drugs, (i.e. collection, analyzing and assessment of ADR data submitted by the pharmaceutical industry, healthcare professionals and patients). The Canada Vigilance Program is Health Canada's PMS program that is entrusted with the responsibility to collect and assess reports of ADRs of health products marketed and sold in Canada. As is the case in most regulated pharmaceutical markets, Health Canada uses the data obtained to conduct a complete analysis of probable safety concerns, recommend pharmaceutical manufacturers to change product labels, and work with manufacturers to enact these changes, communicate new safety information to healthcare professionals and the public.[23] The Canada Vigilance Program, initiated in 1965, operates on the basis of adverse reaction reports submitted by healthcare professionals and consumers. The reports can be submitted on a voluntary basis, either directly to Health Canada or to the market authorization holders. This program applies to a wide range of products including prescription and nonprescription medicines, natural health products, biological and radiopharmaceuticals. At the regional level, the program is ably supported by the presence of seven Canada Vigilance Regional Offices, who act as the point of contacts for ADR reporters. These regional offices collect reports and forward these to the Canada Vigilance National Office for further assessment. In addition to the Canada Vigilance Program, Health Canada formed the Drug Safety and Effectiveness Network (DSEN) as a reaction to the introduction of the Food and Consumer Action Plan. The DSEN, in joint collaboration with the Canadian Institute for Health Research, initiated the Canadian Network for Observational Drug Effect Studies (CNODES) in 2011. CNODES built a network comprising researchers and databases from across Canada with the aim of coordinating drug safety and efficacy-based research for drugs marketed in Canada. A key aspect of CNODES was its access to the UK's Clinical Practice Research Data link, as it enabled CNODES to analyze drugs marketed in the UK before they were approved in Canada. CNODES was preceded by the Vaccine and Immunization Surveillance in Ontario (VISION), which was operated by the Institute for Clinical Evaluative Sciences. However, this program was intended to primarily function as a vaccine vigilance setup.

Current Post Marketing Surveillance System: In 2002, Health Canada formed the Marketed Health Products Directorate, which was apart of the broader Canada Vigilance Program, with a specific decree for PMS. The Marketed Health Products Directorate (MHPD), operating under the aegis of the Health Products and Food Branch (HPFR), monitors the activities associated with the assessment of safety trends and risk communication regarding marketed drug products. The MHPD is involved in the development of regulations concerned with reporting of adverse reactions. For this, it coordinates with international organizations which enhances the ease with which information and data can be shared across different regions. The core responsibilities of the MHPD are as follows:

- Collection and monitoring of ADRs and drug incident data.
- Review and analysis of health product safety information.
- Conduct a risk–benefit analysis of approved healthcare products.
- Communicate drug-related risks to healthcare professionals.
- Develop and implement policies to efficiently regulate healthcare products.
- Monitor the regulatory advertising schemes.

In 2005, the Canada Vigilance Program was renamed MedEffect Canada. MedEffect Canada acted as a comprehensive tool that ensured improved access to ADR information. Initially, MedEffect Canada was established as a partnership initiative between professional healthcare organizations and consumer groups. It was envisioned as a 5-year pilot project to ensure that access to safe and effective healthcare products was available to all. The MedEffect program was introduced by the MHPD with the following goals:

- To enable centralized access to reliable and accurate drug product safety data as and when they are made available.
- To put in place a simple and efficient system for healthcare professionals and other ADR reporters to file ADR reports *via* phone, email or mail.
- To generate awareness about the necessity of reporting ADRs to Health Canada.
- To help identify and communicate potential risks.

A key aspect of the MedEffect program is the Adverse Reaction Online database, where data for ADRs for all health products are readily available including drugs, biologics, prescription and nonprescription drugs and natural health products.

ADR Reporting Requirements: The Canadian ADR reporting program include shealth care professionals as well as consumers as recognized reporters and thereby lets them report ADRs directly to Health Canada and marketing authorization holders. In this manner, PV can be observed efficiently as manufacturers are furnished with sufficient time to understand the ADRs and report them to Health Canada within the stipulated duration of 15 days. Health Canada stipulates that the reporter of an ADR must mandatorily include specific information in the form while submitting the report. Patient information must be filled in that includes the physical features of the patient such as height, weight and age. The patient name is not included in the form for reasons of confidentiality. The form must also provide a description of the reaction experienced by the patient along with the therapy dates, (i.e. the date the ADR occurred/resolved and the date the drug therapy commenced/stopped). Lastly, Health Canada requires the reporter to include contact information of the patient as well as the reporter, in case Health Canada requires any additional information with regard to the adverse reaction. In some cases, relevant tests/lab data, as well as concomitant health product data, may be provided.

Data Assessment and Management: Health Canada makes use of MedDRA terminology for coding ADR reports that are submitted as a part of the Canada Vigilance Program. It has introduced the technology to facilitate the electronic transfer of adverse reaction data efficiently, between the marketing authorization holder and the regulatory authorities. This entire setup has been implemented keeping in mind International Council for Harmonization of Technical Requirements for Pharmaceuticals for Human Use (ICH) directives and standards. An electronic gateway has been introduced for the benefit of large industrial companies, whereas small and medium-scale manufacturers can operate the system by means of a web- based portal. Once the reports are collected, the reports are assessed for integrity and completeness, and then forwarded for further processing. It is the responsibility of the marketing authorization holders (MAHs) to collect follow-up data *via* telephone calls, site visits, and written requests. During the assessment, the identity of the reporter and the patient is kept confidential as per the provisions of the PrivacyAct.[30]

The reports submitted to Health Canada are assessed by employing the WHO-defined causality categories, thereby determining the causal relationship. Signals from the vigilance database are discerned through a systematic and periodic review of ADR reports, by employing appropriate statistical tools. The MHPD staff assesses and reviews adverse reaction reports, either individually or as a summary of collective reports. As per the Canadian Vigilance System, the process of providing personalized feedback to reporters on the association of drugs and ADRs does not exist. The reporters are instead provided with receipt of adverse reaction reports along with links to electronic monthly bulletins published by Health Canada and MHPD.

Risk Minimization: Health Canada has implemented a number of initiatives to ensure that the rate of incidence of ADRs is kept at a minimum.

- Health Canada has always laid emphasis on educating healthcare professionals and patients/consumers with regards to pharmacovigilance. The availability of suitable tools on the MedEffect Canada website has helped realize this goal to a certain extent.
- In addition, Health Canada organizes various outreach programs for healthcare professional groups nationally. These programs are aimed at imparting ADR reporting information for all pharmaceutical products.
- Over the years, Health Canada has developed various bilateral international agreements with several foreign agencies. This has enabled the continuous flow of data on ADRs across the world, thereby permitting Health Canada to monitor all international safety concerns.
- In Canada, pharmaceutical manufacturers are required to submit periodic safety update reports as well as risk management plans at predefined intervals to Health Canada, thereby providing evidence of the continued safety of the drug product.

Risk Communication

- Health Canada publishes a monthly adverse reaction bulletin/newsletter, *Health Product Info Watch*, that it distributes among healthcare professionals including physicians and pharmacists. This newsletter provides clinically relevant safety information on pharmaceutical products including biologics, medical devices and natural health products.[33] It also posts risk communications such as warnings, recalls, advisories and foreign product alerts on the MedEffect website. This website is regularly updated, to provide valuable information on health products to Canadians.
- Another initiative undertaken by Health Canada is the Dear Healthcare Professionals (DHP) letters initiative. A DHP letter is a correspondence usually in the form of emails, posts or fax, sent from the regulatory authority or the MAH of a pharmaceutical product. These letters are intended for healthcare professionals and contain important new safety information. These letters provide recipients with information concerning action(s) or practices that have been suggested to reduce particular risks of ADRs associated with a pharmaceutical product.[34]

PMS and PV are based on the core principle that patient health and patient safety are critical factors to be considered when manufacturing and marketing pharmaceutical products. Hence, while PV in a broader sense focuses on adverse reaction reporting along with disseminating knowledge among the healthcare community and patients in order to minimize risks, PMS fulfils the post-approval requirements of assessing and monitoring the potential risks associated with the use of pharmaceutical products in a larger patient population. In addition to potential risks, hitherto unknown adverse reactions can also be recognized during the PMS of drugs. In the UK, spontaneous reporting of ADRs is an integral mechanism of PMS and PV, and the same is achieved through the presence of the Yellow Card Scheme, operated by the MHRA, which has developed into a robust adverse reaction reporting system over the years. The adverse reaction reports collected through the Yellow Card scheme can be directly submitted to the MHRA *via* post, telephone or the internet. On the other hand, in Canada, the Canada Vigilance Program (now known as

MedEffect), an initiative of Health Canada, is entrusted with the responsibility to collect and assess reports of ADRs of health products marketed and sold in Canada. In 2005, the MedEffect Canada program brought about key changes to the Canada Vigilance Program, keeping in view the needs and goals for patient safety in current times, which crucially included centralized access to reliable and accurate drug product safety data.

For Further Reading

1. Huang YL, Moon J, Segal JB. A comparison of active adverse event surveillance systems worldwide. Drug Saf 2014; 37: 581–596. [PMC free article] [PubMed] [GoogleScholar]
2. VlahovicV, Mentzer D. Postmarketing surveillance. HandbExpPharmacol 2011; 205: 339–351. [PubMed] [GoogleScholar]
3. Edwards IR, Aronson JK. Adverse drug reactions: definitions, diagnosis and management. Lancet Respir Med 2000; 356: 1255–1259. [PubMed] [Google Scholar]
4. Lunevicius R, Haagsma JA. Incidence and mortality from adverse effects of medical treatment in the UK, 1990–2013: levels, trends, patterns and comparisons. Int J Qual Heal Care 2018; 30: 558–564. [PMC free article] [PubMed] [GoogleScholar]
5. Adverse Drug Reaction Canada. Working to Prevent Canada's 4th Leading Cause of Death, https://adrcanada.org/ (2018, accessed 8 June2019).
6. Avery A, Anderson C, Bond C, et al. Evaluation of patient reporting of adverse drug reactions to the UK's 'YellowCard scheme': literature review, descriptive and qualitative analyses, and questionnaire surveys. Health Technol Assess (Rockv) 2011; 15: 1–234. [PubMed] [GoogleScholar]
7. Anderson C, Gifford A, Avery A, et al. Assessing the usability of methods of public reporting of adverse drug reactions to the UK Yellow Card Scheme. Heal Expect 2012; 15: 433–440. [PMC free article] [PubMed] [GoogleScholar]
8. Metters J. Report of an independent review of access to the yellow card scheme. London: TSO National Audit Office, 2004. [GoogleScholar]
9. Marketed Health Products Directorate. Yellow Card Scheme - MHRA, https://yellowcard.mhra.gov.uk/monitoringsafety (accessed 8 June2019).
10. Rabbur RSM, Emmerton L. An introduction to adverse drug reaction reporting systems in different countries. Int J Pharm Pract 2005; 13: 91–100. [Google Scholar]
11. Tomorrow's Pharmacist. Yellow Card reporting scheme: what to report and where to? Pharm J 2005. [GoogleScholar]
12. BMA Board of Science. Reporting adverse drug reactions: a guide for healthcare professionals. London: British Medical Association, 2006. [Google Scholar]
13. Black Triangle: Additional Monitoring of Medicines,www.rpharms.com/resources/quick-reference-guides/black-triangle-additional-monitoring-of-medicine (accessed 8 June 2019).

14. The Yellow Card Scheme: guidance for healthcare professionals, patients and the public,www.gov.uk/guidance/the-yellow-card-scheme-guidance-for-healthcare professionals (2015, accessed 8 June2019).
15. Blenkinsopp A, WilkieP, Wang M, et al. Patient reporting of suspected adverse drug reactions: a review of published literature and international experience. Br J ClinPharmacol 2007; 63: 148–156. [PMC free article] [PubMed] [GoogleScholar]
16. Drug Safety Update-GOV.UK, www.gov.uk/drug-safety-update (accessed 8 June2019).
17. Hillman D, Ryder C. Applying for an EU marketing authorisation: a pharmacovigilance perspective. Regulatory Rapporteur 2019; 16: 23–27. [Google Scholar]
18. Gough S. Post-marketing surveillance: a UK/European perspective. Curr Med Res Opin 2005; 21: 565–570. [PubMed] [GoogleScholar]
19. French DD, Margo CE, Campbell RR. Enhancing postmarketing surveillance: continuing challenges. Br J ClinPharmacol 2015; 80: 615–617. [PMC free article] [PubMed] [GoogleScholar]
20. Health Products and Food Branch Inspectorate.www.canada.ca/en/health-canada/services/drugs-health-products/drug-products/applications-submissions/guidance-documents/clinical-trials/drugs-health-products-inspectorate.html (accessed 8 June 2019).
21. Good pharmacovigilance practices. Guidelines (GUI-0102) - Canada.ca,www.canada.ca/en/health-canada/services/drugs-health-products/compliance- enforcement/good-manufacturing-practices/guidance-documents/pharmacovigilance-guidelines-0102.html#a41 (accessed 8 June2019).
22. Cheung RY, Goodwin SH. An overview of Canadian and US approaches to drug regulation and responses to postmarket adverse drug reactions. J Diabetes SciTechnol 2013; 7: 313–320. [PMC free article] [PubMed] [GoogleScholar]
23. Health Canada. Chapter 4 Regulating Pharmaceutical Drugs. 2011 Fall Report of the Auditor General of Canada, www.oag-bvg.gc.ca/internet/English/parl_oag_201111_04_e_35936.html (2011, accessed 8 June 2019). [Google Scholar]
24. Health Canada. Canada Vigilance Program,www.canada.ca/en/health-canada/services/drugs-health-products/medeffect-canada/canada-vigilance-program.html (accessed 8 June2019).
25. Health Canada. Health Product Vigilance Framework,www.canada.ca/content/dam/hc-sc/migration/hc-sc/dhp-mps/alt_formats/pdf/pubs/medeff/fs-if/2012- hpvf-cvps/dhpvf-ecvps-eng.pdf (2012, accessed 8 June2019).
26. Wilson K, Ducharme R, Hawken S. Association between socioeconomic status and adverse events following immunization at 2, 4, 6 and 12 months. Hum Vaccines Immun other 2013; 9: 1153–1157. [PMC free article] [PubMed] [Google Scholar]
27. Health Canada. An overview of the Marketed Health Products Directorate, http://publications.gc.ca/site/archivee-archived.html?

url=http://publications.gc.ca/collections/collection_2011/sc-hc/H164-2-2008-eng.pdf (2012, accessed 8 June2019).

28. Health Canada. MedEffect Canada, www.canada.ca/en/health-canada/services/drugs-health-products/medeffect-canada.html (accessed 8 June2019).

29. Health Canada. Adverse reaction reporting and health product safety information,www.canada.ca/content/dam/hc-sc/migration/hc-sc/dhp-mps/alt_formats/pdf/pubs/medeff/fs-if/2011-ar-ei-guide-prof/2011-ar-ei-guide-prof-eng.pdf (2011, accessed 8 June2019).

30. Health Canada. Adverse reaction and medical device problem reporting,www.canada.ca/en/health-canada/services/drugs-health-products/medeffect-canada/adverse-reaction-reporting.html (accessed 8 June 2019).

31. vanHunselF, Härmark L, Pal S, et al. Experiences with adverse drug reaction reporting by patients. Drug Saf 2012; 35: 45–60. [PubMed] [GoogleScholar]

32. Kaur SD. A comparative analysis of post-market surveillance for natural health products (NHPs). MSc Thesis, University of Ottawa, UK, 2013. [Google Scholar]

33. Health Canada. Health Product InfoWatch,www.canada.ca/en/health-canada/services/drugs-health-products/medeffect-canada/health-product-infowatch.html (accessed 8 June2019).

34. Dear Health Care Professional Letter - OPDIVO®, www.canada.ca/content/dam/hc-sc/migration/hc-sc/dhp-mps/alt_formats/pdf/prodpharma/notice-avis/conditions/opdivo_dhcpl_lapds_183397-eng.pdf (2016, accessed 8 June 2019).

Chapter 9

Abbreviated New Drug Application (ANDA) Submissions

Learning Objectives

To understand

- How Drugs are Developed and Approved
- Types of Drug Approval Applications
- Investigational New Drug (IND)
- New Drug Application (NDA)
- Abbreviated New Drug Application (ANDA)
- Over-the-Counter Drugs (OTC)
- Biologic License Application (BLA)
- Abbreviated New Drug Application (ANDA): Generics
- Components of Regulatory Filing and Data Requirements
- ANDA Submissions
- CTD FORMAT
- Generic drug approval process in USA
- Hatch-Waxman Act
- Abbreviated New Drug Applications (ANDA)

TYPES OF CERTIFICATIONS

- ANDA approval process in USA
- Withdrawal of Approval of an ANDA
- Generic drug approval process in EU
- Centralized Procedure
- Letter of intent to submit

- Generic Medicinal Product
- Hybrid Medicinal Product
- Generic Drug Entry Prior to Patent Expiration
- Hatch Waxman Act
- STATUTORY PROVISIONS
- Principle provisions of Hatch-Waxman Act
- Generic Drug Approval Process
- Generic Drug Competition Provisions
- ANDA Stay Provision and Preliminary Injunction Practice
- Tactical Use of the Thirty-Month Stay Provision
- Generic Drug Competition Provisions:
- Statutory 30 months stay on ANDA approval
- Generic Drug Competition Provisions
- Options Available To ANDA Applicants
- Incentives of Patent Law
- Federal Trade Commission Study
- FDA Rulemaking
- 30-Month Stay Provisions
- Requirements for Drug Patent Submissions
- Initiative on Improving Access to Generic Drugs
- ANDA Stay Provision and Preliminary Injunction Practice
- Tactical Use of the Thirty-Month Stay Provision
- Generic Drug Competition Provisions:
- Statutory 30 months stay on ANDA approval
- Generic Drug Competition Provisions
- Options Available To ANDA Applicants
- Incentives of Patent Law
- Federal Trade Commission Study
- FDA Rulemaking
- 30-Month Stay Provisions
- Requirements for Drug Patent Submissions
- Initiative on Improving Access to Generic Drugs

INTRODUCTION

A new drug is defined as one that is not generally recognized as safe and effective for the indications proposed. However, this definition has much greater reach than simply a "new" chemical entity. The term "new drug" also refers to a drug product already in existence, though never approved by the FDA for marketing in the United States; new therapeutic indications for an approved drug; a new dosage form; a new route of administration; a new dosing schedule; or, any other significant clinical differences than those approved. A Generic Drug Product is one that is comparable to an Innovator Drug Product in dosage form, strength, and route of administration, quality, performance characteristics and intended use.

How Drugs are Developed and Approved: The mission of FDA's Center for Drug Evaluation and Research (CDER) is to ensure that drugs marketed in this country are safe and effective. CDER does not test drugs, although the Center's Office of Testing and Research does conduct limited research in the areas of drug quality, safety, and effectiveness. CDER is the largest of FDA's five centers. It has responsibility for both prescription and nonprescription or over-the-counter (OTC) drugs.

Types of Drug Approval Applications

Investigational New Drug (IND): Current Federal law requires that a drug be the subject of an approved marketing application before it is transported or distributed across state lines. Because a sponsor will probably want to ship the investigational drug to clinical investigators in many states, it must seek an exemption from that legal requirement. The IND is the means through which the sponsor technically obtains this exemption from the FDA.

New Drug Application (NDA): When the sponsor of a new drug believes that enough evidence on the drug's safety and effectiveness has been obtained to meet FDA's requirements for marketing approval, the sponsor submits to FDA a new drug application (NDA). The application must contain data from specific technical viewpoints for review, including chemistry, pharmacology, medical, biopharmaceutics, and statistics. If the NDA is approved, the product may be marketed in the United States. For internal tracking purposes, all NDA's are assigned an NDA number.

Abbreviated New Drug Application (ANDA): An Abbreviated New Drug Application (ANDA) contains data that, when submitted to FDA's Center for Drug Evaluation and Research, Office of Generic Drugs, provides for the review and ultimate approval of a generic drug product. Generic drug applications are called "abbreviated" because they are generally not required to include preclinical (animal) and clinical (human) data to establish safety and effectiveness.

Over-the-Counter Drugs (OTC): Over-the-counter (OTC) drugs play an increasingly vital role in America's health care system. OTC drug products are those drugs that are available to consumers without a prescription. There are more than 80 therapeutic categories of OTC drugs, ranging from acne drug products to weight control drug products.

Biologic License Application (BLA): Biological products are approved for marketing under the provisions of the Public Health Service (PHS) Act. The Act requires a firm who manufactures a biologic for sale in interstate commerce to hold a license for the product.

Abbreviated New Drug Application (ANDA): Generics

An Abbreviated New Drug Application (ANDA) contains data which when submitted to FDA's Center for Drug Evaluation and Research, Office of Generic Drugs, provides for there view and ultimate approval of a generic drug product. Once approved, an applicant may manufacture and market the generic drug product to provide a safe, effective, low cost alternative to the American public. A generic drug product is one that is comparable to an innovator drug product in dosage form, strength, and route of administration, quality, performance characteristics and intended use. All approved products, both innovator and generic, are listed in FDA's *Approved Drug Products with Therapeutic Equivalence Evaluations*[1] (*OrangeBook*).

Table 9.1 Different types of ANDA Applications in US

Subsection of 505(j)	Products type
Paragraph I	For the products for which no patent information is available in the orange book
Paragraph II	Used for the products for which all the applicable patents are expired
Paragraph III	Used for the products for which the some or all the applicable patents are valid and the applicant confirms that the product will not be placed in the market till such patents are expired
Paragraph IV	Used for the products for which some or all the applicable patents are valid and applicant try to file the product which does not infringe those patents or applicant invalidates the granted patents. That the patent is invalid, unenforceable, or will not be infringed by the manufacture, use, or sale of the drug product for which the ANDA is submitted On successful outcome, the generic applicant enjoys the six month exclusivity in the market

In Canada, the manufacturer may seek authorization to sell the product in Canada by filing a New Drug Submission with Health Products and Food Branch (HPFB). A New Drug Submission (NDS), typically contains scientific information about the product's safety, efficacy and quality.

Different procedures in Europe: A medicinal product may only be placed on the market in the European Economic Area (EEA) when a marketing authorization has been issued. The marketing authorization holder must be established within the EEA. European Medicines Agency regulates the medicinal products marketing authorization through various committees.

Japan: Japan is the world's second largest market next to the US. With USD 52 billion drug market, it represents 11% of global sales. The Ministry of Health, Labour, and Welfare

(MHLW) is in charge of pharmaceutical regulatory affairs in Japan and the Pharmaceutical and Medical Devices Agency (PMDA, KIKO) undertakes main duties and functions of the Ministry: it handles clinical studies, approval reviews and post-marketing safety measures i.e. approvals and licensing.

Indian Regulations: India being the leading supplier of API and generic drugs to the world, it is important to understand the Indian requirements and regulations associated with pharmaceuticals. When the applicant intends to develop and export the pharmaceuticals, it is necessary to comply with regulations set forth in the Drugs and Cosmetics Act 1940 and Rules 1945.

Emerging Nations: Rest of the World: This region consists of mainly the countries from Asia pacific, Latin America, Eastern Europe, Africa and Gulf countries. While countries from Asia pacific and Gulf have almost harmonized their regulatory environment through the Association of Southeast Asian Nations (ASEAN) and Gulf Co-operation Council (GCC) organizations, rest of the regions are yet to come up with the harmonized regulations in their respective regions.

Components of Regulatory Filing and Data Requirements: The US, EU and Japan are a part of International Conference on Harmonization (ICH), hence the technical requirements for registration of Pharmaceuticals follow the ICH recommendations. These countries require data as per the requirements of Common Technical Document (CTD).

ANDA Submissions: Procedures for ANDAs submissions are set forth in FDA's regulations in part 314 (21 CFR part 314). An ANDA is usually submitted for a drug product that is the same as an already approved drug or listed drug. A *listed drug* is defined in 314.3(b) as a new drug product that has an effective approval under section 505(c) of the FD&C Act for safety and effectiveness or under section 505 (j) of the FD&C Act, which has not been withdrawn or suspended under section 505(e)(1) through (e)(5) or (j)(5) of the FD&C Act, and which has not been withdrawn from sale for what FDA has determined are reasons of safety or effectiveness (§ 314.161). An applicant submits an ANDA based on a listed drug, and the previously approved drug product on which the ANDA relies is officially known as the *reference listed drug* (RLD). A reference listed drug (RLD) is defined as the listed drug identified by FDA as the drug product upon which an applicant relies in seeking approval of its abbreviated application (§ 314.3(b)). FDA lists approved drugs that may be referenced in an ANDA in the *Approved Drug Products with Therapeutic Equivalence Evaluations* (the Orange Book). The Orange Book is updated by a monthly cumulative supplement. On July 9, 2012, GDUFA was signed into law by the President to speed the delivery of safe and effective generic drugs to the public and reduce costs to industry. Under GDUFA, FDA agreed to meet certain obligations as laid out in the GDUFA Commitment Letter.5 Among these obligations is FDA's commitment to performance metrics for the review of new ANDAs that are submitted electronically following the electronic CTD (eCTD) format. For example, FDA has committed to review and act on 90 percent of original ANDA submissions within 10 months from the date of submission in Year 5 of the program, which begins on October 1, 2016. To meet these performance goals, FDA is issuing this guidance to assist ANDA applicants in improving the quality of submissions, to increase the number of original ANDAs acknowledged for receipt upon initial submission, and to decrease the number of review cycles. FDA is committed to providing comprehensive assistance in the early stages of the application process so that an original ANDA will contain all information necessary for FDA to complete its review in one review cycle.

CTD FORMAT: The CTD format was developed by the International Conference on Harmonization (ICH) in an attempt to streamline the variability of submission requirements among Japan, the European Union, and the United States. The CTD collects quality, safety, and efficacy information into a common format that has been adopted by ICH regulatory authorities. As previously stated, only ANDA submissions made electronically following the eCTD format on the date of submission will be subject to the review metric goals described in the GDUFA Commitment Letter. Section 745A (a) of the FD&C Act, added by section 1136 of the Food and Drug Administration Safety and Innovation Act (FDASIA) (Pub. L. 112-144), requires that submissions under section 505(b), (i), or (j) of the FD&C Act and section 351(a) or (k) of the Public Health Service Act (42 85 U.S.C. 262(a) or (k)) be submitted in electronic format specified by FDA, beginning no earlier than 24 months after FDA issues a final guidance specifying an electronic submission format.

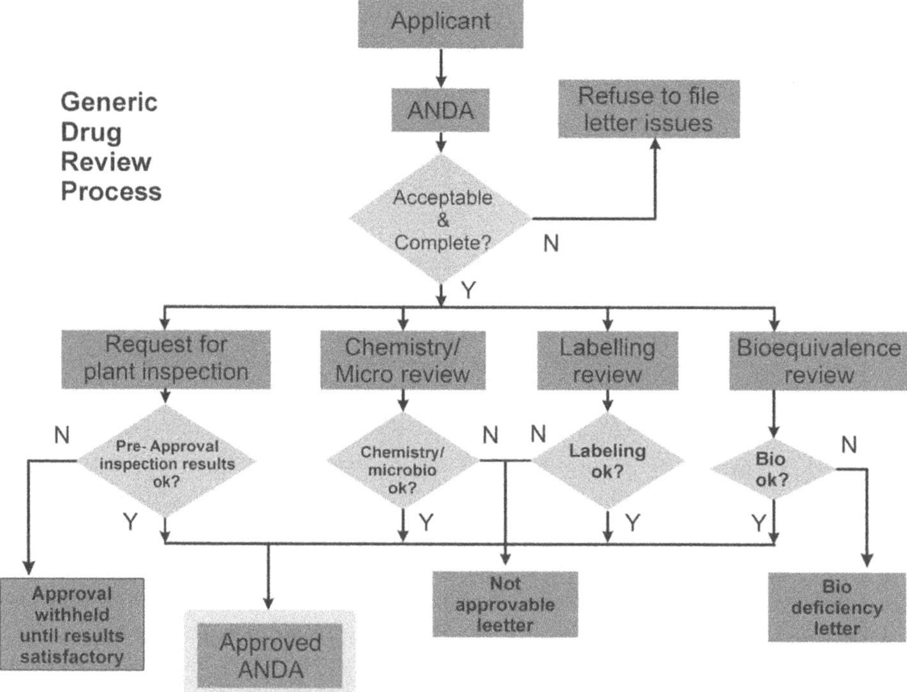

Fig. 9.1 Generic Drug Review Process.

The CTD is comprised of the following modules:

- Module 1: Administrative information;
- Module 2: CTD Summaries;
- Module 3: Quality;
- Module 4: Nonclinical study reports; and
- Module 5: Clinical study reports.

The sections that follow in this guidance detail the information to be submitted in the applicable Modules, sections and subsections.

Generic drug approval process in USA

Hatch-Waxman Act: Intended to balance interests of consumers, the brand name pharmaceutical industry (innovator) and the generic drug industry to "make available more low cost generic drugs and to create a new incentive for increased expenditures for research and development of certain products which are subject to pre-market approval. In fewer than 20 years since enactment of the statute, generic drugs increased from 19% to 47% of prescriptions.

Title I of Hatch-Waxman Act: Authorized marketing of generic drugs upon approval of Abbreviated New Drug Application (ANDA). Under this ANDA can be approved upon submission of evidence that the active ingredient of the generic drug is the "bioequivalent" of a drug previously approved by USFDA after submission of a full NDA without having to submit studies establishing the safety and efficacy of drug.

Title II of Hatch-Waxman Act: This section provided specific extensions of patents covering drugs and other products subject to "regulatory review" by the FDA and government agencies. This provision was intended to balance the benefits of ANDA practice by providing brand name drug companies with the restoration of portions of the terms of their drug patents lost during the testing period required for the approval of the drugs. These patent term adjustments as well as patent extensions implemented 10 years after the enactment of Hatch-Waxman Act.

Abbreviated New Drug Applications (ANDA): Under section 505 (j) of Hatch-Waxman Act, an ANDA may be filed for a generic version of any "listed drug".

Listed Drug: Any drug for which an NDA has previously been approved is deemed to be a listed drug and is listed by FDA in the orange book. Drugs previously approved under ANDA's and Antibiotics are also regarded as listed drugs. An ANDA must include all information required in an NDA except full reports of investigations demonstrating that the drug is safe and effective in use.

ANDA additionally must show: Labeling of the drug for which ANDA is sought is same as the approved labeling for the listed drug. b) Its route of administration, dosage form and strength are the same as the listed drug or supply such information respecting any differences as FDA may require bioequivalence reports c) Status of orange book listed patents on the approved drug.

TYPES OF CERTIFICATIONS

An applicant for ANDA must certify to FDA that in its opinion and to the best of its knowledge, with respect to each listed patent that claims the drug or use of the drug for which the applicant seeking approvals are: Paragraph I; Paragraph II; Paragraph III; Paragraph IV. The Hatch- Waxman act has undertaken necessary considerations to prevent litigations between generics and NDA applicants[6]. The act is successful in making a pathway for approval of generics without infringing the original patent. The pathway for approval of generics by the Hatch-Waxman begins with the certification procedures. Hatch-Waxman proposed four options for application for generic approval. The first three options avoid litigation.

PARAGRAPH I: That the patent information relating to innovator patent has not been filed

PARAGRAPH II: That relevant patent has already expired

PARAGRAPH III: That the generic will not market the drug until after the patent expires

PARAGRAPH IV: The generic manufacturer should certify that an applicable patent is invalid or will not be infringed by the generic product.

ANDA approval process in USA: Initially, an ANDA filer must show that the conditions of use identified in its proposed labeling have been previously approved for the listed drug on which the ANDA is based. According to this statute, ANDA must incorporate the same labeling as that of previously approved for the listed drug except for any changes required because of the differences are approved on the basis of a suitability petition.

Withdrawal of Approval of an ANDA: FDA may withdraw/suspend approval of an ANDA when the approval of the listed drug on which the ANDA relies is either withdrawn or suspended. Further, an approval of an ANDA or 505 (b)(2) application may be withdrawn on the basis of evidence showing that the drug is unsafe for use or ineffective or that the ANDA or 505 (b)(2) application contains any untrue statement of material fact. FDA must withdraw approval of an ANDA if it finds that the approval "was obtained, expedited or otherwise facilitated through bribery, payment of an illegal gratuity, or fraud or material false statement", or may withdraw approval of an ANDA if it finds that the applicant has "repeatedly demonstrated a lack of ability to produce drug, and has introduced or attempted to introduce, such adulterate dorm is branded drug in to commerce".

Generic drug approval process in EU: As for all medicines, generic medicines must obtain marketing authorization before they can be marketed. Marketing authorizations are granted after a regulatory authority, such as the European Medicines Agency, has conducted a scientific evaluation of the medicine's efficacy (how well it works as measured in clinical studies), safety and quality. Applicant shall not be required to provide the results of pre-clinical tests and clinical trials if he can demonstrate that the medicinal product is a generic medicinal product of a reference medicinal product.

Centralized Procedure: Generic/Hybrid medicinal product applications of the medicinal products authorized via the centralized procedure have automatic access to the centralized procedure under article 3(3) of the regulation (EC) number 726/2004. For generic/hybrid applications of a centrally authorized product, the application should state in their "Letter of intent to submit" that they have automatic access to the centralized procedure under article3 (3).

Letter of intent to submit: Before submission of the dossier, applicants should notify the agency of their intention to submit an application, preferably 6-18 months in advance and indicate that the application is generic/hybrid medicinal product application of a medicinal product authorized via centralized procedure. EMA (European Medicines Agency) will inform the applicant on the outcome of the eligibility request.

Generic Medicinal Product: A medicinal product that has; the same qualitative and quantitative composition in active substances as the reference product. The same pharmaceutical form as the reference medicinal product. And whose bioequivalence with the reference medicinal product has been demonstrated by appropriate bioavailability studies.

Hybrid Medicinal Product: Hybrid applications differ from the generic applications in that the results of appropriate pre-clinical tests and clinical trials will be necessary in the following 3 circumstances: Where strict definition of a "generic medicinal product" is not met, Where the bioavailability studies cannot be used to demonstrate bioequivalence, Where the changes in active substance(s), therapeutic indications, strength, pharmaceutical form or route of administration of the generic product compared to the reference medicinal product.

Generic Drug Entry Prior to Patent Expiration: The Drug Price Competition and Patent Term Restoration Act of 1984, otherwise known as the *Hatch-Waxman Act*, have been quite successful in increasing the availability of generic drugs to consumers. By 1996, forty-three percent of the prescription drugs sold in the United States was generic compared to just nineteen percent in 1984[1], and at present it is 70% of prescription drugs. Despite the Act's overall success in promoting increased availability of generic drugs, the Act's provisions relating to patent certification actually delayed approval of generic drugs. The Hatch-Waxman Amendments were intended to balance two important public policy goals. First, Congress wanted to ensure that brand-name (also known as innovator) drug manufacturers would have meaningful patent protection and a period of marketing exclusivity to enable them to recoup their investments in the development of valuable new drugs. Second, Congress sought to ensure that, once the statutory patent protection and marketing exclusivity for these new drugs has expired, consumers would benefit from the rapid availability of lower priced generic versions of innovator drugs.

Hatch Waxman Act: The Drug Price Competition and Patent Term Restoration Act of popularly known as the Hatch-Waxman Act. The act is codified in various sections of Titles 15, 21, 28, and 35 of U.S.C. The informal name comes from two sponsors of this Act, Henry Waxman, representative of California and Senator Orrin Hatch of Utah.

Primary Objective behind this act:

- To encourage greater public access to generic drugs (in favor of generic drug manufacturers)

➢ To spur new pharmaceutical development (in favor of branded drug manufacturers)

In order to reach its objective, Congress used this Act to create a delicate balance between the rights of research-based firms and generic firms, a balance crucial to the American pharmaceutical industry and the public alike.

❖ Prior to Hatch-Waxman Act 1984, generic manufacturers had to file their own "New Drug Application" (NDA) for regulatory approval, either relying on already published scientific literature or with the support of clinical data, to demonstrate the safety and efficacy of their product, even though it was identical to that of previously approved drug. Such generic versions were known as "paper" NDA.

❖ Thus approval of a generic drug was a costly, duplicative and time-consuming process.

❖ Congressional testimony prior to Hatch-Waxman reported that there were 150 off-patent drugs for which no generic existed because the cost of FDA approval was too high.

❖ In 1984, Court of Appeals for the Federal Circuit, in *Roche v. Bolar,* concluded that experimental use i.e. formulation development to obtain stability data, dissolution profile and bioequivalence data for regulatory submission, during the patent term, is an act of infringement.

❖ This decision created a situation of de facto patent term extension which was not supported by Food, Drug and Cosmetic Act, 1938 and Patent Act, 1952.

STATUTORY PROVISIONS: The Hatch-Waxman Amendments amended the Federal Food, Drug, and Cosmetic (FD&C) Act and created a statutory generic drug approval process with section 505(j). Section 505(j) established the abbreviated new drug application (ANDA) approval process, which permits generic versions of previously approved innovator drugs to be approved without submitting a full new drug application (NDA). An ANDA refers to the clinical research and data in a previously approved NDA (the "listed drug") and relies on the Agency's finding of safety and effectiveness for the listed drug product.

Principle provisions of Hatch-Waxman Act: To overcome the above mentioned problems as well as to address the inadequacies in the pharmaceutical regulatory system, on September 24, 1984, President Ronald Reagan signed into law the Drug Price Competition and Patent Term Restoration Act of 1984 ("the Hatch-Waxman Act") having three titles:

Title I: Abbreviated New Drug Application Provisions

Title II: Patent Term Restoration Provisions

Title III: Amendments to the Textile Fiber Products Identification Act and the Wool Products Labeling Act of1939

Generic Drug Approval Process

❖ ANDA process was created to encourage greater access to lower-priced drug products, and to shorten the time it took for generics to reach the market.

- ❖ The ANDA process does not require the generic manufacturer to repeat costly animal (preclinical) and human (clinical) research on ingredients or dosage forms already approved for safety and effectiveness.
- ❖ Drug companies must submit an ANDA for approval to the FDA's Office of Generic Drugs in the Center for Drug Evaluation and Research, wherein, a generic drug must meet the following criteria:
- ✓ Contain the same active ingredient(s) as the innovator drug (inactive ingredients may vary).
- ✓ Be identical in strength, dosage form, and route of administration.
- ✓ Have the same indications.
- ✓ Be bioequivalent (performs in the same manner as the innovator drug).

Generic Drug Competition Provisions

- ❖ **Orange Book:** Approved Drug Products with Therapeutic Equivalence Evaluations, commonly known as the "Orange Book," is compiled by the USFDA and lists all approved drugs. Each holder of an approved NDA must list patents, which he believes would be infringed if a generic drug were marketed before the expiration of these patents. NDA holder should list patent(s) in OB, within 30 days of NDA approval or within 30 days of patent grant.

The statute requires the NDA applicant to:

(a) Submit patents, by patent number, expiration date, and use codes; and

(b) The submitted patent must claim the drug that is the subject of the NDA or must claim a method of using such drug.FDA also publishes a list of exclusivity(s) pertaining to the specific product in OB. Once approved by the FDA, all products, both innovator as well as generic, are listed in OB.

ANDA Stay Provision and Preliminary Injunction Practice:

The scope of exclusivity granted by the FDA's thirty month stay provision under 21 C.F.R. § 314.107 (b) (3) (i) (A) has the same effect as a preliminary injunction because the provision prevents the ANDA applicant from producing, selling, or using its applied for drug product until a trial decision is made in the ANDA applicant's favor. Because of the statute has a similar result to a preliminary injunction, it is useful to compare the differences in how these to results are obtained.

A patent holder seeking a preliminary injunction against an alleged infringer must demonstrate:

- a reasonable likelihood of success on the merits;
- irreparable harm if an injunction is not granted
- a balance of hardships tipping in its favor

- the injunction's favorable impact on the public interest. The factors taken individually are not dispositive; instead, a district court in its discretion "must weigh and measure each factor against the other factors and against the form and magnitude of there life requested.

Showing the first two factors, likelihood of success and irreparable harm, are essential if a preliminary injunction is to be granted.[16]The preliminary injunction should not issue if the alleged infringer raises an infringement or invalidity defense that the plaintiff cannot prove "lacks substantial merit. In contrast to the requirements for issuance of a preliminary injunction, the FDA's thirty- month stay provision under 21 C.F.R. § 314.107 takes effect regardless of likelihood of success or irreparable harm. If a NDA holder files suit, the ANDA applicant's entry into the market is delayed for thirty months or until the ANDA applicant receives a favorable verdict even where the NDA holder has a very small chance of success on the merits of the suit. The ANDA applicant's barrier to entry remains absolute even where the ANDA holder presents powerful defenses that either tend to show non-infringement or presents serious challenges to validity of the NDA holder's patents.

Tactical Use of the Thirty-Month Stay Provision: Because the thirty-month stay provision takes effect automatically, NDA holders have a very significant incentive to file suit against ANDA applicants even where the merits of the case are weak. Additionally, the power of the thirty-month stay provision provides incentive for NDA holders to list as many patents as possible in the Orange Book in order to ensure that competitors will need to make a paragraph IV certification even after a primary patent covering the NDA product has expired. The practice of prosecuting and listing secondary patents is referred to as "ever greening" or "trip wire" listing of patents.

Generic Drug Competition Provisions

Statutory 30 months stay on ANDA approval: Generic applicant, who files paragraph IV in its ANDA, has to notify the patent holder and NDA filer about the ANDA submission with PIV certification, when FDA accepts his ANDA for filing. If the patent holder files an infringement suit against the generic applicant within 45 days of the PIV notification, FDA approval to market the generic version is automatically postponed for 30 months. The 30-month stay was meant to allow time for the patent holder to litigate and resolve the PIV issues. The district court dismissed Abbott's case pursuant to FRCP 12(b)(6) on March 16, 1996, and the Federal Circuit affirmed this dismissal in a succinct January 14, 1997 opinion[23], Here, the ANDA applicants had a clear cut case (clear enough to win the case on a motion to dismiss), but the barest legal argument as to why Abbott's patent should have expired in January 21, 1997 allowed Abbott to trigger the thirty-month stay provision and perpetuate the monopoly on its NDA product for over a year past the expiration date of their patent. The problem is exacerbated by the FDA's apparent lack of review or understanding of the patent laws in that it blindly accepted for the Orange Book Abbott's assertion that its patent would expire in 1997 and used this assertion to deny ANDA approval to two competitors. The Federal Circuit upheld summary judgment in favor Elan and found that Bayer's patent could not possibly cover Élan's product literally or under the doctrine of equivalents because Bayer had "made statements of clear and unmistakable surrender of subject matter outside the claimed SSA range of 1.0 to 4 m^2/g.[26]Despitethe fact that Bayer's patent clearly did not cover Elan's product, Bayer's strained argument for a broad scope of its claims triggered the thirty-month stay provision and delayed Elan's ANDA application at least until March 16, 1999 when the district court granted summary judgment in Elan's favor.

The possible scenarios and tactical litigation moves that can arise are further complicated by the fact that the first ANDA applicant to make a paragraph IV certification is granted 180 days of exclusive production before a second ANDA applicant can gain approval for its application *Mova Pharmaceuticals v. Shalala* illustrates the kind of situation that may arise Mova filed an ANDA application to produce a generic diabetes drug in December 1994.

A paragraph IV certification, however, begins a process in which the question of whether the listed patent is valid or will be infringed by the proposed generic product may be answered by the courts before the expiration of the patent. The submission of an ANDA for a drug product claimed in a patent is an infringing act if the generic product is intended to be marketed before expiration of the patent. This 30-month stay will delay approval of the generic drug product unless the court reaches a decision earlier in the patent infringement case or otherwise orders a longer or shorter period for the stay. Under FDA's traditional interpretation of the Hatch-Waxman Amendments, multiple 30-month stays have been possible. Submission of newly issued patents after an ANDA application has been filed with FDA has required the appropriate certification and notice to the NDA holder and patent owner with the possibility of a 30-month stay if patent infringement litigation resulted. As a result, there have been a number of instances in which delays in ANDA approval have exceeded 30-months. A recent review of FDA's records indicates that of the 442 active ANDAs that contained paragraph IV certifications, only 17 have had multiple 30-month stays, representing 3.8 percent of all applications with patent challenges. However, we note that a significant number of these products have high dollar value annual sales, and we are aware of some instances where multiple stays have resulted in the delay of a generic drug approval for a number of years.

180-Day Exclusivity: The Hatch-Waxman Amendments provide an incentive of 180 days of market exclusivity to the "first" generic applicant who challenges a listed patent by filing a paragraph IV certification and thereby runs the risk of having to defend a patent infringement suit. The statute provides that the first applicant to file a substantially complete ANDA containing a paragraph IV certification to a listed patent will be eligible for a 180-day period of exclusivity beginning either from the date it begins commercial marketing of the generic drug product, or from the date of a court decision finding the patent invalid, unenforceable or not infringed, whichever is first. These two events first commercial marketing and a court decision favorable to the generic are often called "triggering" events, because under the statute they can trigger the beginning of the 180-day exclusivity period. Only an ANDA containing a paragraph IV certification may be eligible for exclusivity. If an applicant changes from a paragraph IV certification to a paragraph III certification, for example, upon losing its patent infringement litigation, the ANDA will no longer be eligible for exclusivity. The 180-day exclusivity provision has been the subject of considerable litigation and administrative review in recent years, as the courts, industry, and FDA have sought to interpret it in a way that is consistent both with the statutory text and with the legislative goals underlying the Hatch-Waxman Amendments. A series of Federal court decisions beginning with the 1998 Mova[2] case describe acceptable interpretations of the 180-day exclusivity provision, identify potential problems in implementing the statute, and establish certain principles to be used by the Agency in interpreting the statute. As described in June 1998 guidance for industry, FDA currently is addressing on a case-by-case basis those 180-day exclusivity issues not addressed by existing regulations. One of the most fundamental changes to the 180-day exclusivity program, resulting from the legal challenges to FDA's regulations, is the determination by the courts of the meaning of the phrase "court decision." The courts have determined that the "court decision" that can begin the running of the 180-day exclusivity period may be the decision of the district court, if it finds that the patent at issue is invalid, unenforceable, or will not be infringed by the generic drug product. FDA had previously interpreted the "court decision" that could begin the running of 180-day exclusivity (and the approval of the ANDA) as the final decision of a court from which no appeal can be or has been taken - generally a decision of the Federal Circuit. FDA had taken this position so that the generic manufacturer would not have to run the risk of being subject to potential treble damages for marketing the drug, if the appeals court ruled in favor of the patent holder.

Generic Drug Competition Provisions: The 180-day exclusivity is the so called incentive for generic companies to step forward and challenge patents. The first applicant to submit a paragraph IV certification ANDA to the FDA has the exclusive right to market the generic drug for 180 days. "First applicant As used in this subsection, the term 'first applicant' means an applicant that, on the first day on which a substantially complete application containing a certification described in paragraph (2)(A)(vii)(IV) is submitted for approval of a drug, submits a substantially complete application that contains and lawfully maintains a certification described in paragraph (2)(A)(vii)(IV) for the drug."

The 180-day market exclusivity period begins on earlier of two dates:

(i) Date of first commercial marketing of approved ANDA; and

(ii) Date of court decision holding that the patent which is the subject of the certification is invalid or not infringed.

The FDA granted the one hundred eighty day exclusivity period to Mylan instead of Mova since Mylan had not yet "successfully defended" itself against Upjohn.[34]Mova challenged this decision and ultimately prevailed in April 1998 when the D.C. Circuit held that the FDA's successful defense requirement was unsustainable based on Congress's statutory language. The complicated statutory construction issues surrounding the 180-day exclusivity period addressed by the D.C. Circuit obscures the overall picture of what happened in this case. Upjohn used Mylan in February 1997, and the trial court ruled that Upjohn's patent was *invalid* and not infringed on March 31, 1998.The problematic interaction between the thirty-month stay provision and 180-day exclusivity period is illustrated by a footnote in the *Mova*case.[37] An *amicus* brief by Biovail Corporation reveals that it was the second applicant to file a paragraph IV certification for a heart medication. The incentive of NDA holders to list as many patents in the Orange Book as possible ("land mine" patents) exacerbates thirty-month stay provision problems. Regulations allow "drug substance (ingredient) patents, drug product (formulation and composition) patents, and method of use patents" to be listed in the Orange Book.[41] Thus, pharmaceutical companies often list "unapproved uses, special crystalline forms of the active ingredient, specific formulations, tablet shape or other subject matter.

Options Available To ANDA Applicants: An ANDA applicant who wants to avoid the thirty-month stay provision and faces patents listed in the Orange Book which do not cover the NDA drug itself but instead cover narrow forms of the drug or irrelevant uses for the drug (unapproved uses) has a very limited number of undesirable legal options available to it. The applicant either must argue to the FDA or to a court that paragraph IV certification should not be required or must certify against all the patents listed in the Orange Book and hope to have the inevitable lawsuit by the NDA holder dismissed on the merits as soon as possible to end the thirty-month stay. The ANDA regulations require that certifications be made only against patents "which claims the reference [Orange Book] listed drug or that claims a use of such listed drug.[47] To "claim" the drug, according to the patent law definition of "claim," a patent's claim section would have to include every element directed at the drug and no other elements. For example, a patent having claims that include elements of the drug and elements of packaging does not "claim" the drug.[48] The code suggests that the term "drug" includes only drug products (dosage forms) and drug substances (active ingredients). FDA regulation interpretations indicate that, in the FDA's view, an ANDA applicant must certify against every patent listed in the Orange Book. The FDA has "determined that 'Congress intended that an ANDA applicant need only consult the Orange Book to determine the existence of an applicable patent claiming the listed drug or use of the listed drug. The FDA's view is supported by the regulations' mechanism for challenging disputed patent. Existence of a formal procedure for disputing an Orange Book listing implies that third parties would have a reason, such as required certification, to dispute a listing.

Incentives of Patent Law: Exclusive rights granted for the originator of an invention or creative work, intellectual property rights, are well recognized in the modern laws of nearly every nation.64 In fact, the Constitution specifically allows Congress "to promote the Progress of Science and useful Arts, by securing for limited Times to Authors and Inventors the exclusive Right to their respective Writings and Discoveries. A number of principle philosophical foundations for privileging intellectual property rights exist. The foundations can help inform policy makers on what extent of intellectual property rights should be granted. Specifically, the ANDA thirty-month stay provision can be evaluated on the basis of how well the provision furthers the goals addressed by these philosophical foundations. The United States patent law regime, according to most courts, is primarily concerned with providing an economic incentive for invention. The U.S. Supreme Court has stated that, "The patent monopoly was not designed to secure to the inventor his natural right in his discoveries. Rather, it was a reward, an inducement, to bring forth new knowledge. People are more likely to invent new products if they get an award in the form of the exclusive right to sell the product because the exclusive right to sell often translates into the ability to charge significant royalties for the invention compared to the price that would be charged if competition existed. The ability of the patent law to encourage development of knowledge through incentives must be weighed against the harm caused by the "patent monopoly. Ultimately, the inventor's royalty results in higher prices for consumers of the invention and perhaps a reduced output of production of the invention. Applying a utilitarian or economic standard to drug patents is an especially delicate balance. Obviously, for utilitarian and humanitarian reasons, the development of promising new drugs should remain a very high priority, and the government should maximize incentives for developing these new drugs. On the other hand, the costs of one inventor maintaining a monopoly on a drug are also quite high. Patient demand for a much needed drug is relatively inelastic, so the royalty on a drug monopoly can be very costly to consumers. The ANDA thirty-month stay provision is problematic from an economic or utilitarian perspective for several reasons. First, an NDA holder may sue an applicant based on any patent listed in the Orange Book for which it can make even the most strained argument for infringement. Many of these patents cover "unapproved uses, special crystalline forms of the active ingredient, specific formulations, tablet shape or other subject matter" which may or may not be truly useful or practical in a real world setting. Thus, the thirty-month stay provision extends the patent monopoly on a drug sold by the NDA holder while potentially only encouraging the NDA holder to prosecute and file suit on patents that disclose inventions that really do not help society at all. In these cases, the stay provision clearly is not supported by an economic or utility maximizing approach to patent laws ince the provision does not hing to encourage useful drug development while society suffers all the costs of the patent monopoly. Secondly, the thirty- month stay provision encourages drug companies to file suit against an ANDA applicant based on unsustainably broad interpretations of their patent claims. For example, Bayer was able to utilize the thirty-month stay provision to prevent Elan from selling a drug with a measured SSA of 6.15 m^2/g on the basis of a Bayer patent listed in the Orange Book which only claimed a range of 1.0 to 4 m^2/g.[72] Bayer's patent is the only legal instrument which documents what Bayer has invented and what knowledge Bayer has contributed to the world in exchange for a patent monopoly, and according to this document, Bayer did not invent any variant of the drug having a SSA greater than 4 m2/g. Third, the thirty-month stay provision does not particularly encourage patents on the core commercial drug invention but instead encourages the practice of listing "ever greening" and "trip wire" patents.[73] In order to promote maximum utility and economic efficiency in society, it would be far better to encourage development on useful core drug inventions instead of encouraging drug companies to spend resources devising and identifying non-useful sub-inventions that may act as "trip wire" patents. A fourth problem with the thirty-month stay provision from an economic or utility maximizing perspective is that it encourages drug company emphasis on profits through patents in general. One problem with patents is that their power to encourage invention is limited by the ability of consumers to pay monopoly rents. The most economically efficient system would encourage that drugs be developed that will help society the most for the minimum research costs, rather than encouraging development of drugs that help the wealthy segment of the population slightly at greater research expense. To reach greater efficiency than the patent system allows, the public could, for example, divert funds from monopoly rents paid to patent holders toward direct government subsidies for drug researchers developing drugs which attack the most devastating diseases that affect the greatest number of people. The thirty-month stay provision enhances the value of patents in a vague way by allowing the patent to be used to significantly delay ANDA approval regardless of whether the patent actually covers the ANDA drug as long as some argument for infringement can be made. By enhancing the value of patents, the stay provision encourages drug companies to focus on the kind of drugs that are made most valuable by patents, namely those drugs which are marketable to people have the money to pay monopoly rents. A fifth problem with the thirty-month stay provision is that any gains it may provide to a company are too unpredictable and speculative to be substantial incentive for research and development. The drug company's primary patent on a new drug protects the company's monopoly on the NDA product for at least twenty years from the date the patent is filed. "Ever greening" or "trip wire" patents which might trigger the thirty-month stay of ANDA approval would not have value until after the primary patent which prevents others from manufacturing and selling the drug has expired. During the twenty-year life of the primary patent, a better drug or treatment technology could potentially be developed thus making the potentiality of a thirty-month stay of competing ANDAs worthless. The thirty-month stay provision could be rescinded or reinterpreted not to be triggered upon suits based on "trip wire" patents again making the stay provision worthless. After twenty years, there may be no need to exclude ANDA competitors as it could be that no significant competitor exists. Since, ex ante, a drug company or inventor is likely to consider the potential gains from the thirty-month stay provision merely speculative rather than significant, the stay provision provides very little incentive for new drug manufacture.

There more efficient possibilities for encouraging research and development of new drugs rather than allowing new drug applicants to block ANDA applications based on patents which would not meet a preliminary injunction standard. One possibility, mentioned above, is that the public's payments toward patent monopoly rents could be shifted towards direct research for the most needed drugs. In this scenario, the thirty-month stay provision would decrease in importance as drug patents in general decrease in importance to drug companies.

Federal Trade Commission Study: In response to reports of brand-name and generic drug companies engaging in anti-competitive behavior, the FTC conducted a study to determine if the 180-day exclusivity and the 30-month stay provisions of the Hatch-Waxman Amendments have been used strategically to delay consumer access to generic drugs. In July 2002, FTC published the findings of their study and provided two primary recommendations. FTC recommended that only one automatic 30-month stay per drug product per ANDA be permitted to resolve infringement disputes over patents listed in the "Orange Book" prior to the filing date of the generic applicant's ANDA. FDA agrees with FTC's conclusion that recently, more ANDAs have been subject to 30-month stays, and more multiple 30-month stays, than in years past, and more patents on average are now being litigated per generic drug application than in the past. FTC's second recommendation was to pass legislation to require brand-name companies and first generic applicants to provide copies of certain agreements to FTC. This is a response to FTC's finding that brand-name companies and first generic applicants have on occasion entered into agreements to delay generic competition. FDA has no objection to this recommendation. FDA agrees with many of the conclusions of the FTC study and has found the factual information provided in the report to be extremely valuable in our own deliberations regarding the generic drug approval process. One example of this is the compilation of information on the disposition of litigation surrounding patents filed after NDA approval. Finally, we note that FTC's report recognized that FDA does not have the capacity to review the appropriateness of patent listings.

FDA Rulemaking: On June 12, 2003, President Bush, HHS Secretary Thompson and FDA Commissioner McClellan announced a new regulation to be effective in 60 days that will streamline the process for making safe, effective generic drugs available to consumers. This rule was first proposed on October 24, 2002, in response, in part, to the FTC recommendations and other changes the Agency identified as being useful in improving generic competition. The new rule will limit an innovator drug company to only one 30-month stay of a generic drug applicant's entry into the market for resolution of a patent challenge. The rule provides a full opportunity for only one 30-month stay per ANDA or 505(b)(2) application; prohibits the submission of patents claiming packaging, intermediates, or metabolites; requires the submission of certain patents claiming a different polymorphic form of the active ingredient described in the NDA; adds a requirement that, for submission of polymorph patents, the NDA holder must have test data demonstrating that a drug product containing the polymorph will perform the same as the drug product described in the NDA; makes changes to the patent information required to be submitted and provides declaration forms for submitting that information to FDA, both with the NDA and after NDA approval; and does not require claim-by-claim listing on the declaration form except for method-of-use patents claiming approved methods of use.

30-Month Stay Provisions: The final rule limits brand-name companies to only one 30-month stay. The rule accomplishes this by establishing when generic companies must provide notice of a paragraph IV patent challenge to a brand-name sponsor and the patent owner (which initiates the 30- month stay process). Notice of a paragraph IV certification must be provided with an initial paragraph IV certification and when a previous certification and notice did not result in a full opportunity for a single 30-month stay. If an ANDA or 505(b)(2) application is amended to include a paragraph IV certification, notice must be provided to the NDA holder and patent owner only if the application did not already contain a paragraph IV certification or there was not a full opportunity for a 30-month stay. If an ANDA or 505(b)(2) applicant changes its paragraph IV certification before the 45-day period after notice to the NDA holder and patent owner has expired, and the NDA holder or patent owner has not initiated patent litigation, such paragraph IV certification and related notice are not considered to have satisfied the requirement of providing one notice of a paragraph IV certification and a full opportunity for a 30-month stay. Generic drug applicants will still have to file paragraph IV certifications to FDA, and the ability of brand-name firms to obtain patents and to challenge alleged infringement in court is undiminished. They will not, however, be able to forestall approval of a generic version of a drug by engaging in submitting later-issued patents or repeated patent filings. These later submissions will no longer result in multiple 30-month stays.

Requirements for Drug Patent Submissions: Under the final rule, drug manufacturers will not be allowed to submit patent information for listing in the Orange Book for drug packaging, drug metabolites, and intermediate forms of a drug. Permitted submissions include patent information on drug product (active ingredients), drug substance (formulation/composition), and approved uses of a drug. In addition, patent submission declarations will be more detailed. There are mandatory forms that must be used to submit patent information to FDA. The forms include a series of questions with check-off boxes to be completed that provide details on the type of patent information submitted. The questions request information on whether the patent is one of the type permitted or not under the regulations, whether the patent is a product-by-process patent and the product claimed is novel, whether the method of use is an approved method of use and the relevant indication included in the approved labeling, and other relevant information. The declarations must be filed with the NDA, amendment, or supplement, and for patent information submitted after NDA approval. The check-off questions are designed so that FDA does not have to do anything more than quickly reviews the form to determine whether the patent information is eligible for listing. A signed attestation is required on the declaration form that requires that the submitter attest to the familiarity with the regulations and the information submitted.

Initiative on Improving Access to Generic Drugs: Concurrent with FDA's June 12, 2003, announcement on publication of its final rule, President Bush announced an initiative on Improving Access to Generic Drugs, which includes the following components:

- A proposed increase of $13 million in Fiscal Year 2004 in FDA resources devoted to improving access to generic drugs.

The proposed addition in the President's fiscal year 2004 budget of an additional $13 million in spending for FDA's generic drug programs would be the largest annual infusion of resources into the generic drug program ever, increasing the program's size by about one-third. FDA will be able to hire about 40 additional staff in generic drugs and expand the new chemistry review division in the Office of Generic Drugs. This expansion should help reduce the average review time by at least two months, increase the percentage of reviews that are completed within 180 days, approach the goal of reviewing 100 percent within 180 days and further reduce the time it takes FDA to review. Beginning in the next fiscal year, FDA will make significant changes in its processes for approving generic drugs. In particular, the FDA will implement early communications with generic drug manufacturers to discuss their applications.

For Further Reading

1. Markman V. West view Instruments holding that the judge must determine the scope of patent claims as a matter of law Inc. 1996; 1384-96.
2. Roberts v. Sears, Roebuck. Drug approval process in the European region, 18th edition, 2002; 6(2):1321-35.

3. Bayer AG. Elan Pharmaceutical Research Corp., 212 F.3d 1241, 1248. http:// openjurist.org/ 212/ f3d/ 1241/2000.
4. Hayes TA. The Food and Drug Administration's regulation of drug labeling, advertising, and promotion: looking back and looking ahead. ClinPharmacolTher. 1998; 63(6):607-616.
5. Derbis J, Evelyn B, McMeekin J. FDA aims to remove unapproved drugs from market: Risk- based enforcement program focuses on removing potentially harmful products. Pharmacy Today. 2008;21-22.
6. David A Donohoe and Maiysha R Branch Akin, Orphan Drug Act. US Food and Drug Administration. 2011;178-192.
7. Georgetown L.J, Justin Hughes. The Philosophy of Intellectual Property.1988; 287-297.

Chapter 10

Guidelines and Principles of Good Clinical Practices (ICH & WHO)

Learning Objectives

To understand

- Overview of the Clinical Research Process

  Key trial activities include:

  (Development of The Trial Protocol, Development of Standard Operating Procedures (Sops), Development of Support Systems and Tools, Generation and Approval of Trial-Related Documents, Selection of Trial Sites and The Selection of Properly Qualified, Trained, and Experienced Investigators and Study Personnel, Ethics Committee Review and Approval of The Protocol, Review by Regulatory Authorities, Enrolment of Subjects in to the Study: Recruitment, Eligibility and Informed Consent, The Investigational Product(S): Quality, Handling and Accounting, Trial Data Acquisition: Conducting The Trial, Safety Management and Reporting, Monitoring The Trial, Managing Trial Data, Quality Assurance of The Trial Performance and Data, Reporting the Trial)

- WHO Principles of GCP
- A Detailed Explanation of the Principles

  (Principle 1: Ethical Conduct, Principle 2: PROTOCOL, Principle3: Risk Identification, Principle 4: Benefit-Risk Assessment, Principle 5: Review by IEC/IRB, Principle 6: Protocol compliance, Principle 7: Informed Consent, Principle8: Continuing Review/Ongoing Benefit-Risk Assessment, Principle 9: Investigator Qualifications, Principle 10: Staff Qualifications, Principle 11: Records, Principle 12: Confidentiality/ Privacy, Principle13: Good manufacturing practice, Principle 14: Quality systems)

Introduction

Good Clinical Research Practice (GCP) is a process that incorporates established ethical and scientific quality standards for the design, conduct, recording and reporting of clinical research involving the participation of human subjects. Compliance with GCP provides public assurance that the rights, safety, and well-being of research subjects are protected and respected, consistent with the principles enunciated in the Declaration of Helsinki and other internationally recognized ethical guidelines, and ensures the integrity of clinical research data. The conduct of clinical research is complex and this complexity is compounded by the need to involve a number of different individuals with a variety of expertise, all of who must perform their tasks skillfully and efficiently.

Overview of the Clinical Research Process

The key activities involved in the conduct of a clinical trial are as follows:

Key trial activities include:

1 **DEVELOPMENT OF THE TRIALPROTOCOL**

Within GCP, clinical trials should be described in a clear, detailed protocol. The sponsor, often in consultation with one or more clinical investigators, generally designs the study protocol; clinical investigators may also design and initiate clinical studies, as sponsor-investigators. Integral to protocol development are the concepts of risk identification, study design and control groups, and statistical methodology. The sponsor and clinical investigator(s) should be aware of any national/ local laws or regulations pertaining to designing, initiating, and con- ducting the study.

(See WHOGCP Principles 2: Protocol; 3: Risk Identification; 4: Benefit- Risk Assessment given below)

2 **DEVELOPMENT OF STANDARD OPERATING PROCEDURES (SOPS)**

All parties who oversee, conduct or support clinical research (i.e., sponsors, clinical investigators, Independent Ethics Committees/Institutional Review Boards [IECs/IRBs] monitors, contract research organizations [CROs]) should develop and follow written standard operating procedures (SOPs) that define responsibilities, records, and methods to be used for study-related activities.

(See WHOGCP Principles 6: Protocol Compliance; 7: Informed Consent; 11: Records; 12: Confidentiality/Privacy; and 14: Quality Systems given below)

Sponsors should consider preparing SOPs for developing and updating the protocol, investigator's brochure, case report forms (CRFs), and other study-related documents; shipping, handling, and accounting for all supplies of the investigational product; standardizing the activities of sponsors and study personnel (e.g., review of adverse event reports by medical experts; data analysis by statisticians); standardizing the activities of clinical investigators to ensure that trial data is accurately captured; monitoring, to ensure that processes are consistently followed and activities are consistently documented; auditing, to determine whether monitoring is being appropriately carried out and the systems for quality control are operational and effective

Similarly, clinical investigators should consider developing SOPs for common trial-related procedures not addressed in the protocol. These may include but are not limited to: communicating with the IEC/IRB; obtaining and updating informed consent; reporting adverse events; preparing and maintaining adequate records; administering the investigational product; and accounting for and disposing of the investigational product.

IECs/IRBs should develop and follow written procedures for their operations, including but not limited to: membership requirements; initial and continuing review; communicating with the investigator(s) and institution; and minimizing or eliminating conflicts of interest.

Regulators should consider developing written procedures for activities pertaining to the regulation of clinical research. These may include but are not limited to: reviewing applications and safety reports; conducting GCP inspections (where applicable) and communicating findings to the inspected parties; and establishing an infrastructure for due process and imposing sanctions on parties who violate national/local law or regulations.

3 DEVELOPMENT OF SUPPORT SYSTEMS AND TOOLS

Appropriate support systems and tools facilitate the conduct of the study and collection of data required by the protocol. Support systems and tools include, but are not limited to, trial-related information documents (e.g., investigator's brochure, case report forms [CRFs], checklists, study flow sheets, drug accountability logs; see *Overview Process 4: Generation and approval of trial-related information documents*), computer hardware and software, electronic patient diaries, and other specialized equipment.

(See WHO GCP Principles 2: Protocol; 11: Records; 14: Quality Systems given below)

The sponsor is generally responsible for developing, maintaining, modifying, and ensuring the availability of support systems and tools for conducting the trial and collecting and reporting required data.

For example, the sponsor may consider developing/designing/providing/ designating: diagnostic or laboratory equipment required by the study protocol, and procedures/schedules for servicing the equipment according to the manufacturer's specifications; computer systems (hardware and software) to be used in the clinical trial (e.g., statistical or other software, electronic patient diaries, coding of personal data), and software validation systems, as needed; facsimile or other communications equipment to facilitate reporting of serious adverse events; Information and training tools for clinical investigators and site personnel

4 GENERATION AND APPROVAL OF TRIAL-RELATEDDOCUMENTS

Development of trial-related documents may facilitate the conduct of the study, collection and reporting of study-related data, and analysis of study results. The sponsor generally develops, designs, and provides various standardized forms and checklists to assist the clinical investigator and his/her staff in capturing and reporting data required by the protocol.

(See WHOGCP Principles 2: Protocol; 7: Informed Consent;11: Records; 14: Quality Systems given below)

Examples of trial information documents include, but are not limited to investigator's brochure; checklists to identify and document the required steps for each of the various clinical trial activities (e.g., investigator selection, approvals and clearances, monitoring, adverse event reporting and evaluation, analysis of interim data); investigational supplies accountability forms to document the amount and source of investigational product shipped and received, the amount dispensed to subjects, and the return/destruction, as appropriate, of any unused product; signature logs and other forms to document by whom activities are completed, when, and the sequence in which they are carried out; case report forms (CRFs) for each scheduled study visit to capture all of the necessary data collected from and reported for each subject; informed consent documents; adverse event or safety reporting forms; Administrative forms to track research funds and expenses; forms to disclose information about the investigator's financial, property, or other interests in the product under study, in accordance with national/local law or regulations; Formats for reports of monitoring visits; Formats for progress reports, annual reports, and final study reports.

5 SELECTION OF TRIAL SITES AND THE SELECTION OF PROPERLY QUALIFIED, TRAINED, AND EXPERIENCED INVESTIGATORS AND STUDY PERSONNEL

Clinical investigators must be qualified and have sufficient resources and appropriately trained staff to conduct the investigation and be knowledgeable of the national setting and circumstances of the site and study population(s). Sponsors should review the requirements of the study protocol to determine the type(s) of expertise required and identify clinical investigators who have the particular medical expertise necessary to conduct the study and who have knowledge, training and experience in the conduct of clinical trials and human subject protection.

(See WHOGCP Principles 2: Protocol; 9: Investigator Qualifications; 10: Staff Qualifications given below)

6 ETHICS COMMITTEE REVIEW AND APPROVAL OF THE PROTOCOL

Within GCP, studies must be reviewed and receive approval/favourable opinion from an Independent Ethics Committee (IEC)/ Institutional Review Board (IRB) prior to enrollment of study subjects.

The investigator generally assumes responsibility for obtaining IEC/ IRB review of the study protocol. Copies of any approval/ favourable opinion are then provided to the sponsor.

(See WHOGCP Principles1: Ethical Conduct; 2: Protocol; 4: Benefit- Risk Assessment; 5: Review by IEC/IRC; 7:Informed Consent; 8: Continuing Review/Ongoing Benefit-Risk Assessment;11: Records; 12: Confidentiality/Privacy given below)

7 REVIEW BY REGULATORYAUTHORITIES

Within GCP, studies must undergo review by regulatory authority (ies) for use of the investigational product or intervention in human subjects and to ensure that the study is appropriately designed to meet its stated objectives, according to national/regional/local law and regulations. [Note: Some countries may not have systems in place for reviewing research or may depend on external review. Also, some countries may have additional requirements for the review and approval of trial sites and/or investigators.]

The sponsor is generally responsible for ensuring that the applicable regulatory authority(ies) review and provide any required authorizations for the study before the study may proceed. The sponsor should also list the trial in applicable and/or required clinical trial registry(ies).

(See WHO GCP Principles 2: Protocol; 4: Benefit-Risk Assessment given below)

8 ENROLEMENT OF SUBJECTS IN TO THE STUDY: RECRUITMENT, ELIGIBILITY AND INFORMED CONSENT

The clinical investigator has primary responsibility for recruiting subjects, ensuring that only eligible subjects are enrolled in the study, and obtaining and documenting the informed consent of each subject. Within GCP, informed consent must be obtained from each study subject prior to enrollment in the study or performing any specific study procedures.

(See WHOGCP Principles 2: Protocol; 6: Protocol Compliance; 7: Informed Consent; 11: Records given below)

9 THE INVESTIGATIONAL PRODUCT(S): QUALITY, HANDLING AND ACCOUNTING

Quality of the investigational product is assured by compliance with Good Manufacturing Practices (GMPs) and by handling and storing the product according to the manufacturing specifications and the study protocol. GCP requires that sponsors control access to the investigational product and also document the quantity(ies) produced, to whom the product is shipped, and disposition (e.g., return or destruction) of any unused supplies. GCP also requires investigators to control receipt, administration, and disposition of the investigational product.

(See WHOGCP Principles2: Protocol; 11:Records; 13: Good Manufacturing Practice; 14: Quality Systems given below)

10 TRIAL DATA ACQUISITION: CONDUCTING THETRIAL

Research should be conducted according to the approved protocol and applicable regulatory requirements. Study records documenting each trial-related activity provide critical verification that the study has been carried out in compliance with the protocol.

(See WHO GCP Principles 2: Protocol; 6: Protocol Compliance; 11: Recordsgiven below)

11 SAFETY MANAGEMENT AND REPORTING

All clinical trials must be managed for safety. Although all parties who oversee or conduct clinical research have a role/responsibility for the safety of the study subjects, the clinical investigator has primary responsibility for alerting the sponsor and the IEC/IRB to adverse events, particularly serious/life-threatening unanticipated events, observed during the course of the research. The sponsor, in turn, has primary responsibility for reporting of study safety to regulatory authorities and other investigators and for the ongoing global safety assessment of the investigational product. A data and safety monitoring board (DSMB) may be constituted by the sponsor to assist in overall safety management.

(See WHOGCP Principles2: Protocol; 3: Risk Identification; 6: Protocol Compliance; 8: Continuing Review/Ongoing Benefit-Risk Assessment; 11: Records; 14:Quality Systems given below)

12 MONITORING THE TRIAL

Sponsors generally perform site monitoring of a clinical trial to assure high quality trial conduct. The sponsor may perform such monitoring directly, or may utilize the services of an outside individual or organization (e.g., contract research organization [CRO]). The sponsor determines the appropriate extent and nature of monitoring based on the objective, purpose, design, complexity, size, blinding, and end- points of the trial, and the risks posed by the investigational product.

The "on site" monitors review individual case histories in order to verify adherence to the protocol, ensure the ongoing implementation of appropriate data entry and quality control procedures, and verify adherence to GCP. In blinded studies, these monitors remain blinded to study arm assignment.

For an investigator-initiated study, the sponsor-investigator should consider the merits of arranging independent, external monitoring of the study, particularly when the study involves novel products or potential significant risks to subjects.

(See WHOGCP Principles2: Protocol; 6: Protocol Compliance; 8: Continuing Review; 11: Records; 14:Quality Systems given below)

13 MANAGING TRIALDATA

Within GCP, managing clinical trial data appropriately assures that the data are complete, reliable and processed correctly, and that data integrity is preserved. Data management includes all processes and procedures for collecting, handling, manipulating, analysing, and storing/archiving of data from study start to completion.

The sponsor bears primary responsibility for developing appropriate data management systems. The sponsor and the investigator share responsibility for implementing such systems to ensure that the integrity of trial data is preserved.

(See WHO GCP Principles 2: Protocol; 6: Protocol Compliance; 11: Records; 14: Quality Systems given below)

(See also Overview Processes1: Protocol development; 2: Development of standard operating procedures; 3: Support systems and tools; 4:Trial information documents; 10:Trial data acquisition given below)

Data management systems should address (as applicable): data acquisition; confidentiality of data/data privacy; electronic data capture (if applicable); data management training for investigators and staff; completion of CRFs and other trial related documents, and procedures for correcting errors in such documents; coding/terminology for adverse events, medication, medical histories; safety data management and reporting; data entry and data processing (including laboratory and external data); database closure; database validation; secure, efficient, and accessible data storage; data quality measurement (i.e., how reliable are the data) and quality assurance; management of vendors (e.g., CROs, pharmacies, laboratories, software suppliers, off-site storage) that participate directly or indirectly in managing trial data.

14 QUALITY ASSURANCE OF THE TRIAL PERFORMANCE AND DATA

Quality assurance (QA) verifies through systematic, independent audits that existing quality control systems (e.g., study monitoring: see GCP Process 12, *Monitoring the trial*; data management systems: see GCP Process 13, *Managing trial data*) are working and effective. Quality assurance audits may be performed during the course of the clinical trial and/or upon trialcompletion.

Sponsors bear primary responsibility for establishing quality systems and conducting quality assurance audits.

(See WHO GCP Principles 11: Records; 14: Quality Systems. See also Overview Processes2: Development of standard operating procedures; 10: Trial data acquisition: conducting the trial; 12; Monitoring the trial; and 13: Managing trial data given below)

15 REPORTING THE TRIAL

The results of each controlled study involving an investigational product should be summarized and described in an integrated clinical study report containing clinical data and statistical descriptions, presentations, and analyses. The report should be complete, timely, well-organized, free from ambiguity, and easy to review.

The sponsor is responsible for preparing clinical study reports. Such reports should generally include:

A description of the ethical aspects of the study (e.g. confirmation that the study was conducted in accordance with basic ethical principles);

A description of the administrative structure of the study (i.e. identification and qualifications of investigators/sites/other facilities);

An introduction that explains the critical features and context of the study (e.g. rationale and aims, target population, treatment duration, primaryendpoints);

A summary of the study objectives;

A description of the overall study design and plan; a description of any protocol amendments;

An accounting of all subjects who participated in the study, including all important deviations from inclusion/exclusion criteria and a description of subjects who discontinued after enrollment;

An accounting of protocol violations; a discussion of any interim analyses;

An efficacy evaluation, including specific descriptions of subjects who were included in each efficacy analysis and listing of all subjects who were excluded from the efficacy analysis and the reasons for such exclusion;

A safety evaluation, including extent of exposure, common adverse events and laboratory test changes, and serious or unanticipated or other significant adverse events including evaluation of subjects who left the study prematurely because of an adverse event or who died;

A discussion and overall conclusions regarding the efficacy and safety results and the relationship of risks and benefits;

Tables, figures, and graphs that visually summarize the important results or to clarify results that are not easily understood;

A reference list;

Where permitted, abbreviated or less detailed reports may be acceptable for uncontrolled or aborted studies.

(See WHO GCP Principles 2: Protocol; 11: Records; see also ICHE3 (Structure and Content of Clinical Study Reports) given below)

WHO Principles of GCP

Principle 1: Research involving humans should be scientifically sound and conducted in accordance with basic ethical principles, which have their origin in the Declaration of Helsinki. Three basic ethical principles of equal importance, namely respect for persons, beneficence, and justice, permeate all other GCP principles.

Principle 2: Research involving humans should be scientifically justified and described in a clear, detailed protocol.

Principle 3: Before research involving humans is initiated, foresee- able risks and discomforts and any anticipated benefit(s) for the individual trial subject and society should be identified. Research of investigational products or procedures should be supported by adequate non-clinical and, when applicable, clinical information.

Principle 4: Research involving humans should be initiated only if the anticipated benefit(s) for the individual research subject and society clearly outweigh the risks. Although the benefit of the results of the trial to science and society should be taken into account, the most important considerations are those related to the rights, safety, and well-being of the trial subjects.

Principle 5: Research involving humans should receive independent ethics committee/institutional review board (IEC/IRB) approval/ favourable opinion prior to initiation.

Principle 6: Research involving humans should be conducted incompliance with the approved protocol

Principle 7: Freely given informed consent should be obtained from every subject prior to research participation in accordance with national culture(s) and requirements. When a subject is not capable of giving informed consent, the permission of a legally authorized representative should be obtained in accordance with applicable law.

Principle 8: Research involving humans should be continued only if the benefit risk profile remains favourable.

Principle 9: Qualified and duly licensed medical personnel (i.e., physicianor, when appropriate, dentist) should be responsible for the medical care of trial subjects, and for any medical decision(s) made on their behalf.

Principle 10: Each individual involved in conducting a trial should be qualified by education, training, and experience to perform his or her respective task(s) and currently licensed to do so, where required.

Principle 11: All clinical trial information should be recorded, handled, and stored in a way that allows its accurate reporting, interpretation, and verification.

Principle 12: The confidentiality of records that could identify subjects should be protected, respecting the privacy and confidentiality rules in accordance with the applicable regulatory requirement(s).

Principle 13: Investigational products should be manufactured, handled, and stored in accordance with applicable Good Manufacturing

Practice (GMP) and should be used in accordance with the approved protocol.

Principle 14: Systems with procedures that assure the quality of every aspect of the trial should be implemented.

A Detailed Explanation of the Principles

Principle 1: Ethical Conduct

Research involving humans should be scientifically sound and conducted in accordance with basic ethical principles, which have their origin in the Declaration of Helsinki. Three basic ethical principles of equal importance, namely respect for persons, beneficence, and justice, permeate all other GCP principles enumerated below Ethical principles have been established by many national and international bodies, including:

1) The World Medical Association Declaration of Helsinki;
2) The Council for International Organizations of Medical Sciences (CIOMS) International Ethical Guidelines for Biomedical Research Involving Human Subjects;

Application

Principle 1 is applied through design and approval of the protocol a favorable risk/benefit assessment fair and transparent procedures and outcomes in the selection of research subjects compliance with national and international laws, regulations, and standards

Implementation

The basic ethical principles of biomedical research are reflected in all GCP principles and processes, impacting on the role and responsibilities of each party within GCP. Each party participating in clinical research has responsibility for ensuring that research is ethically and scientifically conducted according to the highest standards. This includes the investigator(s) and site staff, the sponsor and sponsor's staff (including monitors and auditors), the ethics committee(s), the regulatory authority(-ies), and the individual research subjects.

PRINCIPLE 2: PROTOCOL

Research involving humans should be scientifically justified and described a clear, detailed protocol.

"The experiment should be such as to yield fruitful results unprocurable by other methods or means of study, and not random and unnecessary in nature." (The Nuremburg Code)

"The design and performance of each experimental procedure involving human subjects should be clearly formulated in an experimental protocol." (Declaration of Helsinki)

Application

Principle 2 is applied through development of a clear, detailed, scientifically justified and ethically sound protocol that (1) complies with requirements established by national and local laws and regulations, and (2) undergoes scientific and ethical review prior to implementation.

Implementation

Sponsors are primarily responsible for (a) designing the clinical investigation, (b) developing the study protocol, investigator's brochure, and related materials to describe the procedures that will be followed, study endpoints, and data collection, and other study requirements; and (c) ensuring that the protocol complies with applicable national and local laws and regulations.

Investigators may be consulted by the sponsor during protocol de- sign or, in some cases, may personally contribute to the design of the protocol. Investigators are responsible for familiarizing themselves with the study protocol, investigator's brochure, and related materials to ensure that they are able to carry out the study in compliance with the specifications of the protocol.

ECs/IRBs are responsible for conducting ethical review of the study protocol. This also includes arranging for a scientific review or verifying that a competent body has determined that the research is scientifically sound. (See GCP Principle 5: *Review by IEC/IRB*)

Regulators bear responsibility for allowing a protocol to proceed in accordance with applicable laws and regulations. This may include prospective review of the protocol, the investigator's brochure and other relevant information. Where the protocol or investigator's brochure is inaccurate or materially incomplete, where the protocol does not adequately provide for the protection of subject rights and safety, or where the protocol is deficient in design to meet its stated objectives, the regulatory authority may require protocol modification or take action to disallow the protocol to proceed in accordance with applicable laws and regulations.

Principle 3: Risk Identification

Before research involving humans is initiated, fore see able risks and discomforts and any anticipated benefit(s) for the individual trial subject and society should be identified. Research of investigational products or procedures should be supported by adequate non-clinical and, when applicable, clinical information.

"The experiment should be so designed and based on the results of animal experimentation and knowledge of the natural history of the disease or other problem under study that the anticipated results will justify the performance of the experiment." (The Nuremberg Code)

"Medical research involving human subjects must conform to generally accepted scientific principles, be based on a thorough knowledge of the scientific literature, other relevant sources of information, and on adequate laboratory and, where appropriate animal experimentation." (Declaration of Helsinki)

"The assessment of risks and benefits requires a careful arrayal of relevant data, including, in some cases, alternative ways of obtaining the benefits sought in the research. [T]he assessment presents both an opportunity and a responsibility to gather systematic and comprehensive information about proposed research." (The Belmont Report)

Application

Principle 3 is applied through: conducting a thorough search of available scientific information about the investigational product or procedure(s) (including findings from tests in laboratory animals and any previous human experience]; developing the investigator's brochure, the study protocol, and the informed consent document to adequately, accurately, and objectively reflect the available scientific information on foreseeable risks and anticipated benefits.

Implementation

The responsibility for implementing this principle is shared by sponsors, investigators, IECs/IRBs, and regulators:

The **sponsor** generally conducts the literature review to ensure that there is sufficient information available to support the proposed clinical trial in the population to be studied and that there is sufficient safety and efficacy data to support human exposure to the product. The sponsor may need to conduct pre-clinical studies to ensure there is sufficient safety and efficacy data to support human exposure. The sponsor should summarize available information about the procedure/product in the investigator's brochure, and accordingly set forth the design of the study in the protocol. In general, it is important that the sponsor develop a comprehensive, accurate and complete investigator's brochure, as this is a principal means of communicating vital safety and scientific information to the investigator and, in turn, to the IEC/IRB.

Review of the protocol, investigator's brochure, and other relevant formation enables the **ECs/IRBs** to (1) determine whether the benefits outweigh the risks, (2) understand the study procedures or other steps that will be taken to minimize risks, and (3) ensure that the informed consent document accurately states the potential risks and benefits in a way that will facilitate comprehension by all study subjects, with particular attention to vulnerable groups.

Investigators must be knowledgeable of the protocol, investigator's brochure and other relevant information regarding potential risks and benefits, and must be able to adequately, accurately and objectively identify the potential risks and benefits to subjects. Investigators may need to do some additional literature search beyond that provided by the sponsor. Investigators should also be thoroughly familiar with the appropriate use of the trial product(s)/procedures and should take the necessary steps to remain aware of all relevant new data on the investigational product, procedure, or method that becomes available during the course of the clinical trial.

Regulators bear responsibility for allowing a protocol to proceed in accordance with existing national laws/regulations or internationally accepted standards. This may include prospective review of the protocol, the investigator's brochure and other relevant information to ensure that risk(s) and benefit(s) are accurately identified and justify allowing the protocol to proceed. As appropriate, adopted national standards should address additional national or regional racial, cultural, or religious standards/issues not otherwise covered by the international standards. In accordance with national/local laws and regulations, regulators may establish standards for the conduct of non-clinical studies, review non-clinical and clinical data submitted in support of research permits or marketing applications, and/or inspect facilities that conduct non-clinical and clinical studies.

Principle 4: Benefit-Risk Assessment

Research involving humans should be initiated only if the anticipated benefit(s) for the individual research subject and society clearly outweigh the risks. Although the benefit of the results of the trial to science and society should be taken into account, the most important considerations are those related to the rights, safety, and well being of there search subjects.

"The degree of risk to be taken should never exceed that determined by the humanitarian importance of the problem to be solved by the experiment." (The Nuremberg Code)

"Every medical research project involving human subjects should be preceded by careful assessment of predictable risks and burdens in comparison with foreseeable benefits to the subject or to others. This does not preclude the participation of healthy volunteers in medical research." (Declaration of Helsinki)

"For all biomedical research involving human subjects, the investigator must ensure that potential benefits and risks are reasonably balanced and risks are minimized." (CIOMS, International Ethical Guidelines, Guideline8)

"It is commonly said that benefits and risks must be 'balanced' and shown to be 'in a favorable ratio.' Thus, there should first be a determination of the validity of the presuppositions of the research; then the nature, probability and magnitude of risk should be distinguished with as much clarity as possible. The method of ascertaining risks should be explicit. It should also be determined whether estimates of the probability of harm or benefits are reasonable, as judged by known facts or other available studies." (The Belmont Report)

"Risks should be reduced to those necessary to achieve the research objective. It should be determined whether it is in fact necessary to use human subjects at all. Risk can perhaps never be entirely eliminated, but it can often be reduced by careful attention to alternative procedure .When research involves significant risk of serious impairment, review committees should be extraordinarily.

Insistent on the justification of the risk (looking usually to the likelihood of benefit to the subject or in some rare cases, to the manifest voluntariness of the participation)" (The Belmont Report)". Scientific review must consider inter alia, the study design, including the provisions for avoiding or minimizing risk and for monitoring safety." (CIOMS, International Ethical Guidelines, Commentary on Guideline 2)

"Risks and benefits of research may affect the individual subjects, the families of the individual subjects, and society at large (or special groups of subjects in society)." "In balancing these different elements, the risks and benefits affecting the immediate research subject will normally carry special weight." (The Belmont Report)

"In medical research on human subjects, considerations related to the well-being of the human subject should take precedence over the interests of science and society." (Declaration of Helsinki)

Application

Principle 4 is applied through appropriate study design and through ethical, scientific, and, where applicable, regulatory review of the study protocol prior to its initiation.

Implementation

The responsibility for implementing this principle is shared by sponsors, investigators, IECs/IRBs, and regulators.

The **sponsor** should design research studies to ensure that risks to subjects are minimized.

The **investigator(s)** should review the investigator's brochure and other relevant risk and benefit information in making a decision to conduct the study. The investigator is also responsible for providing adequate, accurate, and objective information on risks and benefits during informed consent of study subjects.

Prior to study initiation, the IEC(s)/IRB(s) should review the protocol, investigator's brochure, and other relevant information to (1) understand the study procedures or other steps that will be taken to minimize risks, (2) understand the potential benefits (if any) and determine whether those benefits outweigh the anticipated risks, and

(3) ensure that the informed consent document accurately states the potential risks and benefits in a way that will allow study subjects to understand what they are undertaking.

Regulators bear responsibility for allowing a protocol to proceed in accordance with applicable laws and regulations. This may include prospective review of the protocol, the investigator's brochure, and other relevant information to ensure that risk(s) and benefit(s) are accurately identified and justify allowing the protocol to proceed. The regulatory authority may require modification to a protocol as a condition to its proceeding and/or may suspend or terminate a protocol based on an unacceptable risk/benefit profile in accordance with applicable laws and regulations.

Principle 5: Review by IEC/IRB

Research involving humans should receive independent ethics committee/institutional review board (IEC/IRB) approval/ favourable opinion prior to initiation.

The "... protocol should be submitted for consideration, comment, guidance, and where appropriate, approval to a specially appointed ethical review committee, which must be independent of the investigator, the sponsor, or any other kind of undue influence. This independent committee should be in conformity with the laws and regulations of the country in which the research experiment is per- formed. " (Declaration of Helsinki)

"Failure to submit a protocol to the committee should be considered a clear and serious violation of ethical standards." (CIOMS, International Ethical Guidelines, Commentary to Guideline 2)

Application

Principle 5 is applied through protocol review by an IEC/IRB that is constituted and operating in accordance with GCP and applicable national/local laws and regulations.

Implementation

The responsibility for implementing this principle is shared by IEC(s)/ IRB(s), investigators, sponsors, and regulators.

A properly constituted and operational **IEC/IRB** reviews the protocol (and/or any proposed changes to the protocol) and provides the investigator with a written decision/opinion. IEC/IRB written procedures should ensure that no subject be admitted to a trial and no deviations from, or changes to, the protocol be initiated before the IEC/IRB issues its approval/favorable opinion.

Investigators submit the study protocol their IEC(s)/IRB(s) and are responsible for securing an approval/favorable opinion prior to admitting any subjects to the trial. Investigators should not implement any deviation from, or changes to, the protocol without agreement by the sponsor and prior review and documented approval/favorable opinion from the IEC(s)/IRB(s) of an amendment, except where necessary to eliminate an immediate hazard(s) to trial subjects. (See GCP Principle 6, Protocol Compliance)

The **sponsor** develops the protocol, selects qualified investigators/ institutions, and confirms that each investigator has had the study protocol reviewed by an IEC/IRB and received IEC/IRB approval/favorable opinion.

In accordance with applicable laws/regulations, **regulators** may inspect the investigator(s), sponsor(s), and/or IEC(s)/IRB(s) to ensure compliance with IEC/IRB review requirements. Regulators should also encourage IECs/IRBs to communicate with them directly on is- sues or concerns they may encounter in their review of human trials.

Principle6: Protocol compliance

Research in humans should be conducted in compliance with the approved protocol.

Once the IEC/IRB gives its approval/favorable decision on the protocol, it is essential that the trial be conducted in compliance with that protocol so that the decision on the ethical acceptability of the trial remains valid.

"The investigator should not implement any deviation from, or changes of, the protocol without agreement by the sponsor and prior review and documented approval/favorable opinion from the IRB/IEC of an amendment, except where necessary to eliminate an immediate hazard(s) to trial subjects, or when the change(s) involves only logistical or administrative aspects of the trial (e.g., change of monitor(s), change of telephone number(s))." (ICH E6, Section 4.5)

Application

Principle 6 is applied through: 1) verifiable investigator adherence to the protocol requirements; 2) submission of any protocol changes to the sponsor and to the IEC/IRB (with approval/favorable opinion) prior to their implementation; and 3) effective monitoring of the study by the sponsor.

Implementation

The responsibility for implementing this principle is shared by IEC(s)/ IRB(s), investigators, sponsors, and regulators.

EC/IRB written procedures should ensure that no subject be admit- ted to a trial and no deviations from, or changes of, the protocol be initiated before the IEC/IRB issues its approval/favorable opinion.

Investigators should be thoroughly familiar with the protocol and are responsible for conducting the trial in compliance with the protocol. Investigators should not implement any deviation from, or changes of the protocol without agreement by the sponsor and prior review and documented approval/favorable opinion from the IRB(s)/IEC(s) of an amendment, except where necessary to eliminate an immediate hazard(s) to trial subjects.

The **sponsor** monitors the study to ensure investigator compliance with the protocol and takes action to secure compliance or terminate the trial in the case of noncompliance. If the monitoring and/or auditing identify serious and/or persistent noncompliance on the part of an investigator/institution, the sponsor should terminate the investigator's/institution's participation in the trial. All parties, including the IEC/IRB, should be notified in such cases.

In accordance with applicable laws/regulations, **regulators** may inspect the investigator(s) or sponsor to ensure compliance with protocol adherence requirements. Regulators should be promptly notified when a sponsor identifies serious and/or persistent noncompliance on the part of an investigator/institution leading to termination of the investigator's/institution's participation in a study.

Principle 7: Informed Consent

Freely given informed consent should be obtained from every subject prior to research participation in accordance with national culture(s) and requirements. When a subject is not capable of giving informed consent, the permission of a legally authorized representative should be obtained in accordance with applicable law.

"In particular, no one shall be subjected without his free consent to medical or scientific experimentation." (United Nations International Covenant on Civil and Political Rights)

"The subjects must be volunteers and informed participants in the research project." (Declaration of Helsinki)

"There is widespread agreement that the consent process can be analyzed as containing three elements: information, comprehension, and voluntariness." (The Belmont Report)

"For all biomedical research involving humans, the investigator must obtain the voluntary informed consent of the prospective subject or, in the case of an individual who is not capable of giving informed consent, the permission of a legally authorized representative in accordance with applicable law. Waiver of informed consent is to be regarded as uncommon and exceptional, and must in all cases be approved by an ethical review committee." (CIOMS, International Ethical Guidelines, Guideline 4)

"Obtaining informed consent is a process that is begun when initial contact is made with a prospective subject and continues throughout the course of the study. By informing the prospective subjects, by repetition and explanation, by answering their questions as they arise, and by ensuring that each individual understands each procedure, investigators elicit their informed consent and in so doing manifest respect for their dignity and autonomy." (CIOMS, International Ethical Guidelines, Commentary on Guideline4)

Application

Principle 7 is applied through a process of informing and ensuring comprehension by study subjects (and/or their legally authorized representatives) about the research and obtaining their consent, including appropriate written informed consent.

Implementation

The responsibility for implementing and overseeing the informed consent process is shared by sponsors, clinical investigators, IECs/ IRBs, and regulatory authorities.

IECs/IRBs are responsible for: reviewing the informed consent document to ensure that it is accurate, complete, and written in language that will be understood by the potential study subjects and translated into other languages, as appropriate; requesting modifications to the informed consent document, as appropriate; and at their discretion, observing the consent process and the research **Investigators** are responsible for ensuring that: staff responsible for obtaining informed consent receive appropriate training, both in research ethics and in the requirements of the specific study protocol; the IEC/IRB reviews and approves the informed consent form and other written information to be used in the study prior to its use; and informed consent is obtained from each subject or the subject's representative prior to involving the subject in any study related activities, including diagnostic or other tests that are administered solely for determining the subject's eligibility to participate in the research.

Sponsors are responsible for monitoring the research at study sites to ensure that sites are obtaining informed consent from all study subjects prior to subjects' inclusion in the research study.

Principle8: Continuing Review/Ongoing Benefit-Risk Assessment

Research involving humans should be continued only if the benefit-risk profile remains favourable.

"During the course of the experiment the scientist in charge must be prepared to terminate the experiment at any stage, if he has probable cause to believe, in the exercise of the good faith, superior skill, and careful judgment required of him that a continuation of the experiment is likely to result in injury, disability, or death to the experimental subject." (The Nuremburg Code)

"The ethical review committee should conduct further reviews as necessary in the course of the research, including monitoring of its progress." (CIOMS, International Ethical Guidelines, Guideline 2)

"The committee has the right to monitor ongoing trials" (Declaration of Helsinki)

"Clinical trial sponsors should develop a process to assess, evaluate and act on safety information during drug development on a continuous basis in order to ensure the earliest possible identification of safety concerns and to take appropriate risk minimization steps. Such steps can include modification of study protocols, to incorporate strategies to ensure that clinical trial participants are not exposed to undue risk." (Management of Safety Information from Clinical Trials, Report of CIOMS Working Group VI. Identification and Evaluation of Risk from Clinical Trial Data)

Application

Principle 8 is applied through development and implementation of processes for evaluating risks and benefits of the research as additional information becomes available during the course of the study. Principle 8 encompasses (1) safety monitoring of the study by investigator(s) and sponsor (including use of a data and safety monitoring board [DSMB], where appropriate); (2) reporting serious unexpected adverse events or other unanticipated risks to the sponsor, IEC/IRB, and regulators; (3) review by the IEC/IRB of any unanticipated risks as they occur, or at scheduled intervals appropriate to the degree of risk; (4) revising the protocol, investigator's brochure, and/or informed consent document as needed, and suspending or terminating studies if necessary to protect the rights and welfare of study subjects.

Implementation

Sponsors, IECs/IRBs, DSMBs (if applicable), and regulators share responsibility for ongoing safety evaluations of the investigational product(s). The **investigator** reports unanticipated problems involving risks to subjects and provides periodic progress reports at intervals appropriate to the degree of risk to sponsors and IECs/IRBs in accordance with the national/local laws and regulations. The investigator provides adequate, accurate, and objective information on risks and benefits during informed consent of study subjects, and renews the consent of the subject to continue in the study, as appropriate.

The **sponsor** monitors the study and performs safety evaluations of the investigational product(s) by analyzing data received from the investigator(s) and the DSMB (if one has been appointed). The sponsor also assures reporting (including expedited reporting to investigator(s), IEC(s)/IRB(s), and the regulatory authority(ies) of adverse reactions that are both serious and unexpected.

As the study progresses, the **IEC(s)/IRB(s)** conducts follow-up re- views appropriate to the degree of risk, but generally at least once per year, including review of the investigator's progress reports to determine if the benefits still outweigh the risks.

The **regulatory authority** reviews data submitted in research or marketing permits and may require modification to a protocol as a condition to its proceeding and/or may suspend or terminate a protocol based on an unacceptable benefit-risk profile in accordance with applicable laws and regulations.

Principle 9: Investigator Qualifications

Qualified and duly licensed medical personnel (i.e., physician or, when appropriate, dentist) should be responsible for the medical care of trial subjects, and for any medical decision(s) made on their behalf."The experiment should be conducted only by scientifically qualified persons. The highest degree of skill and care should be required through all stages of the experiment of those who conduct or engage in the experiment." (The NurembergCode)

"Medical research involving human subjects should be conducted only by scientifically qualified persons and under the supervision of a clinically competent medical person... " (Declaration of Helsinki)

Application

Principle 9 is applied through the responsibilities of the clinical investigator to the study subject and through the sponsor's selection of qualified investigator(s).

Implementation

The **investigator** is responsible for providing, or ensuring that subjects have access to, medical care for medical problems arising during their participation in the trial that are, or could be related to the study intervention, and for following the subjects' status until the problem isresolved.

"It is recommended that the investigator inform the subject's primary physician about the subject's participation in the trial if the subject has a primary physician and if the subject agrees to the primary physician being informed."

Primary responsibility for selecting qualified clinical investigators to conduct a study resides with the **sponsor**

The **IEC(s)/IRB(s)** is responsible for ensuring that the rights and welfare of study subjects are protected. Consideration of investigator qualifications and experience and the adequacy of the site (including the supporting staff, available facilities, and emergency procedures) by the IEC/IRB will ensure that subjects have access to appropriate care for medical problems arising during participation in the trial.

National and/or local **regulatory authorities** have indirect responsibility related to clinical investigator qualifications. Regulators

(1) establish licensing and practice standards for physicians and other medical personnel,

(2) enforce compliance with such standards, and

(3) impose disciplinary actions, as appropriate, on physicians and other medical personnel who fail to meet such standards. Different regulatory agencies and authorities may be responsible for the over-sight of clinical research vs. the licensure and oversight of medical professionals; exchange of information among regulatory agencies is encouraged in such circumstances.

Principle 10: Staff Qualifications

Each individual involved in conducting a trial should be qualified by education, training, and experience to perform his or her respective task(s) and currently licensed to do so, where required.

GCP requires that the clinical investigator is appropriately qualified by education, training, and experience to conduct the clinical trial. GCP also requires that each clinical investigator will have adequate resources available, including sufficient staff, who are also appropriately qualified by education, training, and experience, to assist him/ her with the trial and ensure the safety of study subjects.

Application

Principle 10 is chiefly applied through the clinical investigator's selection of appropriate staff to assist with the conduct of the study.

Implementation

The **investigator** bears primary responsibility for (1) selecting qualified staff to assist in the conduct of the investigation; (2) ensuring that study staff receive appropriate training, related to ethics and consent procedures as well as requirements of the specific protocol;

(3) establishing clear procedures for activities related to the conduct of the study; (4) assigning tasks to staff, based on their qualifications, experience, and professional licenses; and (5) personally supervising staff to ensure that they satisfactorily fulfill their study-related duties. Although the investigator may delegate tasks to members of his/her staff, nevertheless, the investigator retains overall responsibility for the study and ensuring that his/her staff complies with applicable laws and regulations for human subject protection and the conduct of clinical research

The **IEC/IRB** is responsible for ensuring that the rights and welfare of study subjects are protected. Consideration of the site's characteristics (e.g., number and qualifications of supporting staff, available facilities and equipment, and emergency procedures) will allow the IEC/IRB to evaluate the adequacy of the site, and ensure that subjects' welfare is not compromised during the trial.

Sponsors have the responsibility for selecting appropriately qualified investigators to conduct the study; part of that consideration is ensuring that investigators have sufficient staff (also with appropriate qualifications) available, who is appropriately trained to conduct all study-related activities, and who understand how to capture and document required observations and data.

In accordance with national and/or local laws and regulations, **regulatory authorities** may inspect study sites to determine if the conduct of the study is in compliance with local laws/regulations. Such inspections would include finding out who was assigned responsibility for conducting various study-related activities (e.g., screening subjects to determine if they meet inclusion/exclusion criteria; obtaining informed consent; conducting physical examinations; collecting and analyzing study data; recording, transcribing, or reporting data to the sponsor; administering the investigational product to subjects), and determining whether these activities were appropriately assigned and within the scope of the staff member's professional license(s).

Principle 11: Records

All clinical trial information should be recorded, handled, and stored in a way that allows its accurate reporting, interpretation, and verification.

Principle 11 embraces the concepts of data quality and data integrity as well as appropriate procedures for data handling and record keeping. Also implicit in this principle is the preparation and maintenance of essential documents: i.e., documents (including source documents) that individually and collectively permit evaluation of the con- duct of a trial and the quality of the data produced.

Application

Principle 11 is applied through: 1) the understanding and application of basic elements of data quality and integrity; 2) adherence to the study protocol as well as applicable written procedures for collecting, recording, reporting, maintaining and analyzing clinical trial information; and 3) the preparation of essential documents (including source documents), at all stages throughout the conduct of the clinical trial.

Implementation

IECs/IRBs, investigators, sponsors, and regulators all bear responsibility for documenting their activities within GCP, and maintaining records pertaining to duties related to the conduct or oversight of the clinical trial for the time required under national or local law and regulations. All parties are responsible for ensuring the accuracy, completeness, legibility and availability (as necessary) of such documents.

ECs/IRBs document their reviews of study protocols and informed consent/recruitment/ advertising materials through minutes that capture the IECs'/IRBs' deliberations and through copies of correspondence with the clinical investigator.

Investigators prepare and maintain case histories that record all observations and other data pertinent to the investigation on each individual administered the investigational drug or employed as a control in the investigation.

Sponsors ensure that study protocols address appropriate data handling and record-keeping requirements and design CRFs appropriately to facilitate the capture of all significant trial-related data and observations. Sponsors also secure the services of monitors to ensure compliance of the clinical investigators, and verify that the study was carried out according to the approved study protocol.

Regulators rely on clinical trial information to support regulatory decision-making and may inspect all of the parties involved in conducting or overseeing research. Critical to regulatory inspection is direct access to and review of existing clinical trial records. As part of an inspection, regulators compare records at the clinical investigator site and sponsor site with data and reports submitted to the regulatory authority to verify the information submitted. Regulators also prepare and maintain records of their inspections and findings.

Principle 12: Confidentiality/ Privacy

The confidentiality of records that could identify subjects should be protected, respecting the privacy and confidentiality rules in accordance with the applicable regulatory requirement(s).

"The right of research subjects to safeguard their integrity must al- ways be respected. Every precaution should be taken to respect the privacy of the subject, the confidentiality of the patient's information and to minimize the impact of the study on the subject's physical and mental integrity and on the personality of the subject." (Declaration of Helsinki)

"The investigator must establish secure safeguards of the confidentiality of subjects' research data. Subjects should be told the limits, legal or other, to the investigators' ability to safeguard confidentiality and the possible consequences of breaches of confidentiality." (CIOMS, International Ethical Guidelines, Guideline 18)

Application

Principle 12 is applied (1) through appropriate procedures to protect the privacy of the subject, and (2) by document and data control to protect the confidentiality of the subject's information.

Principle 12 is also applied through the informed consent process which requires as an essential element that certain explanations be provided to the subject about the confidentiality of the subject's records and about access to those records by monitor(s), auditor(s), the IEC/IRB, and the regulatory authority(-ies).

Implementation

ECs/IRBs review/approve the informed consent procedures and document to ensure, among other things, that there is adequate explanation regarding (1) the risks related to release of the subject's private information, (2) how the confidentiality of the subject's records will be maintained, and (3) persons who may have access to the subject's records (e.g., monitor(s), auditor(s), the IEC/IRB, and the regulatory authority (-ies)).

Investigators should (1) implement procedures to protect and restrict access to study records and private information (e.g., password protection for files, keeping study records in secured areas),

(2) follow national/local laws and regulations relating to privacy and confidentiality, (3) ensure that study staff are aware of and receive appropriate training related to their responsibility and procedures to be used for protecting subjects' private information and records,

(4) ensure that study staff follow the procedures established for this purpose, and (5) ensure that the consent form and process inform study subjects about the procedures to be used to protect their private information and the circumstances under which their medical and study records may be viewed by regulators, sponsors, monitors, and/or the IEC/IRB

Sponsors ensure that sites (1) allow regulators, IECs/IRBs, and monitors direct access to records necessary to verify compliance with national/local laws and regulations pertaining to the conduct of clinical trials, and (2) inform subjects about, and obtain their consent for, such access.

Principle13: Good manufacturing practice

Investigational products should be manufactured, handled, and stored in accordance with applicable Good Manufacturing Practice (GMP) and should be used in accordance with the approved protocol.

"The sponsor should ensure that the investigational product(s). is characterized as appropriate to the stage of development of the product(s), is manufactured in accordance with any applicable GMP, and is coded and labeled in a manner that protects the blinding, if applicable.

Application

Principle 13 is applied through 1) appropriately characterizing the investigational product (including any active comparator(s) and placebo, if applicable), 2) adhering to applicable Good Manufacturing Practice (GMP) standards in the manufacturing, handling and storage of the investigational product, and 3) using the product according to the approved study protocol.

Implementation

Responsibility for implementing this principle is shared by sponsors (or contract manufacturers/ contract research organizations), investigators, and regulators.

Sponsors implement this principle directly or indirectly through con- tract, by developing and characterizing the investigational product.

They make the necessary notifications/submissions to the applicable regulatory authority(ies), identify GMP requirements, if any, that may apply to the manufacturing, handling and storage of the investigational product, and ensure compliance with those requirements. Sponsors manufacture the investigational product directly or have it manufactured under contract at a manufacturing site in accordance with applicable GMP. They are responsible within GCP for the handling, storage, distribution and final disposition of the investigational product(s).

The sponsor also develops the study protocol and investigator's brochure, monitors protocol compliance, and ensures that written procedures include instructions that the investigator/institution should follow for the handling and storage of investigational products for the trial and documentation thereof.

Investigators are responsible for familiarity with the investigator's brochure and for conducting the research in compliance with the protocol, including any instructions for storing and handling investigational products. Investigators are responsible for explaining correct use (including handling and storage) of the investigational product to the study subjects. Investigators also ensure that any un- used investigational products are returned to the sponsor after the trial is completed.

In accordance with national/local laws and regulations, **regulators** may establish GMP requirements for investigational products, review manufacturing data submitted in support of research permits or marketing applications, and/or inspect manufacturing facilities. Because investigational products may be imported, regulators should be familiar with the manufacturing requirements in the country of origin and their conformance with international GMP standards

Regulators may also inspect investigators for compliance with the study protocol, including instructions for storing and handling investigational products.

Principle 14: Quality systems

Systems with procedures that assure the quality of every aspect of the trial should be implemented.

Application

Principle 14 is applied through development of procedures to control, assure, and improve the quality of data and records and the quality and effectiveness of processes and activities related to the conduct and oversight of clinical research.

Implementation

All of the parties who conduct and oversee clinical trials (sponsors, clinical investigators, IECs/IRBs, and regulatory authorities) should adopt and implement quality systems for the processes and activities for which they are responsible.

Sponsors secure the services of monitors to ensure compliance of the clinical investigators and verify that the study was carried out according to the approved study protocol. Sponsors also audit the monitors' performance and other quality control activities and systems to ensure each system's performance.

Monitors review study records at the sites, report their findings to the sponsor, and prepare written reports that document each site visit or trial-related communication

Investigators supervise to ensure that study staff follow established procedures for the conduct of the study, e.g. obtaining IEC/IRB approval of the study, obtaining informed consent from subjects, establishing and maintaining subjects' case histories, transcribing data from subjects' medical files to the CRFs, reporting adverse events and other unanticipated problems, etc.

ECs/IRBs develop and adopt SOPs for reviewing studies and informing the clinical investigator of any required modifications to the study protocol, and for assuring that such modifications are in place before the study proceeds. In accordance with national/local laws and regulations, IECs/IRBs may develop SOPs to allow IEC/IRB members or a third party to observe the consent process to verify that subjects are being provided the opportunity to ask questions about the study and that subjects receive a copy of the informed consent document. IECs/IRBs implement systems to assure that continuing review of the study takes place at intervals appropriate to the degree of risk, and that investigators are notified so that they may provide the necessary documentation to the IEC/IRB in advance of the deadline.

In accordance with applicable laws/regulations, **regulators** may inspect all parties that conduct or oversee research and verify the information submitted to the regulatory authority. Regulators may ask for sponsors' monitoring plans as a condition of allowing a study to proceed. Regulatory authorities also optimally develop SOPs and quality systems for internal regulatory activities, including policies and procedures for reviewing product applications and for the conduct of GCP inspections.

Chapter 11

Comparison of Clinical Trial Regulations in India, Europe and USA

Learning Objectives

To understand

- Clinical Trials Introduction
- Drug Development Process
- Clinical Trial Phases in India, EU and USA

  (Phase I clinical trials: Is the treatment safe, Phase II clinical trials: Does the treatment work, Phase III clinical trials: Is it better than)
- Submission for FDA approval: New drug application (NDA)
- Phase IV clinical trials: What else do we need to know?
- Phase V clinical trials
- Clinical Regulatory Agencies - India

  (Ministry of Health and Family Welfare, Central Drug Standards Control Organization, Indian Council of Medical Research, Ministry of Chemicals and Fertilizers)
- Clinical Regulations in Europe

  (Committee for Medicinal Products for Human Use, Committee for Medicinal Products for Veterinary Use, Committee on Orphan Medicinal Products, Committee on Herbal Medicinal Products, Paediatric Committee, Committee for Advanced Therapies, Pharmacovigilance Risk Assessment Committee)
- Clinical Regulations in USA
- A Comparison of Clinical Trail Regulations in India, Europe and USA

Clinical Trials Introduction

Clinical trials explore how a treatment reacts in the human body and are designed to ensure a drug is tolerated and effective before it is licensed by regulatory authorities and made available for use by doctors. Studies vary in their primary goal or endpoint (i.e. the most important outcome of the trial), the number of patients involved, and the specifics of the study design. However, all clinical studies conform to a strict set of criteria to protect the patients involved and to ensure rigorous evaluation of the drug. (1)

For safety purposes, clinical trials start with small groups of patients to find out whether a new approach causes any harm. In later phases of clinical trials, researchers learn more about the new approach's risks and benefits.

A clinical trial may find that a new strategy, treatment, or device

- improves patient outcomes;
- offers no benefit; or
- Causes unexpected harm. (2)

The goal of clinical trials is to create an environment that is favourable to conducting clinical trials, with the highest standards of safety for participants and increased transparency of trial information.

The regulation will require:

- consistent rules for conducting clinical trials
- information on the authorization, conduct and results of each clinical trial carried out to be publicly available.

This will increase the efficiency of all trials with the greatest benefit for those conducted in multiple Member States. It aims to foster innovation and research, while helping avoid unnecessary duplication of clinical trials or repetition of unsuccessful trials.

Drug Development Process

- New medicines originate in the laboratory where researchers identify, isolate and study thousands of molecules for their potential as future therapies.
- Once a candidate molecule (compound) has been identified in the laboratory, it is subjected to rigorous pre-clinical testing (in the laboratory and/or in animals) to assess its chemical, biological and toxicological properties (how harmful it is).
- These pre-clinical tests allow researchers a snapshot of whether a compound may have pharmacological activity.
- If results of pre-clinical studies are positive, the compound may be entered into a clinical trial program: this involves several 'phases' of study, starting with small studies usually in healthy volunteers and progressing in steps through to evaluation of the drug in people with the disease. At each phase, only those compounds that meet strict criteria for safety and effectiveness (efficacy) advance to the next phase.

- When results of clinical trials indicate the compound being studied is safe and effective the company applies to *regulatory authorities* for marketing authorization (permission to sell. (3)

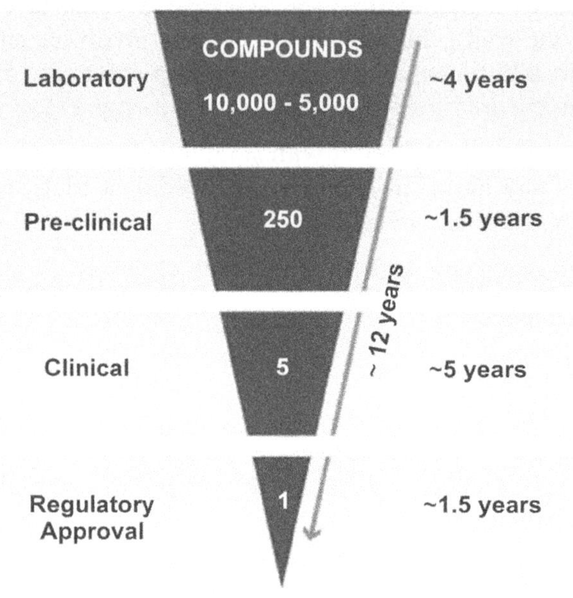

Fig.11.1 Drug Development Process.

CLINICAL TRIAL PHASES IN INDIA, EU AND USA: (1)

The clinical trial phases are same in all the three countries. They are:

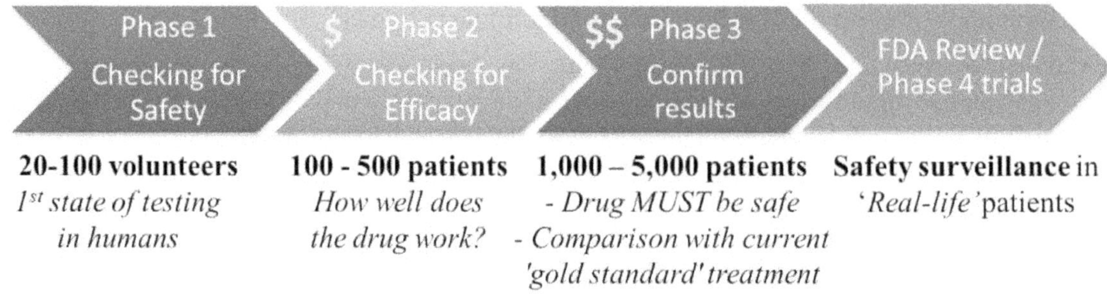

Fig.11.2 Clinical Trial Phases.

Phase 0 Clinical Trial (or) Pre-clinical Trial

Even though phase 0 studies are done in humans, this type of study is not like the other phases of clinical trials. The purpose of this phase is to help speed up and streamline the drug approval process.

Phase 0 studies are exploratory studies that often use only a few small doses of a new drug in a few patients. They test to find out whether the drug reaches the receptor tissue, whether the dose is adequate for the humans (dose standardization in humans), how the drug acts in the human body, and how the human body respond to the drug. The patients in these studies might need extra biopsies, scans, and blood samples as part of the study process. The biggest difference between phase 0 and the later phases of clinical trials is that there is no chance the volunteer will benefit by taking part in a phase 0 trial the benefit will be for other people in the future. Because drug doses are low, there is also less risk to the patient in phase 0 studies compared to Phase I studies. Phase 0 studies help researchers find out whether the drugs do what they're expected to do. If there are problems with the way the drug is absorbed or acts in the body, this should become clear very quickly in a phase 0 clinical trial. This process may help avoid the delay and expense of finding out years later in phase II or even phase III clinical trials that the drug doesn't act as expected to based on lab studies. Phase 0 studies aren't used widely, and there are some drugs for which they wouldn't be helpful. Phase 0 studies are very small, often with fewer than 15 people, and the drug is given only for a short time. They are not a required part of testing a new drug.

Phase I clinical trials: Is the treatment safe?

Phase I studies of a new drug are usually the first that involve people. The main reason for doing phase I studies is to find the highest dose of the new treatment that can be given safely without serious side effects. Although the treatment has been tested in lab and animal studies, the side effects in people cannot always be predicted. These studies also help to decide on the best way to give the new treatment.

Key points of phase I clinical trials

- The first few people in the study often get a low dose of the treatment and are watched very closely. If there are only minor side effects, the next few participants may get a higher dose. This process continues until doctors find the dose that is most likely to work while having an acceptable level of side effects.
- The focus in phase I is looking at what the drug does to the body and what the body does with the drug.
- Safety is the main concern at this point. Doctors keep a close eye on the people and watch for any serious side effects. Because
- of the small numbers of people in phase I studies, rare side effects may not be seen until later.
- Placebos are not part of phase I trials.
- These studies usually include a small number of people (20 to 80).
- Often, people with different types of cancer can take part in the same Phase I study.

- These studies are usually done in major cancer centers.
- These studies are not designed to find out if the new treatment works against cancer.

Overall, phase I trials are the ones with the most potential risk. But phase I studies do help some patients. For those with life-threatening illnesses, weighing the potential risks and benefits carefully is key.

Phase II clinical trials: Does the treatment work?

If a new treatment is found to be reasonably safe in phase I clinical trials, it can then be tested in a phase II clinical trial to find out if it works. The type of benefit or response the doctors look for depends on the goal of the treatment. It may mean the cancer shrinks or disappears. Or it might mean there's an extended period of time where the cancer doesn't get any bigger, or there's a longer time before the cancer comes back. In some studies, the benefit may be an improved quality of life. Many studies look to see if people getting the new treatment live longer than they would have been expected to without the treatment.

Key points of phase II clinical trials

- Usually, a group of 25 to 100 patients with the same type of cancer gets the new treatment in a phase II study. They are treated using the dose and method found to be the safest and most effective in phase I studies.
- In a phase II clinical trial, all the volunteers usually get the same dose. But some phase II studies do randomly assign participants to different treatment groups (much like what's done in phase III trials). These groups may get different doses or get the treatment in different ways to see which provides the best balance of safety and effectiveness.
- No placebo is used.
- Phase II studies are often done at major cancer centers, but may also be done in community hospitals or even doctors' offices.

Larger numbers of patients get the treatment in phase II studies, so there's a better chance that less common side effects may be seen. If enough patients benefit from the treatment, and the side effects are not too bad, the treatment is allowed to go on to a phase III clinical trial. Along with watching for responses, the research team keeps looking for any side effects.

Phase III clinical trials: Is it better than

What's already available?

Treatments that have been shown to work in phase II studies usually must succeed in one more phase of testing before they are approved for general use. Phase III clinical trials compare the safety and effectiveness of the new treatment against the current standard treatment.

Because doctors do not yet know which treatment is better, study participants are often picked at random (called *randomized*) to get either the standard treatment or the new treatment. When possible, neither the doctor nor the patient knows which of the treatments the patient is getting. This type of study is called a *double-blind study*.

Key points of phase* III *clinical trials

- Most phase III clinical trials have a large number of patients, at least several hundred.
- These studies are often done in many places across the country (or even around the world) at the same time.
- Phase III clinical trials are more likely to be offered by community-based oncologists.
- These studies tend to last longer than phases I and II.
- Placebos may be used in some phase III studies, but they are never used alone if there is a treatment available that works.

As with other studies, patients in phase III clinical trials are watched closely for side effects, and treatment is stopped if they're too bad.

Submission for FDA approval: New drug application (NDA)

In the United States, when phase III clinical trials show a new drug is more effective and/or safer than the current standard treatment, a new drug application (NDA) is submitted to the Food and Drug Administration (FDA) for approval. The FDA then reviews the results from the clinical trials and other relevant information.

After review, the FDA may ask for more information or even require that more studies be done. This can extend the approval process to more than 5 years.

On the other hand, based on its review, the FDA can decide that the treatment is OK to be used in patients with the type of illness the drug was tested on. In this case, the new treatment often becomes the standard of care, and newer drugs must then be tested against it before being approved. However, in some cases, the clinical trials are still not over and phase IV trials continue.

Phase IV clinical trials: What else do we need to know?

Drugs approved after phase III trials are often watched over a long period of time in phase IV studies. Even after testing a new medicine on thousands of people, the full effects of the treatment may not be known. Some questions may still need to be answered. For example, a drug may get FDA approval because it was shown to reduce the risk of cancer coming back after treatment. But does this mean that those who get it are more likely to live longer? Are there rare side effects that haven't been seen yet, or side effects that only show up after a person has taken the drug for a long time? These types of questions may take many more years to answer, and are often addressed in phase IV clinical trials.

Key points of phase IV clinical trials

- Phase IV studies look at drugs that have already been approved by the FDA. The drugs are available for doctors to prescribe
- for patients, but phase IV studies are needed to answer important questions.
- May involve at most, a few tens of thousands of people.
- This is the safest type of clinical trial because the treatment has already been studied a lot and used in possibly millions of people. Phase IV is looking at safety overtime.

- These studies may also look at other aspects of the treatment, such as quality of life or cost effectiveness.
- Phase V clinical trials
- This translational research is designed to "move from bench to bedside". Phase V clinical trials refer to comparative effectiveness research and community-based research. Research is done on data collected. All reported uses are evaluated. Patients are not monitored. Its main focus is to determine integration of a new therapy into wide spread clinical practice.

Phases	Dosing	Number of subjects	Main goal of clinical phase
Preclinical	Unrestricted	Not applicable	Testing in non-humans (efficacy, toxicities, pharmacokinetics)
0	Subtherapeutic	About 10	Pharmacokinetics and pharmacodynamics
IA/IB	Ascending doses	20 - 100	Dose-ranging
IIA/IIB	Therapeutic dose	100 - 300	Drug efficacy
IIA/IIB	Therapeutic dose	100 - 2000	Therapeutic effect
iV	Therapeutic dose	Anyone seeking treatment	Log- term effects
V	No dosing	All reported use	Research on data collected

Fig.11.3 Clinical Trial Phases, Subjects and Goal.

CLINICAL REGULATORY AGENCIES - INDIA (4)

The main regulatory agencies for clinical trials in India:

1. Ministry of Health and Family Welfare
2. Central Drug Standards Control Organization
3. Indian Council of Medical Research
4. Ministry of Chemicals and Fertilizers

1. Ministry of Health and Family Welfare

This is the regulatory agency, which is primarily dealing with healthcare. This government body has several bodies under its administrative control. Some of them are:

- Medical Council of India
- Dental Council of India
- Pharmacy Council of India
- Central Drug Standards Control Organization
- Hospital Services Consultancy Corporation Limited

This regulatory agency acts by prescribing the standards in order to ensure the safety, efficacy as well as the quality of the following products:

- Drugs

- Cosmetics
- Diagnostics
- Devices
- In addition, this regulatory agency is also regulating the following aspects of clinical trial
- Market authorization of new drugs
- Clinical trials standards

The role of Ministry of Health and Family Welfare in a clinical trial does not stop with this alone. This body will also supervise the drug imports. Furthermore, it is this regulatory agency, which will approve the license to drug manufacture.

2. Central Drug Standards Control Organization

This national regulatory authority is being operated under the 'Ministry of Health and Family Welfare'. This is the primary regulatory authority for the pharmaceuticals as well as medical devices in the nation. The Central Drug Standards Control Organization is serving the parallel function to the U.S. FDA, Japan's PMDA and European Union's EMA.

With this regulatory agency, it is the Drug Controller General of India who is regulating all the pharmaceuticals and medical devices. As such, the DCGI is being advised by two other bodies, which are:

- Drug Technical Advisory Board
- Drug Consultative Committee

As such, the whole regulatory agency has been divided into zonal offices to perform the following functions:

- Pre-licensing inspections
- Post-licensing inspections
- Post-market surveillance
- Recalls (if required)

The Central Drug Standards Control Organization is maintaining a good track record with 'World Health Organization'. At present, this agency is planning to open its international offices in China.

3. Indian Council of Medical Research

This is one among the oldest research bodies of the country. The Indian Government is funding this agency. The governing body of this organization is presided by the Union Health Minister. In addition, the scientific advisory board is assisting this regulatory agency. Various eminent experts in biomedical disciplines will assist ICMR in both scientific and technical matters. This regulatory agency is acting to promote biomedical research in the country and is considered as the apex body for the following activities:

- Formulation of biomedical research
- Coordination of biomedical research
- Promotion of biomedical research

  ICMR is the regulatory body, which has formulated guidelines for several aspects that are relating to national health. Treatments for conditions like malaria, cancer, type 2 - diabetes and retinoblastoma have been covered by various guidelines by Indian Council of Medical Research.

  The ICMR guidelines that are pertaining to the clinical trial research in the country are:

  - Ethics guidelines for biomedical research: This includes the following information:
  - General research principles for the research works that involve human subjects.
  - Specific research principles for the research works that involve human subjects in specific areas.
  - *Guidelines for Good Clinical Laboratory Practices*: These guidelines are aiming to elucidate the step-wise procedures that are to be followed by the laboratories for strengthening the quality of all the test results. In India, these guidelines must be taken up by all the ICMR labs, which are engaging in clinical trial research. A checklist will be prepared in order to monitor all these ICMR laboratories for compliance with ICMR guidelines.

4. Ministry of Chemicals and Fertilizers

   This ministry in India is the primary administrative unit of the following departments:

   - Department of Chemical and Petrochemicals
   - Department of Fertilizers
   - Department of Pharmaceuticals

   The ministry of chemicals and fertilizers is involved in the following activities:

   - Setting and revising the drug prices
   - Maintaining the data on production/export/import
   - Enforcing and monitoring the availability of medicines
   - Giving options to the parliament
   - This government body is regulating the industrial policy on drugs in the country.

CLINICAL REGULATIONS IN EUROPE

The European Medicines Agency (EMA) is a European Union agency for the evaluation of medicinal products. Prior to 2004, it was known as the European Agency for the Evaluation of Medicinal Products (EMEA). The EU is currently the source of about one-third of the new drugs brought onto the world market each year.

The main regulatory agencies for clinical trials in Europe are:

1. Committee for Medicinal Products for Human Use

   A single evaluation is carried out through the Committee for Medicinal Products for Human Use (CHMP). If the Committee concludes that the quality, safety and efficacy of the medicinal products are sufficiently proven, it adopts a positive opinion. This is sent to the European Commission to be transformed into a marketing authorization valid for the whole of the EU. A special type of approval is the Paediatric-Use Marketing Authorisation (PUMA), which can be granted for medical products intended exclusively for paediatric use.

   The CHMP is obliged by the regulation to reach decisions within 210 days, though the clock is stopped if it is necessary to ask the applicant for clarification or further supporting data. This compares well with the average of 500 days taken by the U.S. Food and Drug Administration.

2. Committee for Medicinal Products for Veterinary Use

   The Committee for Medicinal Products for Veterinary Use (CVMP) operates in analogy to the CHMP as described above.

3. Committee on Orphan Medicinal Products

   The Committee on Orphan Medicinal Products (COMP) administers the granting of orphan drug status since 2000. Companies intending to develop medicinal products for the diagnosis, prevention or treatment of life-threatening or very serious conditions that affect not more than five in 10,000 persons in the European Union can apply for 'orphan medicinal product designation'. The COMP evaluates the application and makes a recommendation for the designation, which is then granted by the European Commission.

4. Committee on Herbal Medicinal Products

   The Committee on Herbal Medicinal Products (HMPC) assists the harmonization of procedures and provisions concerning herbal medicinal products laid down in EU Member States, and further integrating herbal medicinal products in the European regulatory framework since 2004.

5. Paediatric Committee

   The Paediatric Committee (PDCO) deals with the implementation of the paediatric legislation in Europe Regulation (EC) No 1901/2006 since 2007. Under this legislation, all applications for marketing authorization of new medicinal products, or variations to existing authorizations, have to either include data from paediatric studies previously agreed with the PDCO, or obtain a PDCO waiver or a deferral of these studies.

6. Committee for Advanced Therapies

   The Committee for Advanced Therapies (CAT) was established in accordance with Regulation (EC) No 1394/2007 on advanced-therapy medicinal products (ATMPs) such as gene therapy, somatic cell therapy and tissue engineered products. It assesses the quality, safety and efficacy of ATMPs, and follows scientific developments in the field.

7. Pharmacovigilance Risk Assessment Committee

   A seventh committee, the Pharmacovigilance Risk Assessment Committee (PRAC) has come into function in 2012 with the implementation of the new EU pharmacovigilance legislation (Directive 2010/84/EU). The Agency constantly monitors the safety of medicines through a pharmacovigilance network and Eudra Vigilance, so that it can take appropriate actions if adverse drug reaction reports suggest that the benefit-risk balance of a medicine has changed since it was authorized. (5)

   When the Regulation becomes applicable, it will replace the existing EU Clinical Trial Directive (EC) No. 2001/20/EC and national legislation that was put in place to implement the Directive.

   The authorization and oversight of clinical trials remains the responsibility of Member States, with EMA managing the database and supervising content publication on the public website.

Key benefits of the Regulation

- Harmonized electronic submission and assessment process for clinical trials conducted in multiple Member States.
- Improved collaboration, information sharing and decision-making between and within Member States.
- Increased transparency of information on clinical trials.
- Highest standards of safety for all participants in EU clinical trials.

EU Clinical Trial Portal and Database

The portal will be the single entry point for submitting clinical trial information in the EU, which will be stored in the database. EMA will make information stored in the database publicly available subject to transparency rules.

The clinical trial application form and supporting dossier will cover all regulatory and ethics assessments from the Member States concerned. It will also include the public registration of the clinical trial and any subsequent updates.

EMA published the functional specifications for the EU portal and database to be audited in December 2014, following a public consultation:

- Functional specifications for the EU portal and EU database to be audited

The system will contain collaboration tools, workflow and document management capabilities, accessible via individual workspaces.

Sponsor Workspace

A secure workspace will assist clinical trial sponsors in preparing and compiling data to submit to the database for assessment by Member States. It will allow sponsors to:

- search and access clinical trials;

- compile clinical trial application dossiers for new and updated trials;
- cross-reference to product documents in other clinical trials;
- supervise their own clinical trials and check progress;
- receive alerts and notifications for ongoing trials;
- record clinical trial results;
- upload documents for clinical trial application form submission;
- respond to requests for information and view deadlines;
- manage users and user roles. Authority workspace:

A secure workspace will support the activities of Member States and the European Commission in overseeing clinical trials. It will allow Member States to:

- view application dossiers;
- manage tasks related to the assessment of clinical trials;
- collaborate within and between Member States;
- receive alerts and notifications for ongoing trials;
- download documents submitted by clinical trial sponsors;
- record inspections of sites and clinical trials. Public website

Through the website, members of the public can access detailed information on all clinical trials conducted in the EU, in all official EU languages. The website will provide the following features:

- overview of clinical trial statistics;
- advanced search;
- download data and reports;
- site updates and announcements. Implementation

Although the regulation was adopted and entered into force in 2014, the timing of its application depends on confirmation of full functionality of the EU portal and database through an independent audit. The Regulation becomes applicable six months after the European Commission publishes notice of this confirmation. (6)

CLINICAL REGULATIONS IN USA (7)

The **Food and Drug Administration** (**FDA** or **USFDA**) is a federal agency of the United States Department of Health and Human Services, one of the United States federal executive departments. The FDA is responsible for protecting and promoting public health through the control and supervision of food safety, tobacco products, dietary supplements, prescription and over-the-counter pharmaceutical drugs (medications), vaccines, biopharmaceuticals, blood transfusions, medical devices, electromagnetic radiation emitting devices (ERED), cosmetics, animal foods & feed and veterinary products. (5)The FDA was empowered by the United States Congress to enforce the Federal Food, Drug, and Cosmetic Act, which serves as the primary focus for the agency; the FDA also enforces other laws, notably Section 361 of the Public Health Service Act and associated regulations, many of which are not directly related to food or drugs. These include regulating lasers, cellular phones, condoms and control of disease on products ranging from certain household pets to sperm donation for assisted reproduction.

The FDA is led by the Commissioner of Food and Drugs, appointed by the President with the advice and consent of the Senate.

The FDA has its headquarters in unincorporated White Oak, Maryland. The agency also has 223 field offices and 13 laboratories located throughout the 50 states, the United States Virgin Islands, and Puerto Rico. (3) In 2008, the FDA began to post employees to foreign countries, including China, India, Costa Rica, Chile, Belgium, and the United Kingdom.

Clinical trials are conducted by US pharmaceutical and medical device companies in support of an application to the FDA for authorization to market a drug or device. Firstly applicant files the Investigational New Drug applications (INDs) that must be completed to file a New Drug Application (NDA) because most clinical trials conducted by pharmaceutical and biotech companies are undertaken pursuant to an IND.

The federal Food Drug and Cosmetic Act (FD&C) was passed in 1938 after a tragedy involving a deadly sulfanilamide elixir; it required FDA testing for safety for the first time. In 1962, Congress passed significant amendments to the Act adding a requirement for proof of efficacy before marketing of drugs in response to the thalidomide tragedy.

Section 505 of the FD & C provides that no person may introduce a new drug into interstate commerce without first filing an application with the FDA. This section of the law specifies the general content of such an application. The FDA promulgated regulations implementing this section of the FD&C at 21 C.F.R. In 1991, the FDA and the Department of Health and Human Services (DHHS) adopted the so-called "Common Rule" intended to protect the rights of human subjects enrolled in clinical trials. This is codified at 45 C.F.R. Part 46 Subpart A for those clinical studies conducted by or with the support of federal agency or department and at 21 C.F.R.

All clinical trials conducted to secure FDA marketing authorization must adhere to 21 C.F.R. Parts 50 and 56 which are regulations designed to protect the rights of human subjects. Part 50 governs the requirement for securing informed consent from human subjects who participate in clinical trials. This requirement applies not only to drug trials but to any clinical investigation that involves other substances (e.g., food, additives) or medical devices. The general requirement for informed consent is set forth-in 21 C.F.R. Part 50 also includes requirements for documentation of consent and exceptions for the requirement, as well as special safeguards for children and other vulnerable populations.

FDA publishes guidance and information sheets to provide industry and researchers with more information about the agency's views on application of regulations among other topics. The guidance is not binding on the agency but is very helpful to those seeking to conform to the regulations.

21 C.F.R. Part 56 sets forth the legal obligation to secure review of any clinical investigation subject to FDA regulation by an independent body known as an Institutional Review Board (IRB). Under the requirements set forth in 21

C.F.R. Part 56, the IRB must not only approve the investigation before it can commence but also must monitor it and ensure that it is conducted in accordance with the approval given by the IRB. Part 56 also sets forth requirements for the composition and operation of the IRB. IRBs must meet these requirements to be qualified by the FDA. If the FDA determines that a registered IRB is not adhering to the regulations and that the lack of compliance may adversely affect the rights or safety of human subjects, it may disqualify the IRB. In this case, the IRB may not oversee clinical investigations that support FDA marketing authorization or other action.

21 C.F.R. permits waiver of the requirement for IRB review upon application by the sponsor to the FDA; a waiver may be granted by the FDA in circumstances where the agency determines that the rights of the human subjects can be protected by other mechanisms. These alternative mechanisms include review by an independent ethics committee operated under the regulatory framework of another country that adheres to international standards of clinical practice.

21 C.F.R. Part 54 requires certain disclosures regarding financial relationships between sponsors and investigators as a financial relationship may create a conflict of interest for an investigator that could adversely affect the trial outcome.

A Comparison of Clinical Trail Regulations in India, Europe and USA

PARAMETERS	EUROPE	USA	INDIA
1. LEGAL FRAME WORK	• European Union EU Directives applicable to all members • National laws apply • Legal representative required	• Federal statutes and regulations applicableto all 50 states • Inividual state laws apply • Authorized representative	• CDSCO under the aegis of Ministry of Health & Family Welfare have the duty of regulating and ensuring the quality of medicines and pharmaceutical under the Drugs & Cosmetic Act
2. CLINICAL TRIAL APPLICATION	• CTA written approval required • Approval timeframe varies • Annual safety report only required • Format CTD paper or	• IND written approval not required to proceed comment CT • May proceed 30-days after FDA	• Form 44 is an application made for grant of permission to import or manufacture a new drug or to

	electronic • National CTA fees may apply	receives IND unless noticed otherwise • IND annual report required • Format paper or electronic, US format or CTD • No fees Required	undertake clinical trail. • Documents pertaining to chemical and pharmaceutical information, animal pharmacology, toxicology data and clinical pharmacology data. • Investigator's Brochure. Trail protocol, case report form, informed consent form. patient information sheet, investigator's undertaking and IEC approvals (if obtained during review process) • Regulatory status of the trial in other participating countries also needs to be reported. • Fees for phase I application is Rs 50000 • Fees for phase II and III application is 25000
3. INSTITUTIONAL REVIEW BOARD	• EC approval required • ECs appointed or authorized by states	• IRB approval required • IRB registration required	• DCGI approval • IRB/EC approval required
4. FORMS REQUIRED	• Statement of Investigator not required by member states	• Form FDA 1572 is required to be signed by the PI. If study is	• Form no: 44 is required for application of clinical trail.

		conducted in US and submitted to IND	
5. RECORD RETENTION	• Essential Document Record includes CRF excluding medical records ≥5 years • ≥ 15 years or CT discontinuation if data used to support a marketing application	• Record retention 2 years after marketing application is not approved	• Retention of records 3 years after marketing application is approved
6. INVESTIGATIONAL MEDICINAL PRODUCT REQUIREMENTS	• Label must comply with Annex 13 of EU Directive 2001/83/EC • Language requirements varies between member ststes • Sponsor is responsible for destruction of unused and/or retured IMP	• Label must be in English, except for Puerto Rico • The following statement is required: " caution: New Drug Limited by Federal (or United States) law to investugational use"	• Study code • API and formulation • Batch no., expiry date and retest date • Dosage • Direction of Use • Manufactured by • "FOR CLINICAL TRAIL USE ONLY"
7. ADVERSE EVENT REPORTING	• Review and monitors the safety information of IMPs used in clinical trails conducted in their respective territories through the use of the Eudra Vigilance Clinical Trail module (EVCTM) • Report to the sponsors all serious adverse events immediately	• Required to report to the sponsor any adverse events caused by or probably caused by IMP • Notify FDA and all participating investigators in a written IND safety report of : Any adverse experience associated with the use of the drug that is both serious and unexpected. • Required to report	• Upon the discovery of any injury or death related o a clinical trail, sponsor will now be required to inform the DCGI within 24 hours. • Following this reporting line, relevant clinical trail stakeholders will be required to submit individual reports for scrutiny by an independent review committee, due to be created by the DCGI

		unexpected to report unexpected fatal or life threatening experiences ASAP, but not later than 7 days; Follow-up reports ASAP but no later than 15 days of receipt of new information	
8. REGULATORY COMPLIANCE	• Covered under Article 15 of Directive 2001/20/EC CA responsible for implementing provisions for the suspension of a CT • Conducting inspections and verifying compliance Inspection reports may also be made available to sponsor, EC. EMEA and other member states must comply with good distribution practices (GDPs) and Good Laboratory Pratices (GLPs) • No comparable EU regulation specific to Phase1 CGMPs (Annex 13 guideline provides flexibility dependent upon the stge of development of the product)	• All clinical trails must comply with 21 CFR Parts 50, 54, 56 and 312 • Phase 1 IMP are exempt from certain parts of 21 CFR part 211 unless the clinical trial involves a marketed drug product or one that was manufactured in a phase 2 and/or 3 study	• Indian GCP states that if the sponsor is a foreign company. Organization or person(s)-it shall appoint a local representative of CRO to fulfill the appropriate local responsibilities as governed by the Indian regulations

Chapter 12

Challenges in the Implementation of GCP Guidelines

LEARNING OBJECTIVES

To understand

- Challenges in the implementation of GCP guidelines

  (Professional Training on GCP, Infrastructure, Regulatory Environment, ERB / IRB / IEC ICD Administration, Safety Reporting, Investigational Product, Record Keeping/Source Document(s)

  Grants and Payments

  Trial Report or Publication)

  Current Issues and Uncertainties in Clinical Trials In India

Some of the Challenges in the Implementation of GCP Guidelines

1. Professional Training on GCP
2. Infrastructure
3. Regulatory Environment
4. ERB / IRB / IEC
5. ICD Administration
6. Safety Reporting
7. Investigational Product
8. Record Keeping / Source Document(s)
9. Grants and Payments
10. Trial Report or Publication

1. Professional Training on GCP

- The scarcity of GCP trained competent professionals.

- Lack of professional training on GCP across various stakeholders(Sponser, investigator, ERB, patient, regulators etc).
- No Indian University offers a curriculum in this discipline.

2. **Infrastructure**
   - Most of the hospitals in India do not meet the infrastructure requirements as per GCP guidelines.
   - Lack of supportive infrastructure like labs and diagnostics up to the standards of international accreditation.
3. **Regulatory Environment**
   - Biggest challenge is their implementation and adherence.
   - Do not have a regulatory inspection system in place to monitor and adherence and compliance to these guidelines.
   - Mostly the adherence to the GCP guidelines is a matter of self-discipline at the part of Sponsor(s), investigator(s) and ERB(s).
4. **ERB / IRB / IEC**
   - GCP requires written standard operating procedures (SOP) for ERB / IRB / IEC.
   - No standard guidelines on what should be the content of an ideal SOP.
   - Many of the hospitals either do not have written SOP for ERB or have improper guidelines not about all the critical elements of GCP.
   - No provision to check whether the SOP is followed during each meeting or not.
5. **ICD Administration**
   - In India the patient / legal representatives has immense faith on treating doctor that they insist on signing the documents without even reading or after reading it superficially.
   - A layman cannot understand the wording and contents of the majority of the documents.
   - Situation becomes even grim when translations are used, which leads to varied interpretations due to authentic validation.
   - Lack of patient's advocacy group who can be a guardian to the patients' rights and safety, makes poor uneducated masses susceptible to abuse in clinical trials in the name of treatment.
6. **Safety Reporting**
   - Investigator and sponsor have joint responsibility to report all the serious and un expected adverse events to ERB / IRB and regulatory authorities
   - The regulatory pharmacovigilance presently is not optimally implemented for adverse event handling and review.

- In majority of cases sponsor does not even comply with the expedited safety reporting to local regulatory authority and regulators often remain unaware of this fact.

7. **Investigational Product**
   - Investigational product storage, handling and access control is a major challenge.
   - It is difficult to produce an evidence of temperature chain maintained during shipment of investigational product(s) from sponsor's facility to investigator site(s). Eg: Courier, Custom clearance etc.
   - There is no validation and regular standardization of thermometers provided by the sponsor.
   - No standard solutions are available for storing investigational product(s) requiring.

8. **Record Keeping / Source Document(s)**
   - Record retention and retrieval is always a major challenge in majority of hospitals.
   - The document of patient disease, treatment and progress note is not adequate to meet the standards of good documentation practices that ensures data completeness and correctness.
   - Hospitals using electronic records as source data / document compliance to part 11 is a major hurdle.
   - Archival or trial documents for the stipulated time and under proper environment.

9. **Grants and Payments**
   - Trials agreements are based on the institutional practices where the research grants goes to a centralized research account, which in majority of the cases remains un - utilized.
   - No incentive to the investigator(s) for investing extra time, efforts and intellectual capital.

10. **Trial Report or Publication**
    - Negative trials or trials that get terminated prematurely are rarely published.
    - This is a major threat towards validity of Evidence Based Medicine as one gets to know the positive results only.
    - India, no doubt has a talented pool of clinical research professional(s) but the above-mentioned challenges needs to be addressed in order to perform the world class clinical trials in compliance with GCP guidelines.

Current Issues and Uncertainities in Clinical Trials In India

Clinical research in India grew at a fast pace between 1995 and 2008, and by 2008 –2009 there were several hundred projects ongoing across the country. The global financial crisis of 2009 led to as lowing down of that pace, and in 2010 the number of projects submitted for regulatory approval in India shrunk by about 25%. Although the demand has picked up again thereafter, India remains a very small player in the global clinical development effort, with no more than 2% to 3% of the world's trials including India as a location.[8]

Despite great potential, regulatory delays and controversies surrounding clinical trials in India **(Table 2)** threaten to further stagnate the country's transition toward becoming a global hub for drug discovery and development. Misconceptions about clinical trials in India generally stem from ignorance of the processes and safeguards inbuilt into the system. In addition there are gaps in regulatory oversight and enforcement that keep regulators from being able to ensure and certify compliance to guidelines at the site level across a multiplicity of sites. Technicalities involved in the analysis and interpretation of outcomes have often led to misrepresentation of facts. It is hoped that these uncertainties will resolve over time. Much will depend on the development of science-based regulatory reforms and the success of indigenous entrepreneurship.

Current Issues Surrounding Clinical Trials in India

Informedconsent	Sporadic reports of patients signing informed consent without adequate comprehension of the information in the consent form points to the need for closer scrutiny of the process. Video recording of the informed consent discussion between the investigator and patient has been suggested as a means of ensuring that investigators spend time with patients to explain the risks and benefits of participating in a clinical trial
Compensation for trial-related injury	Inadequate process detail and lack of fair balance in the determination of causality and compensation payouts has led to uncertainties that have resulted in sponsors hesitating to include India in their global drug development plans.
Deaths reported from clinical trials	Misinterpretation of figures by the media has led to the impression that clinical trials are to blame for deaths of patients participating in clinical trials. Closer analysis should reveal the potential for clinical trials to reduce mortality not only because commercial incentives drive sponsors toward more effective and safer drugs, but also because in resource-starved situations, clinical trials assure better access to health care.
Financial irregularities at sites	Alleged cases of investigators working in public institutions diverting clinical trial funding into personal accounts has led sponsors to insist on tripartite arrangements with institutional administrators in order to ensure transparency of funding and of the utilization of funds.
Fraud and data manipulation	Occasional cases of fraud by investigator or site staff have been identified by CRO monitors. Cases of fraudulent ethics committees have also come to light. These instances highlight the need for proscriptive regulatory provisions against fraud and a system of approval and accreditation of ethics committees.

Chapter 13

Ethical Guidelines in Clinical Research

LEARNING OBJECTIVES

To understand

- History
- Development of Various Ethical Guidelines - Changing Scenario
- The Indian Perspective
- Ethical Principles:

  (Principle of Essentiality, Principles of Voluntariness, Informed Consent and Community Agreement, Principle of Non-Exploitation, Principle of Privacy and Confidentiality, Principle of Precaution and Risk Minimization, Principle of Professional Competence, Principle of Accountability and Transparency, Principle of the Maximization of the Public Interest and of Distributive Justice, Principle of Institutional Arrangements, Principle of Public Domain, Principle of Totality of Responsibility, Principle of Compliance)
- Informed Consent
- Vulnerable Population
- Therapeutic Misconception
- Post-Trial Access
- Ethics Committee
- The Way Ahead
- Ethical Guidelines as Per ICH

  (Social and clinical value, Scientific validity, Fair subject selection, Favorable risk-benefit ratio, Independent review, Informed consent, Respect for potential and enrolled subjects)

The word 'ethics' is derived from the Greek word, *ethos*, which means custom or character. Ethics is the systematic study of values, so as to decide what is right and what is wrong. In clinical research human beings are involved, as opposed to animals, atoms or asteroids, as the object of study. It focuses on improving human health and well-being, typically by identifying better methods to treat, cure or prevent illnesses. Ethics in clinical research focuses largely on identifying and implementing the acceptable conditions for exposure of some individuals to risks and burdens for the benefit of the society at large.

History

The ethical guidelines in various parts of the world were formulated only after discovery of inhumane behavior with participants during research experiments. In the pre-World War II era, most of the research experiments were carried on own self or on one's own patients. World War II led the states to take more interest in science and research resulting in initiation of larger, systematic clinical investigations to gain knowledge for better treatment of patients, specially the soldiers. Most of the studies were carried out through defence efforts and used mainly the prisoners without concern of their consent and wellbeing. The experiments by the Nazi doctors in their concentration camps were the cruelest of all of them. In some of the most dreadful of these experiments, they kept the prisoners in compression chambers, freezing water, created gunshot wounds and even transplanted grafts among twins to see the body's response in such adverse situations. Death was the end point in most of the experiments and when it was not so, the doctors did antemortem dissection to study changes in the body. The discovery of these experiments stunned the whole world which led to formulation of Nuremberg code[1] in Germany to prevent recurrence of such episodes. It was the first international code for ethics in clinical research laying down the guidelines for research on human subjects. It laid down ten clear principles to be followed by researchers and made voluntary consent essential, allowed subjects to withdraw from the experimentation at any time, banned experiments that could result in major injury or death of the subjects and made mandatory to have preclinical data before experimenting on humans.

Development of Various Ethical Guidelines - Changing Scenario

The Nuremberg code was not honored by some researchers and there continued to be abuses and exploitations of humans in research. The Willow brook State Study [2] to know natural course of infective hepatitis in children and the Jewish Chronic Disease Hospital study[3] to understand body's ability to reject cancer cells in debilitated subjects were examples of unethical research. This led the World Medical Association (WMA) to develop a set of guidelines to safeguard the rights and wellbeing of participants in clinical research. The set of guidelines was adopted by the 18th WMA General Assembly and was called the Declaration of Helsinki[4]. It was revised five times and the latest version was published in 2000 at the 52nd WMA, Edinburgh, Scotland. It contains 32 principles, which stress on informed consent, confidentiality of data, vulnerable population and requirement of a protocol, including the scientific reasons of the study, to be reviewed by the ethics committee.

In the United States the ethical guidelines were setup after the discovery of the Tuskegee Syphilis Study[3]. The study was started in 1932 with 399 syphilitic African American men to see the natural course of syphilis and was supposed to last for about six months but as the researchers were getting “good data” they decided to continue it. The participants were misled and deprived of treatment even after the introduction of penicillin in the 1940s. These ethical atrocities were exposed in 1972 resulting in discontinuation of the study, but till then it had already led to 28 deaths and permanent disability in 100 subjects; moreover 40 patients infected their wives resulting in 19 cases of congenital syphilis. To probe into the study the ‘National Commission for the Protection of Human Subjects of Biomedical and Behavioral Research’ was formed which wrote the Belmont Report[5] in 1979 and laid the foundation for regulations regarding ethics and human subjects’ research in the US. The Belmont report stressed upon three basic ethical principles: respect for person, beneficence and justice. These were applied in the form of informed consent, assessment of risks and benefits by ethics committees and selection of subjects.

With the increasing interest of pharmaceutical industries in carrying out research experiments in the developing and the under developed countries, in 1982, the Council for International Organizations of Medical Sciences (CIOMS)[6] in association with World Health Organization (WHO) developed ‘International Ethical Guidelines for Biomedical Research Involving Human Subjects’. They especially stressed upon ethical issues in less developed countries like investigator's duties regarding consent, appropriate inducements, special/vulnerable populations, therapeutic misconceptions and post-trial access.

The Indian Perspective

The Indian Council of Medical Research (ICMR), in February 1980, released a ‘Policy Statement on Ethical Considerations involved in Research on Human Subjects’. This was the first policy statement giving official guidelines for establishment of ethics committees (ECs) in all medical colleges and research centers. But as with other nations of the world, these guidelines were not respected by many researchers and India was not free of controversial research works. In 1970s and 1980s researchers at the Institute for Cytology and Preventive Oncology in New Delhi, carried out a study on 1158 women patients of different stages of cervical dysplasia or precancerous lesions of the cervix[7]. These patients were left untreated to see how many lesions progressed to cancer and how many regressed. By the end of the study seventy-one women had developed malignancies and lesions in nine of them had progressed to invasive cancer. Sixty-two women were treated only after they developed localized cancer. After the controversy about the study became public in 1997, the ICMR started developing ‘Ethical Guidelines for Biomedical Research on Human Subjects’ and finalized them in the year 2000. These are a set of guidelines which every researcher in India should follow while conducting research on human subjects. Although not a law, these guidelines have been put into force through Schedule Y. With the changing scenario in the research field and development of modern techniques, the guidelines were revised in 2006[8]. These guidelines have elaborated the three basic ethical principles: respect for person, beneficence and justice by inducting twelve general principles as follows:

Ethical Principles

1. **Principle of Essentiality:** The research being carried out should be essential for the advancement of knowledge that benefits patients, doctors and all others in aspects of health care and also for the ecological and environmental well being of the planet.
2. **Principles of Voluntariness, Informed Consent and Community Agreement:** The research participant should be aware of the nature of research and the probable consequences of the experiments and then should make a independent choice without the influence of the treating doctor, whether to take part in the research or not. When the research treats any community or group of persons as a research participant, these principles of voluntariness and informed consent should apply to the community as a whole and also to each individual member who is the participant of the research or experiment.
3. **Principle of Non-Exploitation:** Research participants should be remunerated for their involvement in the research or experiment. The participants should be made aware of all the risks involved irrespective of their social and economic condition or educational levels attained. Each research protocol should include provisions of compensation for the human participants either through insurance cover or any other appropriate means to cover all foreseeable and hidden risks.
4. **Principle of Privacy and Confidentiality:** All the data acquired for research purpose should be kept confidential to prevent disclosure of identity of the involved participant and should not be disclosed without valid legal and/or scientific reasons.
5. **Principle of Precaution and Risk Minimization:** Due care and caution should be taken at all stages of the research and experiment (from its beginning as a research idea, formulation of research design/ protocol, conduct of the research or experiment and its subsequent applicative use) to prevent research participant from any harm and adverse events. EC has to play an active role in risk minimization.
6. **Principle of Professional Competence:** Clinical research should be carried out only by competent and qualified persons in their respective fields.
7. **Principle of Accountability and Transparency:** The researcher should conduct experiments in fair, honest, impartial and transparent manner after full disclosure of his/her interests in research. They should also retain the research data, subject to the principles of privacy and confidentiality, for a minimum period of 5 years, to be scrutinized by the appropriate legal and administrative authority, if necessary.
8. **Principle of the Maximization of the Public Interest and of Distributive Justice:** The results of the research should be used for benefit of all humans, especially the research participants themselves and/or the community from which they are drawn and not only to those who are socially better off.
9. **Principle of Institutional Arrangements:** It is required that all institutional arrangements required to be made in respect of the research and its subsequent use or applications should be duly made in transparent manner.

10. **Principle of Public Domain:** The results of any research work done should be made public through publications or other means. Even before publication, the detailed information of clinical trials should be made public before start of recruitment via clinical trial registry systems that allow free online access like: www.ctri.in/; www.actr.org.au/; www.clinicaltrials.gov/ or www.isrctn.org/.

11. **Principle of Totality of Responsibility:** All those directly or indirectly connected with the research should take the professional and moral responsibility, for the due observance of all the principles, guidelines or prescriptions laid down in respect of the research.

12. **Principle of Compliance:** All those associated with the research work should comply by the guidelines pertaining to the specific area of the research.For research to be conducted ethically we need to follow these twelve general principles laid down by the ICMR. In order to follow these principles we should be aware about the informed consent process, vulnerable population, therapeutic misconception, post trial access and structure and role of ethics committees. These concepts hold special importance in developing countries like ours, as most of the research participants are uneducated and economically backwards, hence we discuss them here.

Informed Consent [8,9]

A well-documented informed consent is the hallmark of any ethical research work. It is the responsibility of the investigator/researcher to obtain the informed consent of the prospective participant or in the case of an individual who is not capable of giving informed consent, the consent of a legal guardian. Informed consent respects individual's autonomy to participate or not to participate in research. Adequate information about the research is given in a simple and easily understandable vernacular language in a document known as the 'Participant/Patient Information Sheet' attached along with the 'Informed Consent Form (ICF)'. The patient information sheet should include: A statement that the study involves research; an explanation of the purpose of the research and the expected duration of the subject's participation; a description of the procedures to be followed and identification of any procedures which are experimental; a description of any reasonably foreseeable risks or discomforts to the subjects; a description of any benefits to the subjects or to others which may reasonably be expected from the research; trial treatment schedule(s) and the probability for random assignment to each treatment (especially in randomized placebo controlled trials); a disclosure of appropriate alternative procedures or courses of treatment, if any, that might be advantageous to the subjects; a statement describing the extent, if any, to which confidentiality of records identifying the subjects will be maintained; for research involving more than minimal risk, an explanation as to whether any compensation and an explanation as to whether any medical treatments are available if injury occurs and, if so, what they consist of, and where further information may be obtained; an explanation of whom to contact for answers to pertinent questions about the research and research subjects' rights, and whom to contact in the event of a research-related injury to the subjects; a statement that participation is voluntary and refusal to participate will involve no penalty or loss of benefits to which the subjects are otherwise entitled, also the subjects may discontinue participation at any time without penalty or loss of benefits.

The ICF should specify that the participant has read and understood the patient information sheet; no further permission is required to look into his health records for study purpose until his identity is not revealed; the results arising from the study can be used only for scientific purposes and he voluntarily agrees to take part in the study. The ICF should have space for signature/thumb print of the participant, the principal investigator, a witness and a legally acceptable representative when required.

The ICF with participant/patient information sheet should be approved by the EC before use. The ICF should have the sign or thumb impression of the prospective participant before start of the experiment. If the participant is illiterate, the document should have the signature of a witness, who has seen that the contents of the patient information sheet were adequately explained to the participant. If the participant is a minor or not capable of giving consent, a verbal assent should be taken from him and the consent form should be signed by his legally acceptable representative. If the treating physician of a prospective participant is also the investigator, the informed consent should be taken by any other neutral physician to prevent biased decision of the participant. Informed consent if properly taken protects the rights of prospective participants and thus forms the basis of ethical research work.

Vulnerable Population

Persons who are relatively or absolutely incapable of protecting their own interests are termed as vulnerable research population. The very poor, illiterate patients, children, individuals with questionable capacity to give consent (including psychiatric patients), prisoners, foetuses, pregnant women, terminally ill patients, students, employees, comatose patients, tribals and the elderly are examples of vulnerable population. Declaration of Helsinki[4] states that 'Medical research involving a underprivileged or vulnerable population or community is only justified if the research is responsive to the health needs and priorities of that population or community and if there is a reasonable likelihood that this population or community stands to benefit from the results of the research.' It is the responsibility of the EC to see whether the inclusion of vulnerable populations in the study is justifiable or the population is just being exploited to generate clinical data. To prevent even minor exploitation the EC should consult the representative of vulnerable population that is to be researched upon while reviewing the protocol.

Therapeutic Misconception [10,11]

The therapeutic misconception (TM) is a vexing ethical issue for obtaining valid informed consent. A patient coming to a physician may misinterpret and enrol in a research study thinking it to be routine medical care without understanding the experimental nature of the treatment given. He may misinterpret the information given about the research, such that he believes that aspects of the research will directly benefit him.

Thus, it is important that investigators should make efforts to dispel the TM in order to promote ethical and valid informed consent. ICFs should clarify the salient features of research: The purpose of randomized controlled trials (RCTs), random selection of treatment, masking of treatment, meaning and rationale of placebo, restrictions on treatment flexibility and how treatment decision making differs in RCTs compared with routine medical care. Thus to safeguard the ethical rights of the participants therapeutic misconception needs to be taken care of.

Post-Trial Access [8,12]

The concept of posttrial access holds special importance for clinical research works in the less developed countries. Pharmaceutical companies from developed countries collect the clinical data for their new and experimental drugs from the population in less developed countries. Most of these drugs would never be used by the communities from where the experimental data are collected and here comes the importance of post trial access for safeguarding the rights of such communities. The Helsinki Declaration of WMA, 2000 states that at the end of the trial, every participant should be assured of access to the best proven prophylactic, diagnostic and therapeutic methods identified by the study. The Declaration of the WMA in 2004 reaffirmed its position that "it is necessary during the study planning process to identify post-trial access by study participants to prophylactic, diagnostic and therapeutic procedures identified as beneficial in the study or access to other appropriate care. Post-trial access arrangements or other care must be described in the study protocol so that ethical review committee may consider such arrangements during its review." Therefore, whenever possible EC should consider such an arrangement in the a *priori* agreement. Sometimes more than the benefit to the participant, the community may be given benefit in indirect way through improving their living conditions, establishing counseling centres, clinics or schools and giving education on maintaining good health practices.

Ethics Committee[8,13]

The first appearance of need of ethics committee (EC) was made in Declaration of Helsinki in 1964, while in India it appeared in 1980 in the ICMR Policy Statement. EC also called as the Institutional Review Board or the Ethics Review Board stands as the bridge between the researcher and the ethical guidelines of the country.

The establishment of EC requires 5-15 members with at least one basic medical scientist (preferably one pharmacologist), one clinician, a legal expert, a social scientist / representative of NGO / philosopher or theologian and a lay person from the community. Every institute, where research is going on should have its own EC with its head preferably from outside the institute.

Individuals carrying out research can approach to independent ECs. The decisions of EC should be taken only after quorum formation with a minimum of five members having at least one basic medical scientist, one clinician and one legal expert or retired judge. The ECs should have independence from political, institutional, professional, and market influences, in their composition, procedures, and decision-making. As there are no laws governing the registration, formation or working of ethics committees in India, each ethics committee should have their own standard operating procedures for proper functioning.

ECs are responsible for carrying out the review of proposed research before the commencement of the research. The basic responsibility of EC is to ensure an independent, competent and timely review of all ethical aspects of the project proposals received in order to safeguard the dignity, rights, safety and well-being of all actual or potential research participants. The scientific design and conduct of the study should also be reviewed at the outset as poor science is poor ethics. The appropriateness of the study design in relation to the objectives of the study, the statistical methodology (including sample size calculation) and the potential for reaching sound conclusions with the smallest number of research participants should be assessed. The EC should also look into matters like informed consent process, qualifications of principal investigator and supporting staff, adequacy of infrastructure and facilities, risk benefit ratio, plans to maintain confidentiality and plans for post trial access and compensations. They also need to ensure that there is regular evaluation of the ongoing studies that have received a positive decision. EC is the most important check point for promoting ethical research in the country.

The Way Ahead

Though we have formulated many ethical guidelines for clinical research, are we adequately following them? The answer is ‘No’. This is because the ethical guidelines in India are just the recommendations and not a law. For proper enforcement of these guidelines should be made a part of the law as has been done in US and other countries of the world. Another issue lies with the training of doctors and research scientists in our institutions. Doctors are specially trained to be good clinicians but are never taught even the fundamentals of ethical clinical research. The post graduate dissertation or the PhD thesis is a precious opportunity to train tomorrow's investigators in the elements of ethical clinical research. Undergraduates should also be involved in simple observational research.

Finally if we can overcome these challenges, we will make India a competent and credible place of ethical clinical research.

Ethical Guidelines as Per ICH

The goal of clinical research is to develop generalizable knowledge that improves human health or increases understanding of human biology. People who participate in clinical research make it possible to secure that knowledge. The path to finding out if a new drug or treatment is safe or effective, for example, is to test it on patient volunteers. But by placing some people at risk of harm for the good of others, clinical research has the potential to exploit patient volunteers. The purpose of ethical guidelines is both to protect patient volunteers and to preserve the integrity of the science.

The ethical guidelines in place today were primarily a response to past abuses, the most notorious of which in America was an experiment in Tuskegee, Alabama, in which treatment was withheld from 400 African American men with syphilis so that scientists could study the course of the disease. Various ethical guidelines were developed in the 20th century in response to such studies.

Some of the influential codes of ethics and regulations that guide ethical clinical research include:

- Nuremberg Code (1947)
- Declaration of Helsinki (2000)
- Belmont Report (1979)
- CIOMS (2002)
- U.S. Common Rule (1991)

Using these sources of guidance and others, seven main principles have been described as guiding the conduct of ethical research:

- Social and clinical value
- Scientific validity
- Fair subject selection
- Favorable risk-benefit ratio
- Independent review
- Informed consent
- Respect for potential and enrolled subjects

1. Social and clinical value

Every research study is designed to answer a specific question. Answering certain questions will have significant value for society or for present or future patients with a particular illness. An answer to the research question should be important or valuable enough to justify asking people to accept some risk or inconvenience for others. In other words, answers to the research question should contribute to scientific understanding of health or improve our ways of preventing, treating, or caring for people with a given disease. Only if society will gain useful knowledge which requires sharing results, both negative and positive can exposing human subjects to the risk and burden of research be justified.

2. Scientific validity

A study should be designed in a way that will get an understandable answer to the valuable research question. This includes considering whether the question researchers are asking is answerable, whether the research methods are valid and feasible, and whether the study is designed with a clear scientific objective and using accepted principles, methods, and reliable practices. It is also important that statistical plans be of sufficient power to definitively test the objective, for example, and for data analysis. Invalid research is unethical because it is a waste of resources and exposes people to risk for no purpose

3. **Fair subject selection**

   Who does the study need to include, to answer the question it is asking? The primary basis for recruiting and enrolling groups and individuals should be the scientific goals of the study not vulnerability, privilege, or other factors unrelated to the purposes of the study. Consistent with the scientific purpose, people should be chosen in a way that minimizes risks and enhances benefits to individuals and society. Groups and individuals who accept the risks and burdens of research should be in a position to enjoy its benefits, and those who may benefit should share some of the risks and burdens. Specific groups or individuals (for example, women or children) should not be excluded from the opportunity to participate in research without a good scientific reason or a particular susceptibility to risk.

4. **Favorable risk-benefit ratio**

   Uncertainty about the degree of risks and benefits associated with a drug, device, or procedure being tested is inherent in clinical research otherwise there would be little point to doing the research. And by definition, there is more uncertainty about risks and benefits in early-phase research than in later research. Depending on the particulars of a study, research risks might be trivial or serious, might cause transient discomfort or long-term changes. Risks can be physical (death, disability, infection), psychological (depression, anxiety), economic (job loss), or social (for example, discrimination or stigma from participating in a certain trial). Has everything been done to minimize the risks and inconvenience to research subjects, to maximize the potential benefits, and to determine that the potential benefits to individuals and society are proportionate to, or outweigh, the risks? Research volunteers often receive some health services and benefits in the course of participating, yet the purpose of clinical research is not to provide health services.

5. **Independent review**

   To minimize potential conflicts of interest and make sure a study is ethically acceptable before it even starts, an independent review panel with no vested interest in the particular study should review the proposal and ask important questions, including: Are those conducting the trial sufficiently free of bias? Is the study doing all it can to protect research volunteers? Has the trial been ethically designed and is the risk–benefit ratio favorable? In the United States, independent evaluation of research projects is done through granting agencies, local institutional review boards (IRBs), and data and safety monitoring boards. These groups also monitor a study while it is ongoing.

6. **Informed consent**

   For research to be ethical, most agree that individuals should make their own decision about whether they want to participate or continue participating in research. This is done through a process of informed consent in which individuals (1) are accurately informed of the purpose, methods, risks, benefits, and alternatives to the research, (2) understand this information and how it relates to their own clinical situation or interests, and (3) make a voluntary decision about whether to participate.

There are exceptions to the need for informed consent from the individual — for example, in the case of a child, of an adult with severe Alzheimer's, of an adult unconscious by head trauma, or of someone with limited mental capacity. Ensuring that the individual's research participation is consistent with his or her values and interests usually entails empowering a proxy decision maker to decide about participation, usually based on what research decision the subject would have made, if doing so were possible.

7. **Respect for potential and enrolled subjects**

   Individuals should be treated with respect from the time they are approached for possible participation even if they refuse enrollment in a study throughout their participation and after their participation ends. This includes:

   1. Respecting their privacy and keeping their private information confidential.
   2. Respecting their right to change their mind, to decide that the research does not match their interests, and to withdraw without penalty.
   3. Informing them of new information that might emerge in the course of research, which might change their assessment of the risks and benefits of participating.
   4. Monitoring their welfare and, if they experience adverse reactions, untoward events, or changes in clinical status, ensuring appropriate treatment and, when necessary, removal from the study.
   5. Informing them about what was learned from the research. Most researchers do a good job of monitoring the volunteers' welfare and making sure they are okay. They are not always so good about distributing the study results. If they don't tell you, ask

For Further Study

1. Nuremberg Military Tribunal. The Nuremberg Code. JAMA. 1996;276:1691. [PubMed] [Google Scholar]
2. Krugman S. The Willowbrook Hepatitis Studies Revisited: Ethical Aspects. Rev Infect Dis. 1986;8:157–62. [PubMed] [Google Scholar]
3. Thatte U. Ethical issues in Clinical Research. In: Gupta SK, editor. Basic Principles of Clinical Research and Methodology. 1st ed. New Delhi: Jaypee Brothers; 2007. pp. 58–73. [Google Scholar]
4. World Medical Association. Declaration of Helsinki-Ethical Principles for Medical Research Involving Human Subjects. 2008. Oct, [Last cited on 2010 Apr 13]. Available from: URL: http://www.wma.net/en/30publications/10policies/b3/index.html .
5. The Belmont Report. Washington DC: US Government Printing Office; 1979. National Commission for the protection of human Subjects of Biomedical and Behavioural Research. [Google Scholar]
6. International ethical guidelines for biomedical research involving human subjects. Geneva: Council for International Organization of Medical Sciences; 1993. Council for International Organizations of Medical Sciences. [Google Scholar]

7. Srinivasan S. Some Questionable Drug Trials. 2005. Nov, [Last cited on2010 April]. Available from: URL http://infochangeindia.org/20051112276/Health/Features/Some-questionable-drug-trials.html .
8. New Delhi: Indian Council of Medical Research; 2006. Ethical Guidelines for Biomedical Research on Human Subjects. [Google Scholar]
9. Kher S. Informed Consent Process: Protecting Subjects Rights. In: Gupta SK, editor. Basic Principles of Clinical Research and Methodology. 1st ed. New Delhi: Jaypee Brothers; 2007. pp. 93–105. [Google Scholar]
10. Melo-Martín I, Ho A. Beyond informed consent: The therapeutic misconception and trust. J Med Ethics. 2008;34:202–5. [PubMed] [Google Scholar]
11. Charles W, Paul S. The Therapeutic Misconception: Problems and Solutions. Med Care. 2002;40:55–63. [PubMed] [Google Scholar]
12. Zong Z. Should post-trial provision of beneficial experimental interventions be mandatory in developing countries? J Med Ethics. 2008;34:188–92. [PubMed] [Google Scholar]
13. Operational Guidelines for Ethics Committees that Review Biomedical Research. Geneva: World Health Organization; 2000. World Health Organization. [Google Scholar]

Chapter 14

Composition, Role and Responsibilities of Institutional Ethics Committee (IEC) in Clinical Trials

LEARNING OBJECTIVES

To understand

- Introduction
- Historical Events
- Composition and responsibilities of IEC
- Functions of IEC
- Record Keeping and Archiving

Introduction

As per the WHO definition, a clinical trial is any research study that prospectively assigns human participants to one or more health related interventions to evaluate the effects on health outcome.

Ethics are concerned with the distinction between Right and Wrong, with moral choices, duties and obligations.

The four main principles of Ethical research are:

1. Autonomy.
2. Non-maleficence.
3. Beneficence.
4. Justice.

Historical Events

Institutional Ethics Committee (IEC) is the committee formed of a group of people who go through the research protocol / proposal and state whether it is ethically acceptable. Looking into the history, ethics in medical practice were addressed in Charaka Samhita in 1600 BC which mentions the code of ethical conduct and also by Hippocrates in 600 AD. In first half of 20th century many medicines, vaccines were developed, based on trials on captive groups and prisoners without their consent with no concern for their health & welfare. Several unfortunate things occurred throughout the world like Nazi War Crimes during World War II where studies were done on prisoners at Nazi Concentration camps. After that in 1946 all Nazi doctors were trialed before international tribunal and also mishaps like the Tuskegee Syphilis Experiment 1932-1972 by U.S. Public Health Service where 399 African-American men in Alabama were experimented for Syphilis necessitated the need for and numerous codes of ethics which were:

1947 – Nuremberg Code of Medical Ethics.

1948 – Universal Human Rights – United Nations.

1956 – Code of Medical Ethics-Medical Council of India

1964 – Declaration of Helsinki. Last revision in 2008 at Seoul, Korea by WMA.

1974 – Belmont Report by National Commission by US, PHS.

1980 – Policy Statement on Ethical Consideration involved in Research on Human Subjects ICMR.

1982 – Proposed International guidelines for Biomedical Research involving Human Subjects-WHO & CIOMS

1991 – International Guidelines for Ethical Review in Epidemiological Studies by CIOMS.

1996 – ICH – GCP Guidelines.

2001 – Directorate of Health Services, Government of India published GCP.

2001 – European Union Directive, 2004- revised.

2006 – Ethical Guidelines for Biomedical Research on Human Participants published by ICMR.

ICMR Code is the statement of Ethical Guidelines for Biomedical Research on Human Participants. These Statements of General and Specific Principles may be varied, amended, substituted and added from time to time.

To safeguard the welfare and the rights of the participants it is mandatory that all proposals on biomedical research involving human participants should be cleared by an appropriately constituted Institutional Ethics Committee (IEC). This is also referred to as Institutional Review Board (IRB).

Composition and responsibilities of IEC:

Institutional Head constitutes an IEC and it is independent, competent and multidisciplinary unit. The number of persons are fairly small. The IEC appoints from among its members a chairperson who should be from outside the Institution and not head of the same Institution, and the Member Secretary from the same Institution who conducts the business of the committee. Members of IEC are:

1. Chairperson.
2. One to two persons from basic medical science.
3. One to two clinicians from various Institutes.
4. One legal expert or retired judge.
5. One social scientist/ representative of non-governmental voluntary agency.
6. One philosopher/ ethicist/ theologian.
7. One lay person from the community.
8. Member Secretary.

The Quorum (i.e. the minimum number of people required to conduct a meeting) has 5 persons minimum. As per revised Schedule Y of Drugs & Cosmetics Act, 1940 which is amended in 2005, they should be as:

1. One basic medical scientist (pharmacologist).
2. One clinician.
3. One legal expert or retired judge.
4. One social scientist/ representative of non-governmental organization/Philosopher/ ethicist/ theologian or a similar person.
5. One lay person from the community.

The members work to safeguard the interests and welfare of all sections of the community. If required, subject experts could be invited to offer their views like a paediatrician for pediatric conditions, a cardiologist for cardiac disorders etc. IEC has its own Standard Operating Procedures (SOPs) according to which it functions. These SOPs are updated periodically, and these ensure smooth functioning also. An IEC must preferably be registered at the National Biomedical Research Authority as per the Bill passed in 2007.

Responsibilities of IEC are to protect the dignity, rights and well-being of the potential research participants, to ensure that universal ethical values and international scientific standards are expressed and to assist in the development and the education of a research community responsive to local health care requirements

Functions of IEC:

The IEC's member-secretary screens the research proposals for their completeness and depending on the risk involved categorize them into 3 types:

1) Exemption from review for proposals that involve less than minimal risk.
2) Expedited review for more than minimal risk proposals, minor protocol amendments, research on disaster management, and research on material collected during routine patient care like CT scans.
3) Full review for more than minimal risk and that involve vulnerable subjects.

The ethical review should be done in formal meetings by all primary reviewers and decision is made only when quorum complete. The committee should meet at regular intervals and should not keep a decision pending for more than 3-6 months. Periodic reviews are done as per the SOPs. All the decisions are communicated in writing to the principal investigator (PI). Members should be encouraged to attend trainings so that they are aware of all new guidelines and developments. lements of review are:

- Scientific design, conduct of the study and approval of review committees.
- Examination of predictable risks and potential benefits.
- Procedure for selection of subjects including inclusion/exclusion, withdrawal criteria and other issues like advertisement details.
- Management of research related injuries, adverse events and compensation.
- Justification for placebo and availability of products after the study.
- Patient information sheet and informed consent form in local language.
- Protection of privacy and confidentiality.
- Plans for data analysis and reporting.
- Adherence to all regulatory requirements and applicable guidelines.
- Competence of investigators, research and supporting staff, and facilities.
- Criteria for withdrawal of patients, suspending or terminating the study.

Record Keeping and Archiving

All documentation & communication of an IEC are dated, filed and preserved up to minimum of three years after completion/termination of the study and strict confidentiality maintained during access and retrieval procedures.

All institutions which carry out any form of biomedical research involving human beings should establish an appropriate IEC that is consistent with international and local guidelines and regulations. They must follow ICMR guidelines in India to protect safety and well-being of all participants and should prevent unethical research.

Chapter 15

Regulatory Environment in US, India and Europe

LEARNING OBJECTIVES

To understand

- Regulatory Environment in US
- Regulatory Authority: U.S – FDA
- USFDA Guidelines for Clinical Research
- Synthesis and Purification
  (Pre-Clinical Research, Animal Testing, Short-Term Testing, Long-Term Testing, Animal Pharmacology and Toxicology Studies)
- Manufacturing Information
- Clinical Protocols and Investigator Information
- Sponsor/FDA Meetings (Pre-IND)
  (Phase 1 Clinical Studies, Phase 2 Clinical Studies, Phase 3 Clinical Studies)
- New Drug Application (NDA)
- Phase 4 Clinical Trials (Post-Marketing Surveillance)
- REGULATORY ENVIRONMENT IN INDIA
- Regulatory Authority: INDIA - CDSCO
- Drug Technical Advisory Board (DTAB)
- Drugs Consultative Committee
- Genetic Engineering Approval Committee (GEAC)
- Clinical trials Guidelines in India
- SCHEDULE Y (Revised-2005) of Drugs and Cosmetics Act, 1940
- Protocol amendments have been classified into three categories
- Ethical Guidelines for Biomedical Research on Human Subjects, 2006
- Biomedical Research Good Clinical Practices, 2001
- REGULATORY AUTHORITY IN EUROPE
  (Regulatory Authority: EUROPE – EMEA, National Authorization Procedures, Decentralized Procedure, Good Clinical Practice - Human Medicinal Products.
- GCP Inspectors Working Group)

Regulatory Environment in US

Regulatory Authority: U.S - FDA

Introduction

The U.S. Food and Drug Administration (FDA or USFDA) is an agency of the United States Department of Health and Human Services and is responsible for regulating and supervising the safety of foods, dietary supplements, drugs, vaccines, biological medical products, blood products, medical devices, radiation-emitting devices, veterinary products, and cosmetics.

The FDA also enforces section 361 of the Public Health Service Act and the associated regulations, including sanitation requirements on interstate travel as well as specific rules for control of disease on products ranging from pet turtles to semen donations for assisted reproductive medicine techniques.

The FDA is an agency within the United States Department of Health and Human Services responsible for protecting and promoting the nation's public health. The FDA is headquartered in Rockville, supported by 13 laboratories located throughout the United States.

The agency is organized into the following major subdivisions, each focused on a major area of regulatory responsibility:

- The Office of the Commissioner (OC)
- The Center for Drug Evaluation and Research (CDER)
- The Center for Biologics Evaluation and Research (CBER)
- The Center for Food Safety and Applied Nutrition (CFSAN)
- The Center for Devices and Radiological Health (CDRH)
- The Center for Veterinary Medicine (CVM)
- The National Center for Toxicological Research (NCTR)
- The Office of Regulatory Affairs (ORA)

The FDA works in conjunction with other Federal agencies by including the Department of Agriculture, Drug Enforcement Administration, Customs and Border Protection, and Consumer Product Safety Commission. The local and state government agencies also work in cooperation with the FDA to provide regulatory inspections and enforcement action.

USFDA Guidelines for Clinical Research

The CDER was developed to prnaviovide a user-friendly resource for obtaining information on the Centre's processes and activities of interest to regulated industry, health professionals, academia, and the general public.

The mission of FDA's Center for Drug Evaluation and Research is to assure that safe and effective drugs are available to the American people.

The CDER Center is involved in 4 important activities like:

- ✓ New Drug Review
- ✓ Generic Drug Review
- ✓ Over-the-Counter Drug Review
- ✓ Post Drug Approval Activities.
- ✓ Post Drug Approval Activities.

New drugs receive extensive scrutiny before FDA approval in a process called a New Drug Application or NDA. New drugs are available only by prescription by default. A change to Over the Counter (OTC) status is a separate process and the drug must be approved through an NDA first.

Synthesis and Purification

The research process is complicated, time Guaranteed. FDA estimates that it takes approximately eight test a new drug be forfeit can be approved for the general public.

This estimate includes early lab human subjects.

Pre-Clinical Research

Under FDA requirements, a sponsor must first submit data showing reasonably safe for use in initial, small-scale clinical studies.

The sponsor may have several options for fulfilling this requirements:

(1) Compiling existing nonclinical data from past in vitro laboratory or animal compound;

(2) Compiling data from previous clinical testing or marketing of the States or another country whose population is relevant to the U.S. population;

(3) Undertaking new preclinical studies designed to provide the evidence necessary to support the safety of administering the compound to humans

During preclinical drug development, a sponsor evaluates the drug's toxic and pharmacologic effects through in vitro and in vivo laboratory animal testing. Genotoxicity screening is performed, as well as investigations on drug absorption and metabolism.

At the preclinical stage, the FDA will generally ask, at a minimum that sponsors:

- Develop a pharmacological profile of the drug.
- Determine the acute toxicity of the drug in at least two species of animals.
- Conduct short-term toxicity studies ranging from 2 weeks to3 months depending on the proposed duration of use of the substance in the proposed clinical studies

Animal Testing

In animal testing, drug companies make every effort to use as few animals as possible and to ensure their humane and proper care. Generally, two or more species (one Rodent, one Non-rodent) are tested because a drug may affect one species differently from another.

Animal testing is used to measure how much of a drug is absorbed into the blood, how it is broken down chemically in the body, the toxicity of the drug and its breakdown products (metabolites), and how quickly the drug and its metabolites are excreted from the body.

Short-Term Testing: Testing in animals ranges in duration from 2 weeks to 3 months, depending on the proposed use of the substance.

Long-Term Testing: Testing in animals ranges in duration from a few weeks to several years. Some animal testing continues after human tests begin to learn whether long-term use of a drug may cause cancer or birth defects.

Much of this information is submitted to FDA when a sponsor requests to proceed with human clinical trials. The FDA reviews the preclinical research data and then makes a decision as to whether to allow the clinical trials to proceed.

After the completion of preclinical testing, the company/sponsor files and IND (Investigational New Drug Application) with the data begin to test the drug in humans. It is the means through which sponsor obtain the legal status to call its new investigational molecule as new drug

Generally, this includes data and information in three broad areas:

Animal Pharmacology and Toxicology Studies

Preclinical data to permit an assessment as to whether the product is reasonably safe for initial testing in humans.

Manufacturing Information

Information pertaining to the composition, manufacture, stability, and controls used for manufacturing the drug substance and the drug product.

This information is assessed as to ensure the company can adequately produce and supply consistent batches of the drug.

Clinical Protocols and Investigator Information

Detailed protocols for proposed clinical studies to assess whether the initial-phase trials will expose subjects to unnecessary risks.

Medical review, Chemistry review, Pharmacology/ Toxicology review, Safety review are carried out on the IND application.

Pharmacology and Drug Distribution are carried according to 21CFR 312. 23(a)(8)(I) rules

Toxicology Data regulations are carried according to 21 CFR312.23(a)(8)(ii)(a) rules

The IND becomes effective if FDA does not disapprove it within30 days.

Sponsor/FDA Meetings (Pre-IND)

Prior to clinical studies, the sponsor needs evidence that the compound is biologically active, and both the sponsor and the FDA need data showing that the drug is reasonably safe for initial administration to humans

Phase 1 Clinical Studies:

Phase 1 includes the initial introduction of an investigational new drug into humans. These studies are closely monitored and conducted in healthy volunteer subjects.

These studies are designed to determine the metabolic and pharmacologic actions of the drug in humans, the side effects associated with increasing doses, and, if possible, to gain early evidence on effectiveness. Phase 1 studies also evaluate drug metabolism, structure-activity relationships, and the Mechanism of action in humans.

During Phase 1, sufficient information about the drug's pharmacokinetics and pharmacological effects should be obtained to permit the design of well-controlled, scientifically valid, Phase 2studies.

Phase 2 Clinical Studies:

Phase 2 includes the early controlled clinical studies conducted to obtain some preliminary data on the effectiveness of the drug for a particular indication or indications in patients with the disease or condition.

This phase of testing helps determine the common short-term side effects and risks associated with the drug. Phase 2 studies are typically well-controlled, closely monitored, and conducted in a relatively small number of patients, usually involving several hundred people. Phase 2 studies lasts from six months to two years.

Phase 3 Clinical Studies:

Phase 3 studies are expanded controlled and uncontrolled trials. They are performed after preliminary evidence suggesting effectiveness of the drug has been obtained in Phase 2, and are intended to gather the additional information about effectiveness and safety that is needed to evaluate the overall benefit-risk relationship of the drug. Phase 3 studies also provide an adequate basis for extrapolating the results to the general population and transmitting that information in the physician labeling. Phase 3 studies usually include several hundred to several thousand people.

New Drug Application (NDA)

An NDA is an application submitted to the USFDA for permission to market a new drug product in the United States. To obtain this permission, company/sponsor submits an NDA form along with nonclinical and clinical test data and analyses, drug information and description of manufacturing procedures.

As outlined in Form FDA-356h, ***Application to Market a New Drug for Human Use*** NDAs can consist of as many as 15 different sections:

- ✓ Index;
- ✓ Summary;
- ✓ Chemistry, Manufacturing, and Control;
- ✓ Samples, Methods Validation Package, and Labelling;
- ✓ Nonclinical Pharmacology and Toxicology;
- ✓ Human Pharmacokinetics and Bioavailability;
- ✓ Microbiology (for anti-microbial drugs only);
- ✓ Clinical Data;
- ✓ Safety Update Report (typically submitted 120 days after theNDA's submission);
- ✓ Statistical;
- ✓ Case Report Tabulations;
- ✓ Case Report Forms;
- ✓ Patent Information;
- ✓ Patent Certification; and
- ✓ Other Information

After a NDA is received by the FDA, it undergoes a technical screening generally referred to as a completeness review. At the conclusion of FDA review, there are three possible action letters that can be sent to the sponsor:

Not Approvable Letter: Lists of deficiencies in the application and reasons why the application cannot be approved.

Approvable Letter: The drug can be approved, with the list of minor deficiencies that can be corrected.

Approval Letter: The drug is approved. It can be issued directly, or it may follow an approvable letter

Phase 4 Clinical Trials (Post-Marketing Surveillance):

Sometimes adverse drug effects of drug come after the drug has been in the market for a long time or been used by very large number of patients. Phase IV clinical trials mainly aim at identifying such problems. Withdrawal of a drug from the mark done based on the results of Phase IV clinical trials

REGULATORY ENVIRONMENT IN INDIA

Regulatory Authority: INDIA - CDSCO

Introduction

Drug Controller General of India (DCGI) under central drug standard control organization (CDSCO) has prime responsibility for regulating clinical trial in India.

Two drug organizations are functioning in India to exercise control over drugs:

➢ Central drug standard control organization (CDSCO)

➢ State drug control organizations

It is the sovereign function of the government to ensure safety, efficacy and quality of drugs supplied to the public. This function is performed by the **Central Drugs Standard Control Organization (CDSCO).**

The role of CDSCO in early stages of drug development is minimal but it becomes more pronounced consequent to the lead obtained from animal pharmacology and toxicological studies and the need for its further testing on humans. The requirements of data submission on animal testing for permission to undertake Phase l, Phase II and Phase Ill clinical trials are laid down in Schedule Y of Drugs & Cosmetics rules.

Central drug standard control organization of the government of India is headed by the drugs controller general (India). The prime responsibilities of this organization are:

✓ Controlling the quality of imported drugs;

✓ Coordinating their activities of the states and advising them on matters relating to the uniform administration of the Act in the country.

✓ Laying down rules and ancillary provisions of drug control and standards of drugs;

✓ Controlling the quality of drugs moving in inter-state commerce jointly with state drug control organizations;

✓ Granting approval to "New Drugs" proposed to be imported manufactured in the country;

✓ Controlling the quality of drugs which are exported from India;

✓ To regulate clinical research in India.

✓ Testing of drugs by Central Drugs Labs.

✓ To approve licenses to manufacture certain categories of drugs as Central License

✓ Approving Authority i.e. for Blood Banks, Large volume parenteral and vaccines & Sera.

✓ Monitoring adverse drug reactions (ADR)

✓ Arranging meetings of the two statutory bodies, namely the Drugs Technical advisory board (DTAB) and the drug consultative committee and also processing all matters connected with their functioning.

Drug Technical Advisory Board (DTAB)

It has technical experts and advises the central and state governments on all technical matters arising out of the enforcement of drug control. No rules can be made by the central government without consulting this board.

Drugs Consultative Committee:

It has the central and state drug control officials as members, and its main function is to ensure that the drug control measures are enforced uniformly in all states.

Genetic Engineering Approval Committee (GEAC):

It is authority to approve rDNA pharmaceutical products. GEAC's role is to assess the bio-safety/environmental safety aspect of the biotechnological products.

Other Functions:

- Guidance on technical matters
- Publication of Indian Pharmacopoeia
- Screening of drug formulations available in Indian market
- Participation in the WHO GMP certification scheme
- Coordinating the activities of the State Drugs Control Organizations to achieve uniform administration of the Act; and policy guidance.

Clinical trials Guidelines in India:

The guidelines that govern the conduct of clinical trials in India include:

- Schedule Y (Revised-2005) of Drugs and Cosmetics Act, 1940
- Ethical Guidelines for Biomedical Research on Human Subjects, 2006
- Good Clinical Practices, 2001

SCHEDULE Y (Revised-2005) of Drugs and Cosmetics Act, 1940

[See rules 122A, 122B, 122D, 122DA, 122DAA and 122E]

- Rule 122 A - Permission to import new drug
- Rule 122 B - Permission to manufacture new drug
- Rule 122 DA - Definition of Clinical trials
- Rule 122 E - Definition of New Drugs*

The requirements and guidelines for permission to import and /or Manufacture of New Drugs for sale or to undertake clinical trials.

122-DAA Definition of Clinical trial: "Clinical trial" means a systematic study of new drug(s) in human subject(s) to generate data for discovering and / or verifying the clinical, pharmacological (including pharmacodynamic and pharmacokinetic) and/or adverse effects with the objective of determining safety and / or efficacy of the new drug. "

Application for the permission of carrying out a clinical trial in India is made to the office of DCGI. General recommendations carrying out clinical trials in India as specified in

Schedule Y

Regulations under schedule Y are as follows

- The requirements for carrying out clinical trials in India before a new drug is approved for marketing depend upon the status of drug in other countries.
- For new drugs approved outside India, Phase-3 trials are required to be conducted in India before permission to market the drug in India is granted. Prior to conduct of Phase-3 studies in India subjects, Licensing Authority may require pharmacokinetic studies to be undertaken to verify that data generated in India population is in conformity with data already generated abroad.
- For new drug substances discovered in India, clinical trials are required to be carried out in India right from phase-I. For new drugs substances discovered in countries other than India, phase-I data should be submitted along with the application. After submission of phase-I data generated outside India to the licensing authority, permission may be granted to repeat phase-I trials and/or to conduct phase-2 trials and subsequently phase-2 trials concurrently with other global trials for that drug.
- Application for permission to import or manufacture new drugs for sale or to undertake clinical trials shall be made in "Form 44 format.
- If the study drug is intended to be imported for the purposes of examination, test or analysis, the application for import of small quantities of drugs for such purpose should also be made in Form 12.
- For drugs indicated in life threatening / serious diseases or diseases of special relevance to the Indian health scenario, the toxicological and clinical data requirements may be abbreviated, deferred or omitted, as deemed appropriate by the Licensing Authority.
- Laboratories used for generating data for clinical trials should be compliant with Good Laboratory Practices (GCP).
- In case of studies prematurely discontinued for any reason a summary report (in specified format) should be submitted within 3 months.
- Any unexpected serious adverse event (SAE) occurring during a clinical trial should be communicated promptly (with in 14 calendar days) by sponsor to the licensing authority and to other investigator(s) participating in the study (appendix-0 9).
- The investigator has to give an undertaking on GCP compliance as per the format specified in appendix -7.
- The investigator has to report all serious and unexpected adverse events to the sponsor within 24 hours and to the Ethics committee within 7 working days of their occurrence.
- Ethics committee should have written standard operating procedures and should maintain a record of its proceedings. In case an ethics committee revokes its approval accorded to

a trial protocol, it must record the reasons for doing so and at once communicate such a decision to the investigator as well as to the licensing authority.

- Geriatric patients should be included in phase-3 clinical trials if the disease intended to be treated is characteristically a disease of aging or when the new drug is likely to the geriatric patient's response compared with that the non- geriatric patient.
- Paediatric subjects are legally unable to provide written informed consent and are dependent on their patient(s)/legal guardian to assume responsibility for participation in clinical studies.
- Subsequent to approval of the product, new drugs should be closely monitored for their clinical safety once they are marketed.
- The Periodic Safety Update Reports (PSURs) shall be submitted every six months for the first two years after approval of the drug is granted to the applicant.
- For subsequent two years PSURs need to be submitted annually.
- Licensing authority may extend the total duration of submission of PSURs if it is considered necessary in the submission of PSURs if it is considered necessary in the interest of public health.
- PSURs due for a period must be submitted within 30 calendar days of the last day of the reporting period.

The global clinical trials are classified into 2 categories on their approval duration:

Category A and Category B

Category A: Clinical trials approved by USA, 0K, Switzerland, Australia, Canada, Germany, South Africa, Japan, and EMEA. DCGI will grant the approved within2-4 weeks.

Category B: Clinical trials approved by other countries not listed under category

A. Regulatory turnaround time would be approx 8-12 weeks.

Protocol amendments have been classified into three categories:

1. Those amendments which do permission, been classified into three not require any information or

   a. Administrative and logistic changes

   b. Minor protocol amendments and additional safety assessments in case the IEC

2. Those amendments which require being informed but need not wait for permission,

   a. Additional investigator sites

   b. Amended investigator's brochure, amended ICD

3. Those amendments which require prior permission before implementation of the amendments,

   a. Changes of principal investigator

b. Additional patients to be recruited

c. Major changes in the protocol with respect to the study design,

*Clinical trial on a new drug shall be initiated only after the permission has been granted by the licensing authority under rule 21 (b), and the approval obtained from the respective ethics committee.

Appendices: Provide a study synopsis, copies of the informed consent documents (patient information sheet, informed consent form etc.); CRF and other data collection forms; a summary of relevant pre-clinical safety information and any other documents referenced in the clinical protocol. has already approved these changes.

APPENDIX I

Data to be submitted along with the application to conduct clinical trials / Import / manufacture of new drugs for marketing in the country

1. Introduction
2. Chemical and pharmaceutical information
3. Animal Pharmacology (refer Appendix 'V)
4. Animal Toxicology (refer Appendix Ill)
5. Human I Clinical pharmacology (Phase l)
6. Therapeutic exploratory trials (Phase II)
7. Therapeutic confirmatory trials (Phase Ill)
8. Special studies
9. Regulatory status in other countries
10. Prescribing information
11. Samples & testing protocol

APPENDIX I-A

Data required to be submitted by an applicant for grant of permission to import and / or manufacture a new drug already approved in the country.

1. Introduction
2. Chemical and pharmaceutical information
3. Marketing information
4. Special studies conducted with approval of Licensing Authority

Appendix II

Structure, contents and format for clinical study reports

Appendix III

Animal toxicology (non-clinical toxicity studies)

Appendix IV

Animal pharmacology

Appendix V

Informed consent

Appendix VI

Fixed dose combinations (fdcs)

Appendix VII

Undertaking by the investigator

Appendix VIII

Ethics Committee

Appendix IX

Stability testing of new drugs

Appendix X

Contents of the proposed protocol for conducting clinical trials

Appendix XI

Data Elements for reporting serious adverse events occurring in a clinical trial

Ethical Guidelines for Biomedical Research on Human Subjects, 2006:

The Indian Council of Medical research brought out the 'Policy Statement on Ethical Considerations involved in Research on Human Subjects' in 1980 and revised these guidelines in 2000 as the 'Ethical guidelines for Biomedical Research on Human subjects'.

This statement of Ethical Guidelines for Biomedical Research on Human Participants shall be known as the ICMR Code and shall consist of the following:-

(a) Statement of General Principles on Research using Human Participants in Biomedical Research

(b) Statement of Specific Principles on Research using Human Participants in specific areas of

Biomedical Research Good Clinical Practices, 2001

Good clinical practice is a set of guidelines for bio medical studies which encompasses the design, conduct, termination, audit, analysis, reporting and documentation of the studies involving human subjects.

REGULATORY AUTHORITY IN EUROPE

Regulatory Authority: EUROPE – EMEA

Introduction:

Regulatory Authority in Europe is **European Medicines Agency (EMEA)**. The European Medicines Agency relies on the results of clinical trials carried out by pharmaceutical companies to reach its opinions on the authorization of medicines. Although the authorization of clinical trials occurs at Member State level, the Agency plays a key role in ensuring that the standards of good clinical practice (GCP) are applied across the European Economic Area (EEA) in cooperation with the Member States. It also manages a database of clinical trials carried out in the European Union.

EMEA

- The European Medicines Agency (EMEA) is a decentralized body of the European Union with headquarters in London
- Medicines can be authorized in the European Union by using either the centralized authorization procedure or national authorization procedures.
- The centralized procedure (also known as the 'Community authorization procedure'). This procedure results in a single marketing authorization (called a 'Community marketing authorization') that is valid across the European Union, as well as in the states Iceland. Liechtenstein and Norway.
- The centralized procedure is compulsory for human medicines that are:
  - Derived from biotechnology processes, such as genetic engineering
  - Intended for the treatment of HIV Aids, cancer, diabetes, neurodegenerative disorders or autoimmune diseases and other immune dysfunctions
  - Officially designated 'orphan medicines' (medicines used for rare diseases)
- For medicines that do not fall within these categories (the 'mandatory scope'), companies have the option of submitting an application for a centralized marketing authorization to the EMEA, as long as the medicine concerned is a significant therapeutic, scientific or technical innovation, or if its authorization would be in the interest of public health
- Applications through the centralized procedure are submitted directly to the EMEA. Evaluation by the Agency's relevant scientific committee takes up to 210 days, at the end of which the committee adopts an opinion on whether the medicine should be marketed or not. This opinion is then transmitted to the European Commission, which has the ultimate authority for making decisions on marketing authorizations in the EU
- Once a Community marketing authorization has been granted, the marketing-authorization holder can begin to make the medicine available to patients and healthcare professionals in all EU countries.

National Authorization Procedures

- Each EU Member State has its own procedures for the authorization, within their own territory, of medicinal products that fall outside the scope of the centralized procedure Information about these national procedures can normally be found on the website of the national competent authority in the country concerned.
- The Heads of Agencies website is a useful entry point for such information
- However, there are also two possible routes available to companies for the authorization of such medicinal products in several countries simultaneously:

a. Decentralized Procedure:

- Using the decentralized procedure, companies may apply for simultaneous authorization in more than one EU country of medicinal products that have not yet been authorized in any EU country and that do not fall within the mandatory scope of the centralized procedure

b. Mutual-recognition procedure:

- In the mutual-recognition procedure, a medicine is first authorized in one EU Member State, in accordance with the national procedures of that country

- Following this, further marketing authorizations can be sought from other EU countries in a procedure whereby the countries concerned agree to recognize the validity of the original, national marketing authorization
- **Good Clinical Practice - Human Medicinal Products**

- Requirements for the conduct of clinical trials in the EU, including GCP and GMP and inspections of these, have been implemented in the Clinical Trial Directive (Directive 2001/20/EC) and the GCP Directive (2005/28/EC)
- Clinical trials included in marketing authorization applications in the European Economic Area (EEA)are required to be conducted in accordance with GCP (Directive 2001/83/EC Annex l, as amended by Directive 2003/63/EC)
- Volume 10, Clinical Trials, of the Rules Governing Medicinal Products in the European Union, brings together information on clinical trial authorization, safety monitoring, GCP inspections and GCP and GMP requirements for clinical trials in the EEA
- Europe has adopted the ICH-GCP in July 1996 and this is published also on the EMEA website (ICH has developed unified standards for Europe, US and Japan)

- **GCP Inspectors Working Group:**

- The Sector draws on the expertise of member states' inspectorates for the fulfilment of many of its GCP related tasks. This is primarily achieved through the GCP Inspectors Working Group

- The GCP Inspectors Working Group meets on a regular basis four times a year, at EMEA with representatives of the GCP inspectorates of the European Economic Area Member States, observers from candidate countries and Switzerland
- The GCP Inspectors Working Group has developed procedures for the coordination, preparation, conduct and reporting of GCP inspections carried out in the context of the Centralized Procedure.

Chapter 16

Role and Responsibilities of Clinical Trial Personnel as per GCP

LEARNING OBJECTIVES

To understand

- Contract Research Organizations (CRO's)
- Role and responsibilities of various bodies and personnel involved in clinical trials
- Assuring Quality and Compliance
- The Large Back Room
- Clinical Research Associate
- Job Summary
- Auditors Roles and Responsibilities
- Types of Audits
  (Investigational sites audits, Clinical department process audits, Data management audits, Safety department audits, GCP laboratory audits, Sponsor central file audits)

Introduction

Clinical trials are integral to the development of new medicines, diagnostics, and medical devices. Because there is no other way to demonstrate the effectiveness and safety of new therapeutic modalities for human use or their equivalence or superiority over existing therapy, regulatory authorities require a series of clinical trials to be conducted and their results analyzed before a new treatment can be introduced for general consumption. Every claim that is made in the package insert of a pharmaceutical product must be backed up with evidence from clinical trials. Consequently, clinical trials account for almost 60% of the time and resources required to bring a new drug to market.[1]Yet most of this investment is wasted, because over 80% of new products tested in clinical trials fail to live up to the promise of improvement over existing therapy, and therefore have to be abandoned.

Indeed, the explosive growth of life science technologies juxtaposed with the growing complexity of the science behind discovery and development of new medicines have led to a situation where, despite the plethora of new leads, the conventional research pathway in the developed world has become too expensive and increasingly unaffordable, even for the largest corporate entities.[2]The lower cost of research talent in developing countries, the larger size of study populations in countries like China and India, and the fact that the pharmaceutical markets in these countries is now approaching the size of historically large markets of Europe and North America, are driving pharmaceutical research to developing countries. In India this trend is further accentuated by public health investments being made by nonprofit organizations and investments in drug development research by the local industry. Indeed, given the fact that India is home to the world's highest disease burden in absolute terms,[3] it is imperative that the country take steps to combat that burden through prowess in the development of break through health care products.

CONTRACT RESEARCH ORGANIZATIONS (CRO's)

The early part of the last decades unsubstantial growth of clinical research capability. Many local and multinational companies set up clinical development units in the country,[4]as did several nonprofit entities and publicly funded research bodies under the Department of Biotechnology and the Indian Council of Medical Research. These units were supplemented by contract research organizations (CROs) companies with specific specialization in the execution of research for the development of health care products. Today there are a variety of CROs operating in India from those involved in discovery research to those specializing in the various aspects of preclinical and clinical research. The clinical CROs are the most numerous because entry barriers are relatively low.

A contract research organization (CRO) is an organization that extends services to the medical device, biotechnology and pharmaceutical companies in the form of expertise in research outsourced on a contract model. A contract research organization may extend such helping hand in biopharmaceutical development, clinical research endeavors, clinical trials conduct, product commercialization, biologic assay development and pharmacovigilance. Contract research organization also extend their services to governmental institutes, foundations, traditional universities in addition to research institutions.

Many CROs entirely provide support with respect to clinical-study conduct for drugs and medical device companies. CROs vary from large, international comprehensive service providers to small, forte specific subject groups. CROs that concentrate on clinical-trials related services can extend their customers the expertise of endorsing a new treatment regime or health care device from its beginning to commercialization, without the sponsor employing the staff for these activities. Though the budgets are thoroughly controlled by the sponsor it is left to the CRO to plan their tasks to ensure trials are carried out tightly sticking to the time lines and to instil confidence in the sponsor and also among each other.

Well-placed and optimally paced mission management will be a certainty when there are explicit requisites enlisted by the sponsor to contract research organization and this will lessen the threat of belated outcomes and subsequently reduce the likelihood of study time lines being failed to spot.

A CRO is thoroughly skilled in handling complex drug development programs demanding new regulatory and clinical approaches and will have know-how in implementing and realizing successful completion of novel drug development.

Clinical CROs undertake execution of clinical projects on behalf of a sponsor. This practice is good for sponsors because the skills necessary to execute a clinical trial are very specific and divorced from the basic research, manufacturing, and marketing competencies that sponsors may have. For smaller sponsors who have a single or small number of products to develop, this partnership ensures that they do not have to hire an army of staff to execute a single project and then lay them off once the project is over. So, once an entrepreneur has translated an original scientific idea into a molecule that can combat disease and has put it through the animal tests required to prove that it can be given to patients without unacceptable safety risks, a CRO can be hired to conduct the clinical trials that will be required to collect the data necessary to define the use of the product by patients. CROs are generally capable of doing the rest, which includes preparing a clinical development plan, writing the clinical protocols, obtaining regulatory approvals to conduct clinical trials, contacting health care practitioners to recruit patients into the study using informed consent procedures approved by an ethics committee, ensuring meticulous documentation of the effects of the drug when administered according to the protocol, collecting and analyzing the data, and writing a final report for regulatory submission.

Role and responsibilities of various bodies and personnel involved in clinical trials:

Parties to a Clinical Trial	The role of various bodies involved in the Clinical Trial Process
Sponsor	Discovers, funds, and develops new therapies from bench to bedside. Has commercial incentives to ensure appropriate funding and progress of each project. Has high stakes in the accuracy and validity of data. Bearshigh reputational risk and financial penalties for misconduct.
Regulator	Reviews protocols and data to ensure compliance to regulations and ethical guidelines for each trial at the national level. Conducts inspections to monitor compliance.
Contract research organization	Coordinates the conduct of clinical trials across sites, countries, and regions. Reviews data to ensure accuracy and eliminate fraud. Organizes and analyses data for reporting and submission toregulators.
Investigator	Supervises the informed consent and patient recruitment process, is responsible for care and well-being of patients and compliance to protocol, regulations, documentation.
Ethics committee	Reviews protocols and safety data to safeguard the rights and well-being of patients locally at the site level.
Data safety monitoring	Periodically reviews data to determine whether it is safe and

board	meaningful to continue with a trial. Recommends changes to the protocol to safeguard patient safety.
Site management organization	Coordinates clinical trial activities at the site level. Ensures appropriate documentation of all trial-related activities
Central laboratory	Used to ensure standardization for key laboratory tests, including pathology, imaging, and electrophysiological studies across multiple sites worldwide.

To accomplish these tasks a CRO usually has several departments of qualified and trained individuals: a regulatory department trained in the rules and regulations governing clinical trials; a site identification and start-up unit that maintains contact with health care professionals and institutions that may serve as investigators and sites for the study and ensures that these sites have the necessary infrastructure and staffing to undertake trials; a clinical operations group that works with the investigators at the site to train the team on the study protocol and ensure that the study is conducted in line with complex Good Clinical Practice[5]guidelines; a quality assurance department that conducts periodic audits of study to point out deficiencies if any and ensure that these are corrected and preventive measures put in place; amedical department to review medical aspects of the protocol and product safety; a data management group that is responsible for designing and commissioning electronic databases for the patient data that would emerge from the study; a biostatistics department that would analyze the data using scientific techniques; and a medical writing group that would prepare the final report in line with regulatory guidance's (**Table 1**).

Assuring Quality and Compliance

An important aspect of the CRO's role is to assure compliance to the myriad rules and regulations governing clinical trials. CROs do this by employing trained monitors (also called clinical research associates or CRAs) who frequently visit the sites and review the documentation at the sites to preclude fraud, ensure that informed consent procedures are followed, ensure that the data captured by the investigators are accurate and verifiable, and ensure that the study drugs are being stored and used in line with the protocol. Site staff often need to be trained on Good Clinical Practice guidelines and other aspects of managing trial activities at the site. In the past CROs have organized such training programs. More recently, public-private partnership initiatives have been put in place with active involvement of federal government agencies toward this end in order to build capacity in clinical development with particular focus on public healthinterventions.[6]

CROs often need to work with other third-party providers. One such is the site management organization, which provides trained staffing resources to guarantee quality of documentation at sites. For busy investigators this function can be the difference between research excellence and a critical audit observation. Many large hospitals set up their own site management department that keeps track of all clinical research activities being undertaken in the hospital and, for a fee, helps sponsors coordinate with investigators, the ethics committee, pathology and imaging departments, and the pharmacy-all within the hospital.

The central laboratory is another such provider. Use of a central laboratory for key laboratory tests, especially when such tests are part of the primary or secondary end-points being studied, ensures that the conduct of these tests is standardized across sites and patients and that accreditation and audit requirements can be applied to a single laboratory rather than a multiplicity of laboratories across sites.

Laboratories that participate as a central laboratory in clinical trials must consistently live up to expectations that go beyond what is usually required in the course of routine clinical care. Central laboratories can expect to receive samples for testing from diverse locations within the country and overseas. They therefore need to collaborate with a courier facility for smooth pick-up and dispatch of samples, with minimal sample miscarriage so that need for resampling is minimized, if not eliminated. This function requires thorough training of site teams on sample collection and storage. Reagents and sampling equipment must be shipped to sites before the start of the study and replenished in a timely manner. The central laboratory must have quicker testing turnaround time, when possible, to make up for time lost in sample transportation because clinicians are loath to have to wait longer for test results. The results themselves must be communicated back to the clinician by swift electronic means. Record-keeping and long-term record traceability are essential. Special foolproof systems are required to avoid sample mixups, and the laboratory must be open to audits and possible inspection by regulatory authorities. Participation in external quality control programs and advanced accreditations are now basic requirements. In India, certification by the National Accreditation Board for Testing and Calibration Laboratories is considered mandatory, and accreditation by the College of American Pathologists is highly desirable.

The Large Back Room

The backend activities of a CRO can be quite extensive. Electronic data capture systems must be programmed to receive data from the sites, a process of data triage and cleaning is necessary to ensure that the data entered into the database are internally consistent and complete. Data sets are then passed on to the biostatisticians who supervise programming of the statistical software and run the programs on the dataset received from the data managers. The tables, lists, and figures thus generated are passed on to the medical writers for preparation of the final report in the exhaustive ICH E3[7] format that is accepted across most of the world. The nonclinical work involved may account for as much as 40% (and sometimes more) of the effort involved in a clinical trial. India has now grown to become an important location for off-shoring such back end work in clinical data management, biostatistics, pharmacovigilance, and medical writing, employing more people than in the core clinical domain.

Clinical Research Associate

Job Summary

Responsible for creating, implementing, and maintaining clinical trials. Writes protocols, case report forms, and consent forms. Recruits and selects investigators and ensures good clinical practices are followed.

Roles and Responsibilities

- Design, implement, and monitor clinical trials.
- Prepare integrated medical reports, periodic reports, New Drug Applications (NDAs) and Biological License Applications (BLAs).
- Recruit and select new investigators.
- Ensure case report forms are reviewed and submitted in a timely manner.
- Contract research organizations and vendors.
- Design and write protocols.
- Create informed consent forms for trials.
- Monitor investigator performance and adherence to protocols.
- Address enrollment problems.
- Write integrated medical reports and clinical sections of INDs, IDEs, New Drug Applications (NDAs) and Biological License Applications (BLAs).
- Prepare and present documents of scientific meetings.
- Set up study centers and ensure each center has the trial materials.
- Visit the study centers throughout the trial on a regular basis.
- Check the patient data in the case report forms (CRFs).
- Validate and collect completed CRFs from hospitals and general practices.
- Discuss results with statistician.
- Close down study centers upon completion of trial.
- Write up reports after analysis has been completed.
- Verify that the rights and well-being of human subjects are protected.

* Ensure the conduct of the trial is in compliance with the currently approved protocol/amendment
* Verify that the investigator followed the approved protocol and all GCP procedures.

Auditors Roles and Responsibilities

Introduction

Audit is a systematic and independent examination of trial-related activities and documents to determine whether the evaluated trial related activities were conducted and the data were recorded, analyzed and accurately reported according to the protocol, sponsor's standard operating procedures (SOPs), good clinical practices(GCP),and the applicable regulatory requirements. Investigator sites, sponsor, CRO, ERB are liable to get audited.

The auditors are independent individuals appointed by sponsors/regulatory authorities to conduct a systematic and in depth examination of trial conducted, and compliance with protocol, SOPs, GCP, GLP, GPP and the applicable regulatory requirements. An audit is separate from routine monitoring or quality control functions.

The regulatory auditor is a suitably qualified employee of the FDA/DCGI/other regulatory bodies whose responsibility is to conduct announced or un announced inspection visits at clinical trial sites as required/instructed by the regulatory bodies. Most auditors visits are prearranged but some may not, especially where there is suspected serious breathes of the GCP or malpractices.

Types of Audits

Regulatory auditor is responsible to perform following types of audits

1. Investigational sites audits
2. Clinical department process audits
3. Data management audits
4. Safety department audits
5. GCP laboratory audits
6. Sponsor central file audits

1. Investigational Site Audits

These audits of study sites can be routine: to assess a site's performance; identify deficiencies and develop a corrective action plan; determine the sponsor's level of risk Audits can be conducted "for cause" that is, when the sponsor believes that a site is non-GCP compliant or is suspicious of investigator gross negligence or fraud.

2. Clinical Department Process Audits

The clinical research departments of clinical trials sponsoring companies and firms responsible for post marketing surveillance are being audited here. Reasons for conducting these audits are:

Potential for a regulatory inspection

Desire to improve effectiveness and efficiency

Benchmarking against other clinical departments

Satisfying concerns of upper level management

3. Data Management Audits

Sponsor companies and CRO's data management departments are being audited during these audits. Some of the objectives of these audits are to:

Compare data in data sets against data in CRFs

Review error programs and the query system

Assess treatment of outlier data

Review data transformation and imputation methods

Review file structure and merger of data sets check security and backup procedures

4. Safety Department Audits

Here auditors examine a sample of serious adverse events, either pre or post marketing for the following criteria:

Accuracy of reports and coding

Timelines of regulatory submission

Completeness and follow-up where necessary

Match with adverse event data

Thoroughness of analysis (signal and trend analysis)

Potential "hidden SAE" within the SAE

Down coding or down grading

Appropriate use of technology in processing events

The audits evaluate departmental processes and procedures with the objective of achieving regulatory and industry standards for making improvements.

5. GCP Laboratory Audits

Clinical, analytic, and reference laboratories often participate in clinical trials by processing blood, urine, and saliva samples. It is vitally important that test results are valid and accurately reported. Regulatory auditors examine data records and record keeping and transmittal procedures at these laboratories to determine if these data are accurate. In part, this review establishes that each sample for each patient is reported correctly. Thus auditor is responsible to establish that research was conducted under proper authority with sound scientific rationale, rights/safety/well-being of research subjects was protected and final study data supports the conclusions.

Thus auditor is responsible to establish that research was conducted under proper authority with sound scientific rationale, rights/safety/well-being of research subjects was protected and final study data supports the conclusions.

6. Sponsor Central File Audits

All inspection of sponsors, CROs are conducted without prior notification unless otherwise instructed by the assigning center.

Inspections are conducted to determine.

How sponsor assure to validity of data submitted to them by Clinical Investigator.

The adherence of sponsors to applicable regulations

Chapter 17

Designing of Clinical Study Documents and Informed Consent Process

LEARNING OBJECTIVES

To understand

- Investigator's Brochure (IB)
- Clinical Study Protocol
- Protocol Amendment
- Informed Consent
- Study Progress Reports
- Case Record Form (CRF)
- Informed Consent Process in Clinical Trials
- Informed Consent Procedure
- The Process of Informed Consent:
- Official Guidelines for Informed Consent
- Informed Consent Document Components
- Informed Consent Revisions

Introduction

A brief review of study essential documents that most often require translation during a clinical is given below.

The essential documents for clinical trials are the following:

- Investigator's Brochure
- Clinical Study Protocol
- Subject Information and Informed Consent Form

- Clinical Study Reports
- Case Report Form (CRF)

1. **INVESTIGATOR'S BROCHURE (IB):** Contains pre-clinical and clinical information related to an investigational drug. The information should be presented in a concise, simple, objective, balanced form that should be taken into account during translation.

   The Investigator's Brochure includes Title Page, which provides the Sponsor's name, the identity of investigational product (products), an edition number and date, and the number and date of the edition it supersedes as well. The Sponsor may wish to include a Confidentiality Statement instructing to treat the IB as a confidential document. A standard Investigator's Brochure usually includes the following sections:

   - List of Abbreviations
   - Contents
   - **Summary:** a brief description of significant physical, chemical and pharmaceutical properties of the investigational product, and also pharmacological, toxicological, pharmacokinetic, metabolic and therapeutic information that is relevant to the appropriate stage of clinical trial.
   - Introduction provides the chemical name (and generic and trade names, if approved) of the investigational product, all active components, pharmacological class, the rationale for performing further research with the investigational product and anticipated indications for its use. This section should provide the general approach to be followed in evaluating the investigational product.
   - Physical, chemical and pharmaceutical properties and formulation of the medicinal product.
   - **Non-clinical studies:** this section provides the data from animal studies regarding non-clinical pharmacological, pharmacokinetic, metabolic and toxicological characteristics of the investigational drug.
   - Clinical studies: this section provides information on pharmacokinetics, biotransformation, safety and efficacy in humans; data on post-marketing experience if the product under investigation has been already approved for use for other indications.
   - Conclusions and Guidance for the Investigator
   - References (the references should be provided at the end of each section)

   The Investigator's Brochure should be reviewed at least annually and revised as necessary in compliance with a standard procedure established by drug development company.

2. CLINICAL STUDY PROTOCOL: After the objectives and design of a clinical study have been determined, these issues should be documented in the Study Protocol. The Study Protocol is a document containing instructions for all the parties involved in the clinical trial that establish specific objectives for each participant and provide guidelines for their performing. The Study Protocol should ensure adequate conduction of the clinical trials and collection and analysis of data that are further submitted to the regulatory authorities for review and consideration.

   The following sections should be included in the Study Protocol:

   - Introduction (brief description of the problem and treatment regimen(s))
   - Objectives and purposes of the study
   - Study duration
   - Number of subjects
   - Informed Consent
   - Opinion of the Ethics Committee
   - Subject selection criteria:
     - Inclusion criteria
     - Exclusion criteria
   - Methodology:
     - Study Plan
     - Study schedule
     - Study Visits
     - Study Assessments / Procedures
     - Definition of efficacy endpoints
     - Treatment cycles
   - Safety Reporting
     - Adverse events (AEs)
     - Serious adverse events (SAEs)
     - Abnormal laboratory test values
     - Abnormal values of other safety parameters
     - Withdrawal from the Study
   - Clinical laboratory parameters
   - Other safety parameters
   - Concomitant medications

- Data analysis
- Appendixes

The following appendixes may be included in the Study Protocol: Patient Information Sheet/Written information and/or Informed consent form (ICF). Instruction sheet (e.g. for study subjects or study site staff).

The terms, which may be difficult for understanding by study subjects (both medical and law terms) should be avoided in translation of the abovementioned documents containing patient information. If special terms are used in the documents, they should be clarified or explained.

3. **PROTOCOL AMENDMENT:** Protocol amendment describes major changes to the initial Study Protocol. Protocol amendment must be again approved by the Ethics Committee.

4. **INFORMED CONSENT:** Informed consent is one of the most important elements of system ensuring the ethics of medical experiments and protection of the rights of the study subjects.

   Informed consent is a process by which a subject voluntary confirms his/her willingness to participate in one or another clinical trial, after having been informed of all aspects of the study. Informed consent should be documented by means of a written, signed and dated Informed Consent Form (ICF).

   Potential subjects should be informed of the objectives and methods of the study, the drug product and treatment regimen, the available alternative treatments, potential risks and benefits, and of possible complications and discomforts, which may arise from participation in the study.

   Based on information that he/she had received and understood, the potential subject freely gives consent to participate in a study. The informed consent should not be obtained through inducement or coercion. The subject should be aware that he/she may withdraw from the study at any time, and this will not affect his/her future medical care in any way.

   The main principles of Informed consent

   The subject should be informed of the following:

   - the purposes of the trial;
   - the methods of the trial;
   - the study drug(s) and treatment regimens;
   - available alternative treatment(s);
   - the potential risks and benefits, and possible discomforts.

   The subject should understand:

   - that informed consent should be given freely;

- that consent should not be obtained through inducement or coercion;
- that he/she may withdraw from the study at any time;
- that withdrawal from the study will not affect his/her future medical care.

5. **STUDY PROGRESS REPORTS:** The Investigator should provide written reports on study progress to the Ethics Committee. These may be the **Interim report** on the interim results of the study and their assessment based on the analysis conducted in the course of the study, or the **Final report** - full, comprehensive description of the study including description of investigational materials, study design, and presentation and assessment of results of statistical analysis. Additionally, the Investigator should prepare the written reports on all major changes that might affect study conduction and/or increase risk to study subjects. These are the following: Adverse Event Report or Adverse Drug Reaction Report, Patient Entry Form (Patient Entry Card/Patient Notification Form) and Patient Withdrawal Form, Protocol Deviation/Violation Report, Study Termination Report etc.

   Reporting on study progress is not only responsibility of the Investigator, but also the Study Monitor should provide the written reports on each Study Monitoring Visit (Monitor Report). The Expert Report is prepared for the regulatory authorities by an expert in the appropriate field (company officer or independent person) and covers different aspects of drug development.

6. **CASE RECORD FORM (CRF):** Case record form is a paper or electronic document designed to record all the information for an individual study subject required by the Study protocol.

   The Case record form is used for several purposes:

   - to ensure data collection in accordance with the Study protocol;
   - to ensure fulfilling of the regulatory authorities' requirements for data collection;
   - to facilitate the effective, comprehensive data processing and analysis, results reporting, and to promote the safety data sharing between the study team and other departments of the institution.

     The data collected in the study site during the course of a study should be comprehensive and provide true and fair information on what happened to each study subject. Only if the above criteria are met, the study will reliably answer the questions concerning the efficacy and safety of the investigational drug.

   All CRF's should include the following data:

   - study title and number;
   - Investigator's name;
   - study subject/patient ID (number and initials);
   - inclusion / exclusion criteria;
   - demographic data;

- detailed description of dosage regimens of investigational drug;
- concomitant treatment;
- adverse events (side effects and intercurrent diseases);
- conclusion on subject's health;
- Investigator's signature and date.

Additionally, the CRF's should include special pages to record the following information:

- past medical history;
- results of physical examination;
- primary and secondary diagnoses;
- relevant previous treatment;
- baseline characteristics, results of interim assessments, evaluation of efficacy endpoints, laboratory tests, description of study procedures etc.

All CRF's should be legible and suitable for duplication and possible additional sharing.

Informed Consent Process in Clinical Trials

Informed Consent Procedure

Before a clinical trial the researcher and participant engage in an agreement called an informed consent. The informed consent is firstly a written document outlining the procedure and possible effects and risks to the participant. It also describes the liability of the researcher and that of the volunteer. Any aftercare is also laid out in the initial text.

The informed consent does not stop at this first paper, though. It must continue as a dialogue between the participant and the investigator throughout the clinical trial.

The Process of Informed Consent:

Firstly, the principal investigator (PI) exposes the possible benefits and risks to the volunteer, and if necessary, their legal counsel, before the onset of the clinical trial.

Secondly, the volunteer is encouraged to ask questions and discuss any concerns he or she may have. They are also asked to talk the process over with their families.

Lastly, upon agreeing to the procedures and process involved, the participant signs and dates a consent form, of which he or she receives a copy. Any volunteer may withdraw from the trial at any time for any reason, without ramification. It is the legal responsibility of the PI to ensure the informed consent process is accomplished correctly.

Official Guidelines for Informed Consent

The International Council on Harmonization (ICH) provides parameters to be followed for obtaining informed consent. Under the heading of good clinical practices (GCP) the guidelines for informed consent are outlined in section 1.28. Section 4.8 describes the process of obtaining informed consent from a potential participant.

Researchers are also obligated to observe all federal and local governing guidelines, including personal information and privacy laws in the country in which the study is being conducted. The sponsor may also have regulations that must be respected.

Before its use, the informed consent document must be approved and accepted by an Institution Review Board (IRB), or an independent ethics committee (IEC).

Informed Consent Document Components

The ICH requires the informed consent to contain 20 separate components, as outlined in section 4.8.10 of the GCP. Included in these elements are a description of the study process, the reason for the study, how long it will last, what the possible risks and benefits are, and costs or expenses the volunteer may encounter. Also outlined are any alternative options the participant may have access to, and lastly the participants' rights in the study. This legal document requires two signatures with dates, one of the participants and the other of the administrator conducting the informed consent process. The participant must be fully able to understand the language and all its meanings in the written and verbal consent procedure. The language must be documented on the form.

Informed Consent Revisions

Whenever there is a change of any kind in the clinical trial process a revision must be made to the informed consent. The new form must then be approved by an IRB or IEC. Also the new form must be signed by any new researchers involved and the participants.

These changes can include but are not limited to: additional safety information is revealed, alterations in trial procedures, investigators are added or removed from the trial or volunteer compensation is revised.

For Further Study

- Cochrane Collaboration Glossary
- A. Yu. Mel'kov, English-Russian Glossary of terms used in clinical studies of pharmaceutical products, CRO "InnoPharm"
- Rules of Clinical Practice in the Russian Federation Ministry of Health of the Russian Federation.
- M.V. Leonova, I.L. Asetskaya, Development of Study Protocol and Case Record Form Russian State Medical University, Moscow. Article in Russian language.
- T.K. Efimtseva, A.L. Spasokukotsky, O.V. Mironova. Good Clinical Practice. English-Russian glossary. Ukrainian medical Journal - № 2 (28) - III / IV 2002.

Chapter 18

Data Management in Clinical Research

Learning Objectives

To understand

- Tools for CDM
- Regulations, Guidelines, and Standards in CDM
- Clinical Data Interchange Standards Consortium (CDISC)
- The CDM Process
- Review and finalization of study documents
- Database designing
- Data collection
- CRF tracking
- Data entry
- Data validation
- Medical coding
- Database locking
- Roles and Responsibilities in CDM

Introduction

Clinical trial is intended to find answers to the research question by means of generating data for proving or disproving a hypothesis. The quality of data generated plays an important role in the outcome of the study. Often research students ask the question, "what is Clinical Data Management (CDM) and what is its significance?" Clinical data management is a relevant and important part of a clinical trial. All researchers try their hands on CDM activities during their research work, knowingly or unknowingly. Without identifying the technical phases, we undertake some of the processes involved in CDM during our research work. This article highlights the processes involved in CDM and gives the reader an overview of how data is managed in clinical trials.

CDM is the process of collection, cleaning, and management of subject data in compliance with regulatory standards. The primary objective of CDM processes is to provide high quality data by keeping the number of errors and missing data as low as possible and gather maximum data for analysis.[1] To meet this objective, best practices are adopted to ensure that data are complete, reliable, and processed correctly. This has been facilitated by the use of software applications that maintain an audit trail and provide easy identification and resolution of data discrepancies. Sophisticated innovations [2] have enabled CDM to handle large trials and ensure the data quality even in complex trials.

How do we define 'high quality' data? High quality data should be absolutely accurate and suitable for statistical analysis. These should meet the protocol specified parameters and comply with the protocol requirements. This implies that in case of a deviation, not meeting the protocol specifications, we may think of excluding the patient from the final database. It should be borne in mind that in some situations, regulatory authorities may be interested in looking at such data. Similarly, missing data is also a matter of concern for clinical researchers. High quality data should have minimal or no misses. But most importantly, high quality data should possess only arbitrarily 'acceptable level of variation' that would not affect the conclusion of the study on statistical analysis. The data should also meet the applicable regulatory requirements specified for data quality.

Tools for CDM

Many software tools are available for data management, and these are called Clinical Data Management Systems (CDMS). In multicentric trials, a CDMS has become essential to handle the huge amount of data. Most of the CDMS used in pharmaceutical companies are commercial, but a few open source tools are available as well. Commonly used CDM tools are ORACLE CLINICAL, CLINTRIAL, MACRO, RAVE, and eClinical Suite. In terms of functionality, these software tools are more or less similar and there is no significant advantage of one system over the other. These software tools are expensive and need sophisticated Information Technology infrastructure to function. Additionally, some multinational pharmaceutical giants use custom made CDMS tools to suit their operational needs and procedures. Among the open source tools, the most prominent ones are Open Clinica, open CDMS, TrialDB, and PhOSCo. These CDM software are available free of cost and are as good as their commercial counterparts in terms of functionality. These open source software can be downloaded from their respective websites.

In regulatory submission studies, maintaining an audit trail of data management activities is of paramount importance. These CDM tools ensure the audit trail and help in the management of discrepancies. According to the roles and responsibilities (explained later), multiple user IDs can be created with access limitation to data entry, medical coding, database designing, or quality check. This ensures that each user can access only the respective functionalities allotted to that user ID and cannot make any other change in the database. For responsibilities where changes are permitted to be made in the data, the software will record the change made, the user ID that made the change and the time and date of change, for audit purposes (audit trail). During a regulatory audit, the auditors can verify the discrepancy management process; the changes made and can confirm that no unauthorized or false changes were made.

Regulations, Guidelines, and Standards in CDM

Akin to other areas in clinical research, CDM has guidelines and standards that must be followed. Since the pharmaceutical industry relies on the electronically captured data for the evaluation of medicines, there is a need to follow good practices in CDM and maintain standards in electronic data capture. These electronic records have to comply with a Code of Federal Regulations (CFR), 21 CFR Part 11. This regulation is applicable to records in electronic format that are created, modified, maintained, archived, retrieved, or transmitted. This demands the use of validated systems to ensure accuracy, reliability, and consistency of data with the use of secure, computer generated, time stamped audit trails to independently record the date and time of operator entries and actions that create, modify, or delete electronic records.[3] Adequate procedures and controls should be put in place to ensure the integrity, authenticity, and confidentiality of data. If data have to be submitted to regulatory authorities, it should be entered and processed in 21 CFR part 11-compliant systems. Most of the CDM systems available are like this and pharmaceutical companies as well as contract research organizations ensure this compliance.

Society for Clinical Data Management (SCDM) publishes the Good Clinical Data Management Practices (GCDMP) guidelines, a document providing the standards of good practice within CDM. GCDMP was initially published in September 2000 and has undergone several revisions thereafter. The July 2009 version is the currently followed GCDMP document. GCDMP provides guidance on the accepted practices in CDM that are consistent with regulatory practices. Addressed in 20 chapters, it covers the CDM process by highlighting the minimum standards and best practices.

Clinical Data Interchange Standards Consortium (CDISC)

Multidisciplinary non-profit organization, has developed standards to support acquisition, exchange, submission, and archival of clinical research data and metadata. Metadata is the data of the data entered. This includes data about the individual who made the entry or a change in the clinical data, the date and time of entry/change and details of the changes that have been made. Among the standards, two important ones are the Study Data Tabulation Model Implementation Guide for Human Clinical Trials (SDTMIG) and the Clinical Data Acquisition Standards Harmonization (CDASH) standards, available free of cost from the CDISC website (www.cdisc.org). The SDTMIG standard [4] describes the details of model and standard terminologies for the data and serves as a guide to the organization. CDASH v 1.1[5] defines the basic standards for the collection of data in a clinical trial and enlists the basic data information needed from a clinical, regulatory, and scientific perspective.

The CDM Process

The CDM process, like a clinical trial, begins with the end in mind. This means that the whole process is designed keeping the deliverable in view. As a clinical trial is designed to answer the research question, the CDM process is designed to deliver an error free, valid, and statistically sound database. To meet this objective, the CDM process starts early, even before the finalization of the study protocol.

Review and Finalization of Study Documents

The protocol is reviewed from a database designing perspective, for clarity and consistency. During this review, the CDM personnel will identify the data items to be collected and the frequency of collection with respect to the visit schedule. A Case Report Form (CRF) is designed by the CDM team, as this is the first step in translating the protocol specific activities into data being generated. The data fields should be clearly defined and be consistent throughout. The type of data to be entered should be evident from the CRF. For example, if weight has to be captured in two decimal places, the data entry field should have two data boxes placed after the decimal as shown in Figure 1. Similarly, the units in which measurements have to be made should also be mentioned next to the data field. The CRF should be concise, self-explanatory, and user friendly (unless you are the one entering data into the CRF). Along with the CRF, the filling instructions (called CRF Completion Guidelines) should also be provided to study investigators for error free data acquisition. CRF annotation is done wherein the variable is named according to the SDTMIG or the conventions followed

Figure 1: Annotated sample of a Case Report Form (CRF). Annotations are entered in coloured text in this figure to differentiate from the CRF questions. DCM = Data collection module, DVG = Discrete value group, YNNA [S1] = Yes, No = Not applicable [subset 1], C = Character, N = Numerical, DT = Date format. For example, BRTHDTC [DT] indicates date of birth in the date format internally. Annotations are coded terms used in CDM tools to indicate the variables in the study. An example of an annotated CRF is provided in Figure 1. In questions with discrete value options (like the variable gender having values male and female as responses), all possible options will be coded appropriately.

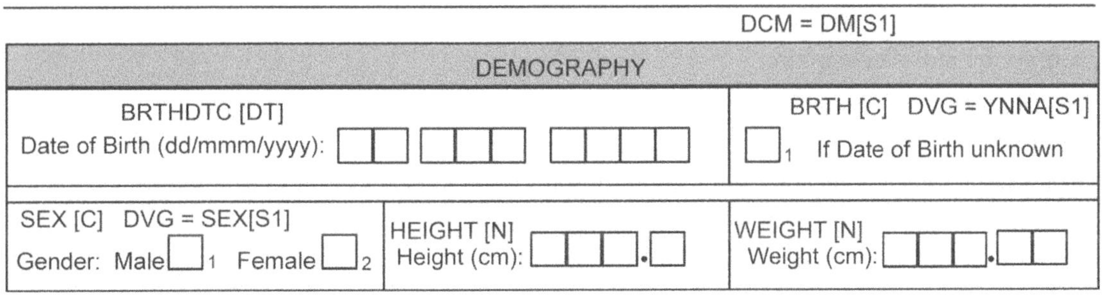

DCM = DM[S1]

DEMOGRAPHY		
BRTHDTC [DT] Date of Birth (dd/mmm/yyyy): ☐☐ ☐☐☐ ☐☐☐☐		BRTH [C] DVG = YNNA[S1] ☐1 If Date of Birth unknown
SEX [C] DVG = SEX[S1] Gender: Male ☐1 Female ☐2	HEIGHT [N] Height (cm): ☐☐☐.☐	WEIGHT [N] Weight (cm): ☐☐☐.☐☐

Table 18.1 List of Clinical Data Management Activities

Data collection
CRF tracking
CRF annotation
Database design
Data entry
Medical coding
Data validation
Discrepancy management
Database lock

Based on these, a Data Management Plan (DMP) is developed. DMP document is a road map to handle the data under foreseeable circumstances and describes the CDM activities to be followed in the trial. A list of CDM activities is provided in Table 1. The DMP describes the database design, data entry and data tracking guidelines, quality control measures, SAE reconciliation guidelines, discrepancy management, data transfer/ extraction, and database locking guidelines. Along with the DMP, a Datam Validation Plan (DVP) containing all edit checks to be performed and the calculations for derived variables are also prepared. The edit check programs in the DVP help in cleaning up the data by identifying the discrepancies.

Database Designing

Databases are the clinical software applications, which are built to facilitate the CDM tasks to carry out multiple studies.[6] Generally, these tools have built-in compliance with regulatory requirements and are easy to use. "System validation" is conducted to ensure data security, during which system specifications,[7] user requirements, and regulatory compliance are evaluated before implementation. Study details like objectives, intervals, visits, investigators, sites, and patients are defined in the database and CRF layouts are designed for data entry. These entry screens are tested with dummy data before moving them to the real data capture.

Data Collection

Data collection is done using the CRF that may exist in the form of a paper or an electronic version. The traditional method is to employ paper CRFs to collect the data responses, which are translated to the database by means of data entry done in-house. These paper CRFs are filled up by the investigator according to the completion guidelines. In the e-CRF based CDM, the investigator or a designee will be logging into the CDM system and entering the data directly at the site. In e-CRF method, chances of errors are less, and the resolution of discrepancies happens faster. Since pharmaceutical companies try to reduce the time taken for drug development processes by enhancing the speed of processes involved, many pharmaceutical companies are opting for e-CRF options (also called remote data entry).

CRF Tracking

The entries made in the CRF will be monitored by the Clinical Research Associate (CRA) for completeness and filled up CRFs are retrieved and handed over to the CDM team. The CDM team will track the retrieved CRFs and maintain their record. CRFs are tracked for missing pages and illegible data manually to assure that the data are not lost. In case of missing or illegible data, a clarification is obtained from the investigator and the issue is resolved.

Data Entry

Data entry takes place according to the guidelines prepared along with the DMP. This is applicable only in the case of paper CRF retrieved from the sites. Usually, double data entry is performed wherein the data is entered by two operators separately.[8] The second pass entry (entry made by the second person) helps in verification and reconciliation by identifying the transcription errors and discrepancies caused by illegible data. Moreover, double data entry helps in getting a cleaner database compared to a single data entry. Earlier studies have shown that double data entry ensures better consistency with paper CRF as denoted by a lesser error rate.[9]

Data Validation

Data validation is the process of testing the validity of data in accordance with the protocol specifications. Edit check programs are written to identify the discrepancies in the entered data, which are embedded in the database, to ensure data validity. These programs are written according to the logic condition mentioned in the DVP. These edit check programs are initially tested with dummy data containing discrepancies. Discrepancy is defined as a data point that fails to pass a validation check. Discrepancy may be due to inconsistent data, missing data, range checks, and deviations from the protocol. In e-CRF based studies, data validation process will be run frequently for identifying discrepancies. These discrepancies will be resolved by investigators after logging into the system. Ongoing quality control of data processing is undertaken at regular intervals during the course of CDM. For example, if the inclusion criteria specify that the age of the patient should be between 18 and 65 years (both inclusive), an edit program will be written for two conditions *viz.* age <18 and >65. If for any patient, the condition becomes TRUE, a discrepancy will be generated. These discrepancies will be highlighted in the system and

Data Clarification Forms (DCFs) can be generated. DCFs are documents containing queries pertaining to the discrepancies identified.

This is also called query resolution. Discrepancy management includes reviewing discrepancies, investigating the reason, and resolving them with documentary proof or declaring them as irresolvable. Discrepancy management helps in cleaning the data and gathers enough evidence for the deviations observed in data. Almost all CDMS have a discrepancy database where all discrepancies will be recorded and stored with audit trail.

Based on the types identified, discrepancies are either flagged to the investigator for clarification or closed in house by Self Evident Corrections (SEC) without sending DCF to the site. The most common SECs are obvious spelling errors. For discrepancies that require clarifications from the investigator, DCFs will be sent to the site. The CDM tools help in the creation and printing of DCFs. Investigators will write the resolution or explain the circumstances that led to the discrepancy in data. When a resolution is provided by the investigator, the same will be updated in the database. In case of e-CRFs, the investigator can access the discrepancies flagged to him and will be able to provide the resolutions online. Figure 2 illustrates the flow of discrepancy management.

The CDM team reviews all discrepancies at regular intervals to ensure that they have been resolved. The resolved data discrepancies are recorded as 'closed'. This means that those validation failures are no longer considered to be active, and future data validation attempts on the same data will not create a discrepancy for same data point. But closure of discrepancies is not always possible. In some cases, the investigator will not be able to provide a resolution for the discrepancy. Such discrepancies will be considered as 'irresolvable' and will be updated in the discrepancy database.

Discrepancy management is the most critical activity in the CDM process. Being the vital activity in cleaning up the data, utmost attention must be observed while handling the discrepancies.

Medical Coding

Medical coding helps in identifying and properly classifying the medical terminologies associated with the clinical trial. For **Figure 2:** Discrepancy management (DCF = Data clarification form, CRA = Clinical Research Associate, SDV = Source document verification, SEC = Self-evident correction)

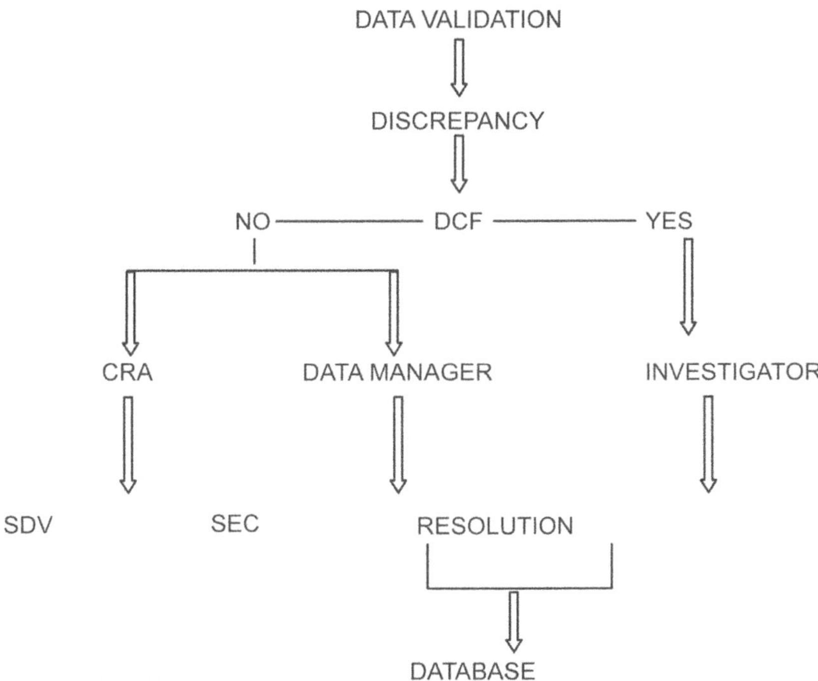

classification of events, medical dictionaries available online are used. Technically, this activity needs the knowledge of medical terminology, understanding of disease entities, drugs used, and a basic knowledge of the pathological processes involved. Functionally, it also requires knowledge about the structure of electronic medical dictionaries and the hierarchy of classifications available in them. Adverse events occurring during the study, prior to and concomitantly administered medications and pre- or co-existing illnesses are coded using the available medical dictionaries. Commonly, Medical Dictionary for Regulatory Activities (MedDRA) is used for the coding of adverse events as well as other illnesses and World Health Organization Drug Dictionary Enhanced (WHO-DDE) is used for coding the medications. These dictionaries contain the respective classifications of adverse events and drugs in proper classes. Other dictionaries are also available for use in data management (eg, WHO-ART is a dictionary that deals with adverse reactions terminology). Some pharmaceutical companies utilize customized dictionaries to suit their needs and meet their standard operating procedures.

Medical coding helps in classifying reported medical terms on the CRF to standard dictionary terms in order to achieve data consistency and avoid unnecessary duplication. For example, the investigators may use different terms for the same adverse event, but it is important to code all of them to a single standard code and maintain uniformity in the process. The right coding and classification of adverse events and medication is crucial as an incorrect coding may lead to masking of safety issues or highlight the wrong safety concerns related to the drug.

Database Locking

After a proper quality check and assurance, the final data validation is run. If there are no discrepancies, the SAS datasets are finalized in consultation with the statistician. All data management activities should have been completed prior to database lock. To ensure this, a pre lock checklist is used and completion of all activities is confirmed. This is done as the database cannot be changed in any manner after locking. Once the approval for locking is obtained from all stakeholders, the database is locked and clean data is extracted for statistical analysis. Generally, no modification in the database is possible. But in case of a critical issue or for other important operational reasons, privileged users can modify the data even after the database is locked. This, however, requires proper documentation and an audit trail has to be maintained with sufficient justification for updating the locked database. Data extraction is done from the final database after locking. This is followed by its archival.

Roles and Responsibilities in CDM

In a CDM team, different roles and responsibilities are attributed to the team members. The minimum educational requirement for a team member in CDM should be graduation in life science and knowledge of computer applications. Ideally, medical coders should be medical graduates. However, in the industry, paramedical graduates are also recruited as medical coders. Some key roles are essential to all CDM teams. The list of roles given below can be considered as minimum requirements for a CDM team:

- Data Manager
- Database Programmer/Designer
- Medical Coder
- Clinical Data Coordinator
- Quality Control Associate
- Data Entry Associate

The data manager is responsible for supervising the entire CDM process. The data manager prepares the DMP, approves the CDM procedures and all internal documents related to CDM activities. Controlling and allocating the database access to team members is also the responsibility of the data manager. The database programmer/designer performs the CRF annotation, creates the study database, and programs the edit checks for data validation. He/she is also responsible for designing of data entry screens in the database and validating the edit checks with dummy data. The medical coder will do the coding for adverse events, medical history, co illnesses, and concomitant medication administered during the study. The clinical data coordinator designs the CRF, prepares the CRF filling instructions, and is responsible for developing the DVP and discrepancy management. All other CDM related documents, checklists, and guideline documents are prepared by the clinical data coordinator. The quality control associate checks the accuracy of data entry and conducts data audits.[10] Sometimes, there is a separate quality assurance person to conduct the audit on the data entered. Additionally, the quality control associate verifies the documentation pertaining to the procedures being followed. The data entry personnel will be tracking the receipt of CRF pages and performs the data entry into the database.

CDM has evolved in response to the ever increasing demand from pharmaceutical companies to fast track the drug development process and from the regulatory authorities to put the quality systems in place to ensure generation of high quality data for accurate drug evaluation. To meet the expectations, there is a gradual shift from the paper based to the electronic systems of data management. Developments on the technological front have positively impacted the CDM process and systems, thereby leading to encouraging results on speed and quality of data being generated. At the same time, CDM professionals should ensure the standards for improving data quality.[11] CDM, being a speciality in itself, should be evaluated by means of the systems and processes being implemented and the standards being followed. The biggest challenge from the regulatory perspective would be the standardization of data management process across organizations, and development of regulations to define the procedures to be followed and the data standards. From the industry perspective, the biggest hurdle would be the planning and implementation of data management systems in a changing operational environment where the rapid pace of technology development outdates the existing infrastructure. In spite of these, CDM is evolving to become a standard based clinical research entity, by striking a balance between the expectations from and constraints in the existing systems, driven by technological developments and business demands.

For Further Study

1. Gerritsen MG, Sartorius OE, vd Veen FM, Meester GT. Data management in multi-center clinical trials and the role of a nation-wide computer network. A 5 year evaluation. Proc AnnuSympComput Appl Med Care 1993:659-62.
2. Lu Z, Su J. Clinical data management: Current status, challenges, and future directions from industry perspectives. Open Access J Clin Trials 2010;2:93-105.
3. CFR - Code of Federal Regulations Title 21 [Internet]. Maryland: Food and Drug Administration; Available from:

   http://www.accessdata.fda.gov/scripts/cdrh/cfdocs/ cfcfr/CFRSearch.cfm?fr=11.10. [Updated 2010 Apr 4; Cited 2011 Mar 1].
4. Study Data Tabulation Model [Internet]. Texas: Clinical Data Interchange
5. Standards Consortium.; c2011. Available from: http://www.cdisc.org/sdtm. [Updated 2007 Jul; Cited 2011 Mar 1].
6. CDASH [Internet]. Texas: Clinical Data Interchange Standards Consortium.; c2011. Available from: http://www.cdisc.org/cdash. [Updated 2011 Jan; Cited 2011 Mar 1].
7. Fegan GW, Lang TA. Could an open source clinical trial data management system be what we have all been looking for? PLoS Med 2008;5:e6.

8. Kuchinke W, Ohmann C, Yang Q, Salas N, Lauritsen J, Gueyffier F, *et al.*Heterogeneity prevails: The state of clinical trial data management in Europe - results of a survey of ECRIN centres. Trials 2010;11:79.
9. Cummings J, Masten J. Customized dual data entry for computerized data analysis. Qual Assur 1994;3:300-3.
10. Reynolds Haertle RA, McBride R. Single vs. double data entry in CAST. Control Clin Trials 1992; 13:487-94.
11. Ottevanger PB, Therasse P, van de Velde C, Bernier J, van Krieken H, Grol R, *et al.* Quality assurance in clinical trials. Crit Rev Oncol Hematol 2003;47:213-35.
12. Haux R, Knaup P, Leiner F. On educating about medical data management - the other side of the electronic health record. Methods Inf Med 2007;46:74-9.

Chapter 19

Safety Monitoring in Clinical Trials

LEARNING OBJECTIVES

To understand

- Common Practice in Safety Monitoring
- Institutional Review Board/Ethics Committee
- Data and Safety Monitoring Board
- Regulatory Authorities
- Medical Community and Patients
- Communicating Safety Information among Stakeholders
- Statistical Methods in Safety Monitoring
- Methods for Single Arm Trials
- Methods for Randomized, Controlled Trials
- A Hypothetical Clinical Trial Example

Introduction

Clinical trials provide the evidentiary basis for regulatory approvals of safe and effective medicines. With long development cycles and ever-increasing costs in conducting clinical trials, both the pharmaceutical industry and regulators are making efforts to be more proactive in safety evaluations. Early safety signal detection not only leads to better patient protection, but also has the potential to save development costs.

Since clinical trials are experiments in humans, they must be conducted following established standards in order to protect the rights, safety and well-being of the participants. These standards include the International Conference on Harmonization Good Clinical Practice (ICH-GCP) Guidelines [1], International Ethical Guidelines for Biomedical Research Involving Human Subjects issued by the Council for International Organizations of Medical Sciences (CIOMS) [2] and the ethical principles set forth in the Declaration of Helsinki [3]. GCP is the "standard for the design, conduct, performance, monitoring, auditing, recording, analyses and reporting of clinical trials that provides assurance that the data and reported results are credible and accurate and that rights, integrity and confidentiality of trial subjects are protected" [1]. The globalization of clinical trials has presented additional challenges to sponsors. Sponsors are held accountable to comply with the relevant local legal and regulatory requirements wherever the clinical trials are conducted. For example, clinical trials conducted in the European Union are required to be conducted in accordance with the Clinical Trials Directive[4].

Safety evaluation is a central component in all stages of the drug development lifecycle. Prior to the marketing authorization of a drug, rigorous safety monitoring and evaluations from preclinical to all stages of clinical trials are required. Pharmaceutical sponsors need to adequately characterize the safety profile of the product in order to obtain regulatory approval and marketing authorization. The approved product label contains the essential information about the product's benefits and risks. The continued vigilance in safety is critical as more data and experience is gathered from a broader patient population once the product is on the market. In some cases, new emerging safety profiles may cast the original benefit-risk assessments in doubt. These are evidenced in some high profile market withdrawals, such as Troglitazone (Rezulin), Rofecoxib (Vioxx) and Rosiglitazone (Avandia). In 2005, the United States Food and Drug Administration (FDA) issued guidance documents on risk management activities, including premarket risk assessment and postmarketing pharmacovigilance and pharmaco epidemiologic assessments [5–7]. Regulatory agencies around the world and the pharmaceutical industry are taking a more comprehensive and holistic approach to safety evaluation in drug development.

This article will focus on safety monitoring during the pre-approval period. Section 2 summarizes the common practice in safety monitoring in clinical trials. Relevant regulatory guidance and industry guidelines are discussed. In Section 3, quantitative safety monitoring methods based on statistical principles are presented. An example is provided to illustrate the applications. We conclude with discussion and recommendations.

Common Practice in Safety Monitoring

Stakeholders in Safety Monitoring

Sponsor

Clinical trial sponsors, usually pharmaceutical companies, are responsible for developing the clinical trial protocol. The protocol describes every aspect of the research, including the rationale for the experiment, objectives, trial population with detailed inclusion and exclusion criteria, administration of the investigational therapies, trial procedures, data collection standards, endpoints and sample size. The protocol also details the safety reporting procedures, specifically on the requirements for expedited reporting of serious adverse events. The Informed Consent Form (ICF) is used to disclose current information about the investigational drug and about the procedures, risks and benefits for subjects who participate in the clinical trial. Informed consent is a vital part of the research process. In addition to the protocol and the ICF, sponsors are responsible for setting up and maintaining clinical databases for the data collected in the trial. Case Report Forms (CRFs) are designed by the sponsor as data collection tools. These tools are increasingly based on electronic data capture modules via the internet rather than the traditional paper-based route. With access to all accumulating data, sponsors are mandated to report key safety information to all stakeholders in a timely fashion. Details of the sponsor's reporting requirements are discussed in Section2.2.

Subjects

Subjects are patients or healthy volunteers who agree to participate in a clinical trial and have signed the ICF. Along with other information, the ICF provides important safety information so the subjects can make an informed decision on whether to participate in the trial. The informed consent must be given freely, without coercion and must be based on a clear understanding of what participation involves. By giving consent, subjects permit the investigators to collect health information and body measurements as per the protocol. While subjects are encouraged to follow the protocol to trial completion, they can withdraw at any time. They do not need to give a reason for withdrawing consent. In a phase 1 clinical trial, when the drug is first used in humans, healthy volunteers are compensated for their time and willingness to be exposed to unknown risks. Later phase trials are mostly conducted in patients with the disease of interest, and payments to these subjects for participation are contentious. The main concern is the payment could be coercive or serve as undue inducement leading to impaired judgment on trial participation[8].

Investigators

Investigators are qualified individuals who are trained and experienced to provide medical care to subjects enrolled in the trial. Investigators identify potential subjects and educate them about the trial participation to ensure that they can make an informed decision. While the trial is ongoing, investigators are expected to adhere to the protocol treatment plan in delivering care. They observe, evaluate, manage and document all effects of treatment, including the reporting of adverse events. They are responsible for notifying their institutional review boards and the sponsor of any issues that pose a threat to the safety and well-being of the trial subjects. Investigators are ultimately accountable and responsible for the conduct of the clinical trial and for the safety of the subjects under their care.

Institutional Review Board/Ethics Committee

The Institutional Review Board (IRB), also known as the ethics committee, is charged with protecting the rights and welfare of human subjects recruited to participate in research protocols conducted under the auspices of the institution to which the IRB is affiliated. The IRB reviews all clinical trial protocols involving human subjects that the particular institution is involved with and has the authority to approve, disapprove or require modifications to the protocols. IRBs bear further the responsibility of reviewing ongoing research to ensure continued diligence that subjects are not placed at undue risk and they give uncoerced, informed consent to their participation. The training and education of investigators at the institution who participate in clinical research is also a responsibility of the IRB. Members of an IRB generally come from a wide range of scientific disciplines and from outside academic communities in which research is being conducted.

Data and Safety Monitoring Board

The Data and Safety Monitoring Board (DSMB), also called data monitoring committee (DMC), is an expert committee, independent of the sponsor, chartered for one or more clinical trials. The mandate of the DSMB is to review on a regular basis the accumulating data from the clinical trial to ensure the continuing safety of current participants and those yet to be enrolled. The DSMB may review efficacy data at pre-defined interim points to assess whether there's overwhelming evidence of efficacy or the lack thereof, such that the clinical equipoise at the beginning of the trial is no longer justified. DSMB has the additional responsibilities to advise the sponsor regarding the continuing validity and scientific merit of the trial. Not all clinical trials require a formal DSMB. DSMBs are most common in double blind randomized phase 3 trials. Members of the DSMB typically include clinical trial experts, including physicians with the appropriate specialty, at least one biostatistician and possibly person(s) from other disciplines, such as biomedical ethics, basic science/pharmacology or law.

Regulatory Authorities

In the US, prior to the initiation of a first in human clinical trial, pharmaceutical sponsors must submit an Investigational New Drug (IND) application to the FDA as required by law. The FDA reviews the IND (typically within 30 calendar days) for safety to ensure that research subjects will not be subjected to unreasonable risk. In 2010, the FDA issued guidance to sponsors and investigators on safety reporting requirements for human drug and biological products that are being investigated under an IND and for drugs that are the subjects of bioavailability (BA) and bioequivalence (BE) studies that are exempt from the IND requirements [9]. The guidance provided the agency's expectations for timely review, evaluation and submission of relevant and useful safety information and implemented internationally harmonized definitions and reporting standards. The European Medicines Agency (EMA) is the European Union's FDA equivalent. The agency has several scientific committees that carry out the evaluation of applications from pharmaceutical companies. In other parts of the world, regulatory authorities will have similar mandates, but may operate under different local laws and regulations.

Medical Community and Patients

Clinical trials generate data that contribute to the body of knowledge about the treatment and the disease that benefit the broader medical community and, ultimately, the patients. Safety information of one product may be informative to other practitioners using a similar class of agents. In 1997, the US Congress passed the Food and Drug Modernization Act (FDAMA), requiring clinical trial registration.

ClinicalTrials.gov was created as a result. The website was further expanded in 2007 after the Congress passed the Food and Drug Administration Amendments Act (FDAAA), which required more types of trials to be registered. In September 2008, as required by FDAAA 801, ClinicalTrials.gov began allowing sponsors and principal investigators to submit the results of clinical studies. Submission of adverse event information was optional when the results database was released and became required in September 2009. The mandatory requirement on clinical trial registration and the disclosure of trial results are significant achievements in advancing science and increasing transparency in clinical research.

Communicating Safety Information among Stakeholders

Timely communication among the various stakeholders is critical to ensure subject safety in clinical trials. Sponsors of clinical trials are accountable for monitoring the subjects appropriately, including the requirement of long-term follow up as appropriate. The protocol (including the ICF) specifies the details of the assessments, the frequency and the length of follow-up. In addition, most pharmaceutical sponsors have Standard Operating Procedures (SOPs) in place to collect, process, review, evaluate, report and communicate accumulating safety data to ensure a systematic approach for safety surveillance and monitoring. In general, safety information, including adverse events and laboratory findings are reported to a sponsor by investigators conducting the clinical trial. However, safety information may come from sources outside the immediate clinical trial. The sponsor is required to promptly review all information relevant to the safety of the drug and to update subjects, investigators, IRBs and regulatory authorities of any new risks associated with the use of the investigational drug that arise from the clinical trial or from other sources.

Amending the clinical trial protocol is one way to implement procedural changes that are necessary given the updated safety information. Another way to communicate the evolving safety information is through the periodic update of the Investigator's Brochure (IB). The IB is a compilation of the clinical and non-clinical data on the investigational drug that are relevant to the study of the drug in human subjects. Its purpose is to provide the investigators and others involved in the trial with the information to facilitate their understanding of the rationale for and their compliance with many key features of the protocol, such as the dose, dose frequency/interval, methods of administration and safety monitoring procedures [1]. The IB should be reviewed at least annually and revised as necessary in compliance with the sponsor's written procedures and the local requirements. A new safety finding that represents a significant risk to study subjects should be communicated to the investigators immediately, along with an update to the IB and possibly to the protocol and the ICF. For trials where DSMBs are in place, sponsors should also communicate significant safety findings to the DSMBs employed to oversee clinical trials of the same or similar investigational drug(s). In other situations, DSMBs may be in possession of critical safety information and they will need to follow the DSMB charter and the protocol to make recommendations to the sponsor with regard to its safety findings and whether the trial should continue as planned.

The goal of safety monitoring in clinical trials is to identify, evaluate, minimize and appropriately manage risks. In Europe, Risk Management Plans (RMPs) are required by the EMA as part of the drug approval process. An RMP includes a summary of important identified risks of the drug, potential risks and missing information, which serves as the basis for an action plan for pharmacovigilance and risk minimization activities. The CIOMS VI working group [10] recommended establishing a multidisciplinary Safety Management Team (SMT) within the sponsor organization to be in charge of safety surveillance and decision making on risk management and minimization activities. The SMT is responsible for coordinating all safety-related activities involving quantitative assessment of risks, signal detection and identification of adverse events of special interest (AESIs). For trials in earlier stages without DSMBs, sponsors may choose to appoint an internal multi-functional data review team removed from the direct day-to-day trial operations related to the investigational drug to perform ongoing review of the safety data. This independent data review team is empowered to perform similar functions as the DSMB on later stage trials.

The CIOMS VI working group endorsed the use of the Development Core Safety Information (DCSI) as the summary of the identified safety issues for an investigational drug. DCSI was recommended to be a part of the IB that defines the list of suspected adverse reactions. Safety issues or adverse drug reactions contained in this document should be considered "expected" for regulatory reporting purposes. Only suspected adverse drug reactions that are both serious and unexpected are subject to expedited case reporting to regulatory authorities in either seven (fatal or life-threatening) or 15 calendar days. Slightly different terminologies exist, including Suspected Unexpected Serious Drug Reaction (SUSAR) [4] or Serious Unexpected Suspected Drug Reaction [9]. Contrary to the routine expedited case reporting to regulatory authorities, the CIOMS VI working group recommended sponsors provide periodic updates of the evolving benefit/risk profile and highlight important new safety information to the participating investigators and IRBs. However, in some regions, expedited case reporting to investigators and IRBs are still required by local regulations.

Regulatory authorities also require reporting of safety information in the aggregate rather than the individual cases. In the US, the FDA IND regulations require annual IND reports, which include aggregate safety information across the entire development program of an investigational drug. CIOMS VI working group recommended defining a single Development Safety Update Report (DSUR) for submission to regulators on an annual basis. For submission of New Drug Applications (NDAs), sponsors aggregate safety information from all relevant trials of the drug to perform integrated safety analyses in support of the filing for marketing authorization. The common data structure using SDTM (Standard Data Tabulation Model) defined by Clinical Data Interchange Standards Consortium (CDISC) has greatly facilitated the safety data integration and analyses. It also enables sponsors to build a safety data warehouse to better respond to safety related queries across the entire drug program. Proactive early planning of safety analyses in a Program Safety Analysis Plan (PSAP) and periodic aggregate safety analyses have been recommended as standard industry practices [11,12]. The PSAP is a living document that will form the basis for integrated safety analyses in an NDA.

Statistical Methods in Safety Monitoring

Methods for Single Arm Trials

With the continued focus on safety monitoring and increased amount of work on case processing and reporting, quantitative approaches to safety evaluations will become increasingly important. Statistical methods can be applied to set up objective criteria in safety assessments and to help detect signals hidden in the volume of safety data. Most phase 2 and phase 3 clinical trials are designed with treatment efficacy as the primary objectives. It is important to consider inclusion of safety assessment criteria in addition to the evaluation of efficacy. In practice, sponsors usually have some ideas about the safety profile based on the mechanism of action of the drug or based on data from preclinical/animal testing, previous trials or data from drugs in a similar class. We recommend sponsors establish upfront safety monitoring criteria to help guide the DSMBs (or the sponsor's independent data review team) on serious adverse events, such as SUSARs or AESIs, even when the trial is not comparative.

As an example, in oncology, it is not uncommon to have a single arm phase 2 trial where all subjects are treated with the same experimental agent. Consider a sequential analysis that the occurrence of an undesirable AESI is evaluated after every subject is treated for a fixed period of time. We assume the probability of the AESI in subjects treated with the agent is π. The sequential probability ratio test (SPRT) introduced by Wald [13,14] can be used to set up a monitoring scheme of the AESI. Let the null and alternative hypotheses be:

$$H_0\text{: } \pi = \pi_0 \text{ and } H_1\text{: } \pi=\pi_1,$$

where π_0 represents the background event rate (*i.e.*, event rate expected of a standard control therapy) considered acceptable and π_1 represent the event rate considered not acceptable.

Let $Y_i = y_i$, $i = 1, 2, \ldots, n$, be the binary indicator of whether the AESI is observed from the *i*-th subject. $\boldsymbol{y}_n = (y_1, y_2, \ldots, y_n)^T$ denotes the vector of n subjects who have already been treated. The sequence of probability ratios (*i.e.*, likelihood ratios) is defined as:

$$\Lambda_n = f(\boldsymbol{y}_n; \pi = \pi_1)/f(\boldsymbol{y}_n; \pi = \pi_0)$$

Let $n_{\max}$ denote the total number of subjects planned for the trial. The monitoring guideline using SPRT is as follows:

- if $\Lambda_n \geq U_n$, conclude π_1;
- if $\Lambda_n \leq L_n$, conclude π_0;
- if $L_n < \Lambda_n < U_n$ and $n < n_{\max}$, then continue the trial.

The upper and lower boundaries in the above monitoring guideline can be solved by specifying the type I (false positive) and type II (false negative) error rates related to the hypothesis testing. The type I error here amounts to falsely identifying a safety problem when none exists, and the type II error means failing to identify a safety problem when one does exist. The type I error may be set at 0.05 and the type II error at 0.2.

While improvements and extensions to the SPRT have been proposed [15], we will examine instead an alternative approach based on the Bayesian framework by Thall and Simon (TS method) [16].

Assuming the prior distributions of π and π_S follow Beta distributions with $\pi \sim$ Beta (a, b) and $\pi_S \sim$ Beta (a_S, b_S), the parameters of the prior distributions can be determined based on either historical data or expert opinions [17]. Unlike in the SPRT, π_S is assumed to follow a distribution based on historical information of the standard control therapy. The posterior distribution of π upon observing x_i events in the first i subjects ($i = 1, \ldots, n_{max}$) is also a Beta distribution:

$$(\pi | X_i = x_i) \sim \text{Beta}(a + x_i, b + i - x_i)$$

It should be noted that during the trial, the parameters characterizing the distribution of π get updated upon observing new data, while those of π_S remain the same, as there is no standard control therapy arm. For any $i = 1, \ldots, n_{max}$, a criterion function is defined as follows:

$$\phi(x_i, i; \pi, \pi_S, \delta) = P(\pi - \pi_S > \delta | i, X_i = x_i)$$

where δ is a positive constant that is pre-specified. Let U_i be the smallest integer, such that $\phi(U_i, i; \pi, \pi_S, 0) \geq p_U$, and $L_i (< U_i)$ be the largest integer, such that $\phi(L_i, i; \pi, \pi_S, \delta) \leq p_L$, where p_U with a large value (e.g., ≥ 0.9) and p_L with a small value (e.g., ≤ 0.05) are predetermined threshold probabilities.

The monitoring guideline after the i-th subject has been treated is as follows:

- if $x_i \geq U_i$, conclude π greater than π_S;
- if $x_i \leq L_i$, conclude π less than $\pi_S + \delta$;
- if $L_i < x_i < U_i$ and $i < n_{max}$, then continue the trial.

The upper boundary implies that any treatment that is highly likely to incur an increased risk over standard treatment is of concern and may not warrant further development. The lower boundary implies that a treatment that is very unlikely to cause an increased risk of at least δ over π_S is considered tolerable.

It should be noted that the monitoring guidelines discussed above for the SPRT and the TS methods are for the general cases. When monitoring safety events, the lower boundaries are usually not relevant and can be ignored. Trials will be stopped when it is considered unsafe to continue. However, whether to stop a trial could depend on many factors, such as other safety observations and efficacy in the context of risk-benefit trade-off. In practice, monitoring guidelines may be considered after a minimum number of subjects have been treated to ensure reliable estimates can be obtained [18]. One important parameter in setting up a monitoring guideline is the specification of π_1 in the SPRT method and δ in the TS method. We recommend close collaboration with clinical experts in soliciting realistic input. Computer simulation of potential outcomes given various scenarios can also help make a decision.

Methods for Randomized, Controlled Trials

For the randomized, controlled clinical trials, we consider similar explicit statistical boundaries for safety monitoring. Here, the monitoring is based on the unblinded aggregate data reviewed regularly by either the DSMB or the sponsor's independent data review team depending on the nature of the trial. We assume the monitoring involves an AESI as in Section 3.1. The event rate in the treated and control arms are π_T and π_C, respectively.

We adopt a Bayesian Beta-Binomial model in setting up the monitoring. At any time point t during the trial, the prior distributions are assumed to be beta distributions with $\pi_T \sim$ Beta (a_T, b_T) and $\pi_C \sim$ Beta (a_C, b_C). The posterior distributions can be expressed as:

$$(\pi_T | X^T = x^T, N^T) \sim \text{Beta}(a_T + x^T, b_T + N^T - x^T)$$

$$(\pi_C | X^C = x^C, N^C) \sim \text{Beta}(a_C + x^C, b_C + N^C - x^C)$$

where x^T and x^C are the numbers of events from the treatment and the control arm and N^T and N^C are the numbers of subjects on the treatment arm and the control arm up to time t.

The criterion function is defined as follows:

$$f(x^T, x^C, N^T, N^C, \pi_T, \pi_C, \delta) = P(\pi_T - \pi_C \Sigma \delta |\ X^T = x^T, X^C = x^C, N^T, N^C)$$

where δ is the pre-specified tolerable risk difference between the two arms on the AESI. When $f(x^T, x^C, N^T, N^C, \pi_T, \pi_C, \delta) > p$, where p is the predetermined upper threshold probability, for example, $p = 0.9$, the risk is considered alarming to warrant considerations of stopping the trial due to imbalance of toxicities.

In situations when additional information regarding exposure in the form of person-time is available, Bayesian methods with the Gamma-Poisson model may be applied instead of the Beta-Binomial model.

A Hypothetical Clinical Trial Example

We apply the methods discussed in Sections 3.1 and 3.2 to a hypothetical clinical trial. Suppose there is a randomized, double blind, controlled clinical trial with planned sample size $n_{max} = 120$. Subjects will be randomized in a 1:1 ratio to the investigational drug arm or the control arm. Based on previous knowledge about the disease and the biological mechanism of action of the investigational drug, the team feels that a serious AESI is a potential risk and requires heightened surveillance. The trial has an independent DSMB.

We first consider a situation where the sponsor monitors the event of the AESI from the combined treatment arms. Suppose an increasing number of observed AESI is reported amidst rapid enrolment, but the next scheduled DSMB meeting is months away. By closely monitoring the overall event rate in the combined arms, the sponsor may be able to decide whether an ad hoc DSMB meeting is warranted. If the pre-determined monitoring boundary is crossed, the team may call the DSMB into an ad hoc session to avoid any delays in waiting for the next scheduled DSMB meeting. Assume the rate of the event from the combined group is deemed acceptable if it's no more than 5% and unacceptable if it is greater than 21%. The boundary to alert the DSMB using the SPRT method is derived using 0.05 type I error and 80% power. The boundary values for the first 10 events are shown in Table 1. For example, if three events of the AESI are observed in 11 or fewer subjects, the boundary is crossed and the team may consider convening an ad hoc DSMB meeting. The boundary values for SPRT can be obtained from the online calculation tool[19].

In addition to the SPRT, Bayesian methods can be used if some knowledge is available to form the prior distributions. We apply the TS method and assume the prior for the AESI in the control arm follows a Beta distribution with Beta (3, 57), and the prior for the AESI in the combined treatment and control group follows Beta(3, 11). Note that the distribution of Beta (3, 57) represents information from prior experiences equivalent to three events from 60 subjects. Similarly, Beta (3, 11) represents prior information equivalent to three events out of 14 subjects. Our choices for the prior distributions assume more knowledge about the control group from historical data, but less knowledge about the experimental group given limited experience. The criterion to alert the DSMB can be established as $P(\pi - \pi_S > 0.1 | i, X_i = x_i) > 0.9$. The derivation of the Bayesian safety boundary follows Section 3.1 or by using the free software Multc Lean, downloadable from the MD Anderson site [20]. The boundary values based on the Bayesian method for the first 10 events are shown in Table 1. They are also plotted in Figure 1. It can be seen that the SPRT method has boundary values that are easier to cross in declaring a safety concern than the Bayesian method, except when only two events are observed.

Table 19.1 Safety Boundary Using Blinded Data Number of Subjects

Number of Events	SPRT	TS
1	n.a.	n.a.
2	2	≤3
3	≤11	≤8
4	≤20	≤13
5	≤28	≤18
6	≤37	≤22
7	≤46	≤27
8	≤55	≤33
9	≤63	≤38
10	≤72	≤43

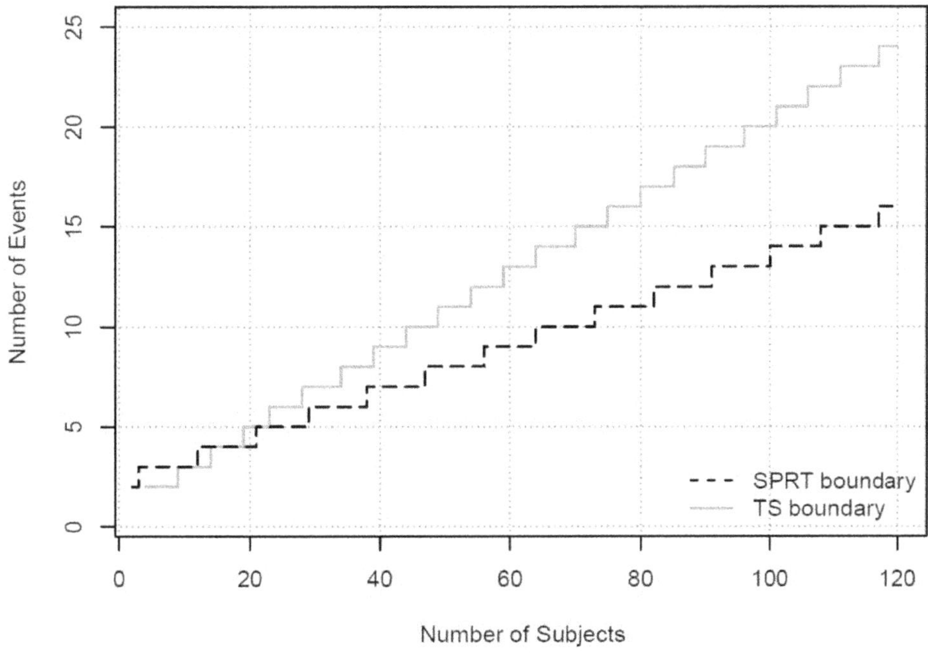

Fig.19.1 Safety Boundaries using Blinded Data.

We now consider setting up the monitoring boundary for the DSMB who has access to the actual treatment assignments. For the same AESI, the Bayesian Beta-Binomial method in Section 3.2 can be used. Assuming the prior distributions are $\pi_T \sim$ Beta (3, 11) and $\pi_C \sim$ Beta (3, 57) and applying the stopping criterion $P(\pi_T - \pi_C \Sigma 0.1 | X^T = x^T, X^C = x^C, N^T, N^C)$ Σ 0.9, the operating characteristics for such a monitoring guideline can be computed through simulations.

The Bayesian boundaries when monitoring the two arms cannot be easily plotted, but the DSMB can use a posterior probability table as a reference. In this example, there are eight subjects in the treatment arm and 11 subjects in the control arm at the analysis time. Table 2 shows the posterior probability table that summarizes the values of the criterion function

$P(\pi_T - \pi_C \Sigma 0.1 | X^T = x^T, X^C = x^C, N^T, N^C)$ under all possible scenarios. In this table, all the bolded numbers highlight the scenarios in which the stopping boundary is crossed. For instance, if at this analysis time there are 3 subjects on the treatment arm who experience the AESI, while none of the subjects on the controlarm has the AESI, then $P(\pi_T - \pi_C \Sigma 0.1 | X^T = x^T, X^C = x^C, N^T, N^C) = 0.92$ and the boundary is crossed.

Table 19.2 An Example of Posterior Probability Table.
Treatment Arm: Events/Subjects

		1/8	2/8	3/8	4/8	5/8	6/8	7/8	8/8
	0/11	0.65	0.82	**0.92**	**0.97**	**0.99**	**1**	**1**	**1**
	1/11	0.58	0.77	0.89	**0.96**	**0.98**	**1**	**1**	**1**
	2/11	0.52	0.71	0.85	**0.94**	**0.97**	**0.99**	**1**	**1**
	3/11	0.45	0.65	0.81	**0.91**	**0.96**	**0.99**	**1**	**1**
	4/11	0.39	0.59	0.76	0.88	**0.94**	**0.98**	**0.99**	**1**
	5/11	0.34	0.53	0.71	0.84	**0.93**	**0.97**	**0.99**	**1**
	6/11	0.29	0.47	0.66	0.81	0.90	**0.96**	**0.98**	**0.99**
	7/11	0.24	0.42	0.60	0.76	0.87	**0.94**	**0.97**	**0.99**
	8/11	0.21	0.37	0.55	0.71	0.84	**0.92**	**0.96**	**0.99**
	9/11	0.17	0.32	0.50	0.67	0.80	0.90	**0.95**	**0.98**
	10/11	0.14	0.27	0.44	0.61	0.76	0.87	**0.93**	**0.97**
	11/11	0.11	0.23	0.39	0.56	0.72	0.84	**0.92**	**0.96**

Monitoring patient safety during clinical trials is a critical component throughout the drug development life-cycle. Pharmaceutical sponsors must work proactively and collaboratively with all stakeholders to ensure a systematic approach to safety monitoring. The regulatory landscape has evolved with increased requirements for risk management plans, risk evaluation and minimization strategies. As the industry transitions from passive to active safety surveillance activities, there will be greater demand for more comprehensive and innovative approaches that apply quantitative methods to accumulating data from all sources, ranging from the discovery and preclinical through clinical and post-approval stages.

We have discussed several statistical methods that can be applied to monitor ongoing clinical trials in either a blinded or an unblended fashion. We recommend the Bayesian approach as the analytical framework for safety monitoring due to its flexibilities in incorporating the 'current' knowledge of the safety profile into the decision making. In addition, Bayesian methods allow sponsors to take advantage of information originating from multiple sources both internal and external to the trial. This is an important advantage, as safety signals identified in clinical trials alone may be limited. The globalization of clinical trials has posed additional challenges. A great deal of coordination is required of sponsors to ensure timely communication of new safety findings among all stakeholders in all regions. Efforts in building a standard safety data warehouse across all trials in a development program will lay a solid foundation for integrated safety analyses. Innovative statistical methods can be applied to increase the efficiency in reviewing a large volume of safety data, to identify safety trends and to establish prospective monitoring guidelines, as described in this article.

For Further Study

1. International Conference on Harmonization (ICH). Guideline for Good Clinical Practice E6(R1), 1996. Available online:

   http://www.ich.org/fileadmin/Public_Web_Site/ICH_Products/Guidelines/Efficacy/E6_R1/Step4/E6_R1 Guideline.pdf (accessed on 8 October2010).

2. Council for International Organizations of Medical Sciences (CIOMS) in collaboration with the World Health Organization (WHO). International Ethical Guidelines for Biomedical Research Involving Human Subjects. CIOMS & WHO: Geneva, Switzerland, 2002.

3. *The Declaration of Helsinki.* World Medical Association: Somerset West, South Africa, 1996.

4. European Clinical Trials Directive 2001/20/EC. Available online: http://eur-lex.europa.eu/LexUriServ/LexUriServ.do?uri=OJ:L:2001:121:0034:0044:en:PDF (accessed on 09 October2012).

5. United States Food and Drug Administration. Guidance for Industry, Premarketing Risk Assessment, 2005. Available online: http://www.fda.gov/downloads/RegulatoryInformation/Guidances/ucm126958.pdf (accessed on 09 October2012).

6. Food and Drug Administration (FDA). Guidance for Industry, Development and Use of Risk Minimization Action Plans, 2005. Available online: http://www.fda.gov/downloads/Regulatory Information/Guidances/UCM126830.pdf (accessed on 09 October2012).

7. Food and Drug Administration (FDA). Guidance for Industry, Good Pharmacovigilance Practices and Pharmaco epidemiologic Assessment, 2005. Available online: http://www.fda.gov/downloads/RegulatoryInformation/Guidances/UCM126834.pdf (accessed on 09 October2012).

8. Grady, C. Payment of Clinical Research Subjects. *J. Clin. Invest.* **2005**, *115*,1681–1687.

9. Center for Drug Evaluation and Research, Center for Biologics Evaluation and Research. Guidance for industry and investigators: Safety reporting requirements for INDs and BA/BE studies, 2010. Available online: http://www.fda.gov/downloads/Drugs/Guidance Compliance Regulatory Information/Guidances/UCM227351.pdf (accessed on 09 October2012).

10. Council for International Organizations of Medical Sciences (CIOMS) Working Group VI. Management of safety information from clinical trials. CIOMS: Geneva, Switzerland,2005.
11. Crowe, B.J.; Xia, H.A.; Berlin, J.A.; Watson, D.J.; Shi, H.; Lin, S.L.; Kuebler, J.; Schriver, R.C.; Santanello, N.C.; Rochester, G.; *et al.* Recommendations for safety planning, data collection, evaluation and reporting during drug, biologic and vaccine development: A report of the safety planning, evaluation and reporting team. *Clin. Trials* **2009**, *6*,430–440.
12. Xia, H.A.; Crowe, B.J.; Schriver, R.C.; Oster, M.; Hall, D.B. Planning and core analyses for periodic aggregate safety data reviews. *Clin. Trials* **2011**, *8*,175–182.
13. Wald, A. Sequential tests of statistical hypotheses. *Ann. Math. Stat.* **1945**, *16*,117–186.
14. Wald, A. *Sequential Analysis.* Wiley: New York, NY, USA, 1947.
15. Goldman, A.; Hannan, P. Optimal continuous sequential boundaries for monitoring toxicity in clinical trials: A restricted search algorithm. *Stat. Med.* **2001**, *20*, 1575-1589.
16. Thall, C.P.; Simon, R. Practical Bayesian guidelines for phase IIB clinical trials. *Biometrics* **1994**, *50*, 337–349.
17. Yin, G. Clinical Trial Design: Bayesian and Frequentist Adaptive Methods. Wiley, Hoboken, NJ, USA,2012.
18. Ball, G. Continuous safety monitoring for randomized controlled clinical trials with blinded treatment information. *Contemp. Clin. Trials* **2011**, *32*,S11–S17.
19. SISA. Wald's Sequential Probability. Available online: http://www.quantitativeskills.com/sisa/statistics/sprt.htm (accessed on 09 October2012).
20. MD Anderson Cancer Center, Software Download Site, Multc Lean. Available online: https://biostatistics.mdanderson.org/SoftwareDownload (accessed on 09 October2012).
21. 2013 by the authors; licensee MDPI, Basel, Switzerland. This article is an open access article distributed under the terms and conditions of the Creative Commons Attribution license (http://creativecommons.org/licenses/by/3.0/).

Chapter 20

Pharmacovigilance

Learning Objectives

To understand

- Importance of PV
- Aims of PV
- Methods used in PV
  (Dangaumou's French method, Kramer *et al.* method, Naranjo *et al.* method (Naranjo scale), Balanced assessment method, Ciba-Geigy method, Loupi*et al.* method, Roussel Uclaf causality assessment method)
- Probabilistic or Bayesian approaches
- WHO-Uppsala monitoring centre (UMC) causality assessment criteria
- Pharmacovigilance Programme of India (PvPI)
- Implementation of PvPI
- Causes of failure of implementation of pharmacovigilance in India
- Pharmacovigilance Methods
- Passive surveillance:
  (Spontaneous reports Case series Stimulated reporting)
- Active surveillance:
  (Sentinel sites Medicine event monitoring Registries Cross-sectional study (survey)
- Case-control study
- Cohort study
- Targeted clinical investigations)
- Adhoc studies
- Descriptive studies
- Natural history of disease
- Medicine utilization study
- Future aspects of pharmacovigilance in India

INTRODUCTION

Pharmacovigilance (PV), also known as drug safety, is the pharmacological science relating to the detection, assessment, understanding and prevention of adverse effects, particularly long term, and short term side effects of medicines [1]. PV is an important and integral part of clinical research [2]. The under reporting of adverse drug reactions (ADRs) is the major setback worldwide which may be attributed to the lack of time and report forms. It has been known that the world health organization (WHO) has initiated the program of reporting all adverse reactions possessed by the drugs [3]. Moreover, its concerns have been widened to include the herbal drug products, traditional and complementary medicines, blood products, biologicals, medical devices, and vaccines. In addition, PV possesses various roles such as identification, quantification, and documentation of drug-related problems which are responsible for drug-related injuries [4-5]. Further, national PV programmes have been introduced which occupies a prime role in increasing the public awareness about drug safety [6-7]. This review article explains the need and importance of PV in daily lives of doctors and patients and the pharmaceutical industry.

Importance of PV

It is the science which deals with the complex process of the understanding and explaining the nature of ADR occurred in a patient taking either oral or parenteral or intravenous (I.V) drugs for an ailment. The drugs being marketed worldwide underwent a whole array of tests and also underwent clinical trials in animals and human subjects to assess the safety of the drug for a particular disease and to know the exact side effects associated with it. Still there is a major part of it goes undetected and some of the ADR are detected in post marketing surveillance. It is estimated that there is significant amount of ADRs which decreases the quality of life, increase hospitalization stay and increases the mortality. A landmark study by Lazarouin 1998 described, ADRs to be the fourth to sixth leading cause of death in the US and ADRs are estimated to cause 3-7% of all hospital admissions[8].

Aims of PV

PV has an important role in the assessment of side effects caused by the drugs whether it is caused by oral drugs; parenteral drugs or I.V. drugs. These drugs are pretested for ADRs before it is being marketed worldwide. PV has a key role in assessment, detection and identification of drugs which caused a particular ADRs and the mechanism by which it caused the injury. But to fulfill these requirements of finding and eliminating, a side effect is the responsibility of the doctors involved in the case; nurses, health workers, residents and proper guidance of the patients themselves help it to alleviate the root cause of ADR.

Current Status and Future Prospects of Pharmacovigilance in India

Many researchers developed different methods of causality assessment of ADRs by utilizing different criteria like chronological relationship between the administration of the drug and the occurrence of the ADR, screening for non-drug related causes, confirmation of the reaction by *in vivo* or *in vitro* tests, and antecedent information on homogeneous events attributed to the suspect drug or to its therapeutic class, etc., to define ADRs in different categories[9]. Currently, there is no universally accepted method for assessing causality of ADRs [10]. Currently, there are many algorithmic methods of causality assessment but no single algorithm is accepted as the gold standard because of the shortcomings and discordances that subsist between them [11]. We would explicate them in short as listed below.

Dangaumou's French Method [12]

This rule of thumb has been used by the French government agency since 1977. The way of doing thing separates an intrinsic imputability (possible case between abused substance and dispassionate event) from an extrinsic imputability (bibliographical data) by the agency of seven criteria (three connected and four semiological) in two different tables. The criteria are (i) drug challenge, (ii) dechallenge, and (iii) rechallenge by the overall score of four possible categories. The semiological criteria are (i) semiology (clinical signs) using per se (suggestive or other), (ii) favoring component, (iii) arbitrary non-drug- related (none or possible), and (iv) laboratory tests show with three possible outcomes (positive, negative or no test for the event-drug pair). Scores are grouped as possible and dubious.

Kramer *et al.* Method [13]

This method applies when the offending drug is administered and a single adverse drug even thus taken place. Each adverse event is assessed independently and assessment is prepared. One of the advantages of this algorithm is its transparency. However, certain levels of experience, expertise, and time are required to use this method effectively.

Naranjo *et al.* method (Naranjo scale) [14]

It is utilized to verify causality in a variety of clinical situations utilizing the categories and definitions of definite, probable, possible, and doubtful. It consists of ten questions which are answered as yes, no and unknown. The event is assigned to a probability category predicated on the total score after totaling. A total score of $\geq$9 is definite, probable is 5-8, possible is 1-4 and doubtful $\geq$ 0. This scale is more powerful when the adverse event is associated with only one drug, but when multiple drugs are involved or there is any interactions between drugs, this scale fails to identify the offending agent.

Balanced assessment method [15]

This method evaluates a case report on various visual analog scale (VAS) models that each criterion is fulfilled individually. It has an added advantage that it considers an alternative causative factor as a possibility and not just as a separate factor. Each case is assessed independently by different assessors and the evaluation depends on the assessor's skills knowledge.

Expert consensus meetings have resulted in Ciba-Geigy method. Experts used their clinical judgment to assess adverse drug events and assign causality on a VAS. This method uses a checklist which is composed of 23 questions, which is split into three sections: (i) History of present adverse reaction, (ii) patient's past adverse-reaction history, and (iii) monitoring-physician's experience. This updated method was found to have a high degree of agreement (62%) when compared with evaluator's assessments.

Loupi*et al.* method [17]

This method developed to assess the teratogenic potential of drug. The first sections of the algorithm sanction for the drug to be omitted if not implicated in the inception of the abnormality. The second section weighs the bibliographical data. The three questions consider alternative etiological candidates other than the drug; chronology of the suspect drug and other bibliographical data, to arrive at a conclusion on causality.

Roussel Uclaf causality assessment method [9]

This method is used in disease states such as liver and dermatological problems. Aretrospect assessment of there producibility of this method among four experts had showed a 37-99% agreementrate.

Australian method [18]

Australian method involves the evidence which helps in to draw the conclusion, such as timing, and laboratory information from case reports presented and the antecedent cognizance on the suspect drug profile is deliberately omitted in the assessment.

Probabilistic or Bayesian Approaches

It utilizes concrete findings in a case to transform a prior into a posterior probability of drug causation [19]. The prior probability is calculated from epidemiological information and the posterior probability cumulates this background information with the evidence in the individual case. It is open-ended approach with no circumscription to the amount of case details that can be assessed utilizing this method. Simultaneous assessment of multiple causes can be assessed[20]. WHO-Uppsala monitoring centre (UMC) causality assessment criteria [21]

The WHO-UMC causality assessment method includes the following criteria

- Certain-adverse event and the time relationship associated with it
- Probable/likely-unlikely to attribute the other drugs or diseases
- Possible-this can be explained by the drug intake or another disease
- Unlikely-adverse event can be explained with the time relationship associated with it but its not impossible
- Conditional/unclassified-more data in needed to make a proper assessment
- Unassessable/unclassifiable-an adverse event is suggested but more data are needed to make an assessment.

PV remains a dynamic part of the clinicians and the general population. After the appearance of these adverse drugs effects, it is very essential that these are reported timely and analyzed. Not only the doctors should be aware of the PV programme but the patients themselves should be made aware of this so self-reporting is increased and the burden on the clinicians is also reduced. India is still in the growing phase of PV and more reporting is necessary to reach the world's standard of reporting these adverse events to provide effective drug use in children's and pregnant women which is one of the most vulnerable populations of all. The PV programme must be able to identify these adverse events timely in the coming years with the help of clinicians, patients, and the pharmaceutical industry to help shape the safety of patients themselves.

Pharmacovigilance Programme of India

Introduction

The world health organization (WHO) initiated a program for reporting all adverse reactions possessed by drugs. Further awareness about adverse drug reactions has resulted in the emergence of the practice and science of pharmacovigilance.[1] The word pharmacovigilance is derived from the Greek word pharmacon meaning 'drug' and the Latin word vigilare meaning 'to keep awake or alert, to keep watch.' Pharmacovigilance is defined as "the pharmacological science relating to the recognition, assessment, understanding and prevention of adverse effects, particularly long term and short term adverse effects of medicines." [2, 3] After discovery and pre-clinical phases, a drug typically undergoes trials in human volunteers. Clinical trials are highly regulated and closely monitored by the investigators and the manufacturing company. It is a mandatory regulatory requirement to report all the adverse events in a clinical trial setting in a given time frame. In the clinical trial setting, "good clinical practice" has moved pharmacovigilance from a reactive to a proactive approach. A robust, well-defined system for monitoring adverse events is in a place for evaluating the safety of the drugs. [4] Pharmacovigilance serves various roles such as identification, quantification and documentation of drug-related problems which are responsible for drug-related injuries. [5, 6]

India is the world's second most populated country with over one billion potential drug consumers. Although, India is participating in the Uppsala monitoring center program, its contribution to this database is relatively small. This problem is essentially due to the absence of a robust adverse drug reaction monitoring system and also the lack of awareness of reporting concepts among Indian health care professionals. In India, it is very important to focus the attention of the medical community on the importance of adverse drug reporting to ensure maximum benefits for public health and safety. For regulatory reporting purposes, if an event is instinctively reported, even if the relationship is mysterious or unstated, it meets the definition of an adverse drug reaction.

An adverse event is any untoward medical occurrence in a patient who is administered a medicinal product and which doesn't necessarily have a causal relationship with this treatment. Adverse drug reactions are noxious and unintended responses to a medicinal product. A reaction, in contrast to an event, is characterized by the fact that a causal relationship between the drug and the occurrence are supposed. [7, 8]

A serious adverse event (SAE) is any untoward medical manifestation, that at any dose:

- Results in death
- Is life-threatening (well-defined as an event in which the subject was at risk of death at the time of the event)
- Requires in-patient hospitalization or causes prolongation of existing hospitalization
- Results in persistent or significant disability/incapacity
- Is a congenital anomaly/birth defect
- Is an important medical event (defined as a medical event(s) that may not be immediately life-threatening or result in death or hospitalization but, based upon suitable medical & scientific judgment, may require intervention to prevent one of the serious outcomes as listed above). [9, 10]

This review article provides a brief overview of the current situation and the future prospects of pharmacovigilance in India.

The Pharmacovigilance exertion in India is organized by The Indian Pharmacopoeia Commission and conducted by the Central Drugs Standard Control Organization (CDSCO). The main responsibility of the IPC is to maintain and develop the pharmacovigilance database consisting of all suspected serious adverse reactions to medicines observed. Indian Pharmacopoeia Commission (IPC) is functioning as a National Coordination Centre (NCC) for Pharmacovigilance Programme of India (PvPI). National Coordination Centre is operating under the observation of steering committee which recommends procedures and guidelines for regulatory interventions. The main duty of National Coordination Centre is to monitor all the adverse reactions of medicines being observed in the Indian population and to develop and maintain its own pharmacovigilance database.

Pharmacovigilance Programme of India (PvPI)

The Central Drugs Standard Control Organization (CDSCO), Directorate General of Health Services under the aegis of Ministry of Health & Family Welfare, Government of India in association with Indian Pharmacopeia commission, Ghaziabad is initiating a nation-wide Pharmacovigilance Programme for protecting the health of the patients by promising drug safety. The Programme shall be coordinated by the Indian Pharmacopeia commission, Ghaziabad as a National Coordinating Centre (NCC). The center will operate under the supervision of a Steering Committee.

The Pharmacovigilance Programme of India (PvPI) was started by the Government of India on 14th July 2010 with the All India Institute of Medical Sciences (AIIMS), New Delhi as the National Coordination Centre for monitoring Adverse Drug

Reactions (ADRs) in the country for safe-guarding Public Health. In the year 2010, 22 ADR monitoring centres including AIIMS, New Delhi was set up under this Programme. To safeguard implementation of this programme in a more effective way, the National Coordination Centre was shifted from the All India Institute of Medical Sciences (AIIMS), New Delhi to the Indian Pharmacopoeia Commission, Ghaziabad, Uttar Pradesh on 15th April 2011.

Before registration and marketing of medicine in the country, its safety and efficacy experience is based chiefly on the use of the medicine in clinical trials. These trials primarily detect common adverse reactions. Some important reactions, such as those, which take a long time to develop, or those, which occur rarely, may not be detected in clinical trials. In addition, the controlled conditions under which medicines are used in clinical trials do not necessarily reflect the way they will be used in practice. For a medicine to be considered safe, its predictable benefits should be greater than any associated risks of harmful reactions. So, in order to gain a complete safety profile of medicine, a continuous post-marketing monitoring system i.e. pharmacovigilance is essential. In order to screen the safety of medicine, information from many sources is used for pharmacovigilance. These include spontaneous (ADRs) reporting mechanism; medical literature published worldwide, action taken by regulatory authorities in other countries, etc. Meanwhile there exist considerable social and economic consequences of adverse drug reactions and the positive benefit/cost ratio of employing appropriate risk management (there is a need to engage healthcare professionals and the public at large, in a well -structured programme to build synergies for monitoring adverse drug reactions in the country). The purpose of the PvPI is to collate data, process and analyze it and use the inferences to recommend regulatory interventions, besides communicating risks to healthcare professionals and the public.

Mission: Safeguard the health of the Indian population by ensuring that the benefits of use of medicine outweigh the risks associated with its use.

Vision: To improve patient safety and welfare in Indian population by monitoring the drug safety and thereby reducing the risk associated with use of medicines.

Objectives

- To create a nation-wide system for patient safety reporting
- To identify and analyze the new signal (ADR) from the reported cases
- To analyses the benefit - risk ratio of marketed medications
- To generate the evidence based information on safety of medicines
- To support regulatory agencies in the decision-making process on use of medications
- To communicate the safety information on use of medicines to various stakeholders to minimize the risk
- To emerge as a national center of excellence for pharmacovigilance activities
- To collaborate with other national centers for the exchange of information and data management
- To provide training and consultancy support to other national pharmacovigilance centers located across globe[11]

Implementation of PvPI

IPC assumed the need for establishing local hospital based centers across the nation for the better patient safety. It was significant to monitor both the known and previously unknown side effects of medicines in order to determine any new information available in relation to their safety profile. In an enormous country like India with a population of over 1.2 billion and with vast ethnic variability, different disease prevalence patterns, practice of different systems of medicines, different socioeconomic status, it was imperative to have a standardized and robust pharmacovigilance and drug safety monitoring programme for the nation.

Short term goals

- To develop and implement pharmacovigilance system in India
- To enroll, initially, all MCI approved medical colleges in the program covering north, south, east and west of India
- To encourage healthcare professionals in reporting of adverse reaction to drugs, vaccines, medical devices and biological products
- Collection of case reports and data

Long term goals

- To expand the pharmacovigilance programme to all hospitals (govt. & private) and centers of public health programs located across India
- To develop and implement electronic reporting system (e-reporting)
- To develop reporting culture amongst healthcare professionals
- To make ADR reporting mandatory for healthcare professionals

Effective communication channels are the key to a successful running of PvPI. The Indian pharmacopoeia commission was summarized in Figure 1. Program communications is described in Figure 2 and ADR monitoring centers are displayed in Figure 3. The functions of the ADR monitoring center are shown in Figure 4 with regional resources for training in India summarized in figure 5. The process of collection, analysis and evaluation of ADRs are described in Figure 6.

Causes of failure of Implementation of Pharmacovigilance in India

Many new drugs are being introduced in the country, so there is a need to improve the pharmacovigilance system in order to protect the Indian population from potential harm that may be caused by some of the new drugs. However, there are numerous issues and problems that have prevented building a robust pharmacovigilance system, which are described below:

1. Pharmacovigilance systems are not well-funded and systematized for a vast country like India to serve patients and the public.
2. The data obtained to date in the zonal centers from various peripheral centers is often poor and not well-analyzed. There is inadequate research on ADRs in India, so the exact incidence of specific ADRs is unknown.
3. Involvement of healthcare professionals (both in rural areas and urban cities and hospitals) and knowledge and motivation for pharmacovigilance is negligible. There little encouragement from the department of health to provide more training and create more awareness amongst them for better reporting.
4. In India, there are several consumers' groups who encourage patients to report any adverse reactions encountered by them, although there is no information for patients to report ADRs directly to the regulatory authority.

Pharmacovigilance Methods

Passive surveillance:

- encompasses all spontaneous AEFI reporting
- from immunization service providers / hospitals / patients
- up to next levels: state/territory then national (TGA) and then global

Active surveillance:

- primarily used for characterization of the AEFI profile, rates and risk factors
- logistical and resource constraints limit wide application
- only for selected AEFI at selected institutions (sentinel) sites
- can also be carried out in the community setting (e.g. cohort event monitoring)

Adhoc studies:

- epidemiological studies (e.g. cohort study, case-control study, case series studies)
- focus on selected vaccine safety concerns (e.g. testing causality hypotheses)
- retrospective or prospective

I. Passive surveillance

a) **Spontaneous reports:** A spontaneous report is a voluntary communication by healthcare professionals or consumers to a company, regulatory authority or other organization that defines one or more adverse drug reactions (ADRs) in a patient who was given one or more medicinal products and that does not originate from a study or any structured data collection scheme. [12] It plays a key role in the identification of safety signals once a medicine is marketed. In various occurrences, spontaneous reports can vigilant a company to rare adverse events that were not noticed in earlier clinical trials or other pre-marketing studies. It can also deliver important information on at -risk groups, risk factors and clinical features of known serious ADRs. [13-16]

Newly, systematic methods for the recognition of safety signals from spontaneous reports have begun to be used. Several of these methods are static in development and their utility for identifying safety signals is being assessed. These methods include the calculation of the proportional reporting ratio, as well as the use of Bayesian and other techniques for signal detection. [17-19] Data mining techniques have also been used to examine medicine-medicine interactions [20], but these techniques should always be used in conjunction with, and not in place of, analyses of single case-reports. Data mining techniques facilitate the evaluation of spontaneous reports by using statistical methods to detect potential signals that merit further evaluation. However, this tool does not quantify the magnitude of risk, and caution should be exercised when comparing medicines. Further, when using data mining techniques, consideration should be given to the threshold established for detecting signals, since this will have implications for the sensitivity and specificity of the method (a high threshold is associated with high specificity and low sensitivity). Confounding factors that influence reporting of spontaneous adverse events are not removed from data mining. The results of data mining should thus be interpreted with the knowledge of the weaknesses of the spontaneous reporting system and, more specifically, the large differences in the ADR reporting rate for different medicines and the many potential biases inherent in spontaneous reporting. All signals should be evaluated while recognizing the possibility of false-positives. In addition, the absence of a signal does not mean that a problem does not exist.

b) **Case series:** A series of case-reports can deliver signs of an association between a medicine and an adverse event, but they are normally more valuable for producing theories than for confirming a relationship between medicine exposure and outcome. [21, 22]

c) **Stimulated reporting:** A number of methods have been used to reassure and simplify reporting by health professionals in definite circumstances for new products or for partial time periods. [23] Such systems comprise on-line reporting of adverse events and methodical motivation of reporting of adverse events based on a pre-designed method. While these methods have been shown to advance reporting, they are not invulnerable to the confines of passive surveillance, particularly discriminating reporting and imperfect information. This should be considered as a procedure of spontaneous event reporting, and thus data acquired from stimulated reporting cannot be used to make precise incidence rates, but reporting rates can be projected.

II) Active surveillance

Active surveillance, in contrast to passive surveillance, pursues to determine the particular number of adverse events through a constant pre-organized process. [24] In common, it is more achievable to acquire wide-ranging data on discrete adverse event reports through an active surveillance system than through a passive reporting system.

a) Sentinel sites: Active surveillance can be attained by revising medical records or questioning patients and/or physicians in a section of sentinel sites to guarantee that comprehensive and precise data on reported adverse events are collected from these sites. The selected sites can deliver information, such as data from specific patient subgroups, which would not be accessible in a passive spontaneous reporting system. [25] The major weaknesses of sentinel sites comprise difficulties with selection bias, small numbers of patients and augmented costs. Active surveillance with sentinel sites is most effective for those medicines used primarily in institutional settings such as hospitals, nursing homes and haemodialysis centers. Institutional settings may use certain medicinal products more commonly and can deliver an arrangement for enthusiastic reporting. Intensive monitoring of sentinel sites can also be supportive in recognizing risks among patients taking orphan medicines followed over time and included in a cohort study to collect data on adverse events using standardized questionnaires. Single cohort studies can quantity incidence, but, without a comparison group, cannot deliver proof of association. This type of registry can be very valuable when examining the safety of an orphan medicine indicated for a specific condition. Customary epidemiological methods are a key constituent in the evaluation of adverse events. There are numerous of observational study designs that are valuable in validating signals from spontaneous reports, case series or medicine event monitoring. The most imperative of these designs is cross -sectional studies, case-control studies and cohort studies. 33' [34]

d) Cross-sectional study (survey)

b) Medicine event monitoring

This is a process of active Pharmacovigilance surveillance. Studies using this process are cohort-based and prospective and observational. For medication event monitoring, patients can be acknowledged from electronic or automated health insurance claims. A single prescription or a series might be composed over the period of monitoring. A follow-up questionnaire can then be sent to each prescribing physician or patient at pre-specified intervals to acquire outcome data. Requests for data on patient demographics, indication for treatment, duration of therapy, dosage, clinical events, reasons for termination and applicable past history can be involved in the questionnaires. 26-30 The restrictions of medicine event monitoring can comprise the poor physician and patient reply rates. 31, 32.

c) Registries:

A registry is a list of patients presenting with the identical representative(s). This representative can be a disease (disease registry) or a specific exposure (medicine registry). Both types of registrations, which vary only by the type of patient data of interest, can gather a cordless of information using standardized questionnaires in a prospective fashion. Disease registries, such as registries for blood dyscrasias, severe cutaneous reactions, or congenital malformations can help to gather data on medicine exposure and other factors related to a clinical condition. A disease registry might also be used as a veil for a case control study associating the medicine exposure of cases recognized from the registry with controls selected either from patients with another condition within the registry, or from patients outside the registry. Exposure (medicine) registries address populations exposed to the medicines of interest to govern if a medicine has a distinct influence on this group of patients. Some exposure (medicine) registries address drug exposures in specific populations, such as pregnant women.

e) Case-control study

In a case-control study, cases of disease (or events) are recognized. Controls, or patients in whom the disease or event of interest has not happened, are then carefully chosen from the source population that gave rise to the cases. The controls should be selected in such a way that the prevalence of exposure among the controls exemplifies the prevalence of exposure in the source population. The exposure status of the two groups is then paralleled using the odds ratio, which is an estimate of the relative risk of disease in the two groups. Patients can be acknowledged from an existing database or using data collected unambiguously for the purpose of the study. If safety data is sought for special populations, the cases and controls can be stratified according to the population of interest. For rare adverse events, prevailing large population-based databases are a useful and efficient means of providing the necessary data on medicine exposure and medical outcome relatively quickly. Case-control studies are predominantly useful when the goal is to examine whether there is a relationship between a medicine (or medicines) and one specific rare adverse event, as well as to identify risk factors for adverse events. Risk factors can include conditions, such as renal and hepatic dysfunction, which might modify the relationship between the medicine exposure and the adverse event. Under particular conditions, a case-control study can deliver the complete incidence rate of the event.

f) Cohort study

In a cohort study, a population at risk for the disease (or event) is monitored over time to record the occurrence of the disease (or event). Information on exposure status is accessible during the follow-up period for each patient. A patient might be exposed to a medicine at one time during follow-up, but not exposed at another time. Meanwhile the population exposure during follow-up is acknowledged, incidence rates can be calculated. In many cohort studies concerning medicine exposure, appraisal cohorts of interest are selected on the basis of medicine use and monitored over time. Cohort studies are useful when there is a requisite to know the incidence rates of adverse events in addition to the relative risks. Multiple adverse events can also be scrutinized using the similar data source in a cohort study. Conversely, it can be problematic to recruit adequate numbers of patients who are exposed to the medicine of interest or to study very rare outcomes. Similar to case-control studies, patients in cohort studies can be recognized from large automated databases or from data collected precisely for the study at hand. In addition, cohort studies can be used to scrutinize safety issues in special populations through oversampling of these patients or by stratifying the cohort if adequate numbers of patients are included. There are numerous automated databases obtainable for pharmaco epidemiological studies.35, 36, 37 They consist of databases that contain automated medical records or automated accounting/billing systems. Databases that are fashioned from accounting/billing systems might be connected to pharmacy claims and medical claims databases. These datasets may contain millions of patients. Subsequently, they are fashioned for administrative or billing purposes; they might not have all the detailed and precise information needed for some research, such as authenticated diagnostic information or laboratory data. Even though medical records can be used to establish and authenticate test results and medical diagnoses, one should know about the privacy and privacy regulations that apply to patient medical records.

g) Targeted clinical investigations

When significant risks are identified from pre-approval clinical trials, further clinical studies might be called in to evaluate the mechanism of action for the adverse reaction. In some instances, pharmacodynamics and pharmacokinetic studies might be conducted to define whether a particular dosing instruction can put patients at an increased risk of adverse events. Moreover, based on the pharmacological properties and the predictable use of the medicine in general practice, conducting specific studies to scrutinize potential medicine-medicine interactions and food-medicine interactions might be entitled to. These studies can comprise population pharmacokinetics studies and medicine concentration monitoring in patients and normal volunteers. One drawback of this method is that the outcome measure might be too shortened and this might have an influence on the quality and eventual usefulness of the results of the trial. Large, simplified trials are similarly resource-intensive.

Descriptive Studies

Descriptive studies are a vital component of Pharmacovigilance, even though not for the recognition or authentication of adverse events related to medicine exposures. These studies are principally used to acquire the circumstantial rate of outcome events and/or to inaugurate the prevalence of the use of medicines in specified populations.

a) Natural history of disease

The discipline of epidemiology initially concentrated on the natural history of disease, including the features of diseased patients and the dissemination of disease, in particular populations, as well as appraising the incidence and prevalence of possible outcomes of interest. These outcomes of interest currently comprise a narrative of disease treatment outlines and adverse events. Studies that scrutinize precise facts of adverse events, such as the contextual incidence rate of, or risk factors for, the adverse event of interest, can assist in placing spontaneous reports into viewpoint. 38

b) Medicine utilization study

Medicine utilization studies (DUS) define how a medicine is marketed, prescribed and used in a population, and how these factors affect outcomes (including clinical, social and economic outcomes). 39 These studies deliver data on definite populations, such as the elderly, children, or patients with hepatic or renal dysfunction, habitually stratified by age, sex, concomitant medication and other characteristics. It can be used to define if a product is being used in these populations. It has been used to define the effect of regulatory actions and media courtesy on the use of medicines, as well as to improve evaluations of the economic burden of the cost of medicines. It can also be used to scrutinize the relationship between optional and definite clinical practice. These studies can help to govern whether a medicine has the probable for abuse by inspecting whether patients are taking mounting doses or whether there is an indication of incorrect duplication

Future aspects of Pharmacovigilance in India

A suitably working pharmacovigilance system is vital if medicines are to be used safely. It will advantage all parties including healthcare professionals, regulatory authorities, pharmaceutical companies and the consumers. It aids pharmaceutical companies to monitor their medicines for risk and to devise and implement effective risk management plans to save their drugs in difficult circumstances. Having considered the problems and challenges facing the development of a robust pharmacovigilance system for India, the following proposals 40 might be follows:

- Making pharmacovigilance reporting mandatory and introducing pharmacovigilance inspections.
- High-level discussions with various stakeholders
- Creating a single country-specific adverse event reporting form to be used by all.
- Creating a clinical trial and post marketing database for SAEs / SUSARs and ADRs for signal detection and access to all relevant data from various stakeholders.
- List all new drugs / indications by maintaining a standard database for every pharmaceutical company.
- Education and training of medical students pharmacists and nurses in the area of pharmacovigilance.
- Collaborating with pharmacovigilance organizations in enhancing drug safety with advancements in information technology, there has been the emergence of new opportunities for national and international collaborations.
- Building a network of pharmacovigilance and pharmacoepidemiologic in India.
- Pharmacovigilance systems are needed to safeguard public health. Diminutive prominence has been put into engendering information that can assist a healthcare professional or a patient in medication decision-making processes. The collecting and dissemination of this information is a chief goal of Pharmacovigilance.

For Further Study

1. Pipasha B, Biswas A K. Setting standards for proactive pharmacovigilance in India: The way forward. Indian J Pharmacol 2007; 39(3):124-8.
2. WHO. Pharmacovigilance: Ensuring the Safe Use of Medicines. Geneva: WHO;2004.
3. WHO. Policy Perspectives on Medicines. Geneva: WHO; 2004.
4. SkalliS, Soulaymani Bencheikh R. Safety monitoring of herb-drug interactions: A component of pharmacovigilance. Drug Saf2012;35(10):785-91.
5. ArnottJ, HesselgreavesH, NunnAJ, Peak M, Pirmohamed M, Smyth RL, *et al.* What can we learn from parents about enhancing participation in pharmacovigilance? Br J Clin Pharmacol2013;75(4):1109-17.
6. Gerritsen R, Faddegon H, DijkersF, van Grootheest K, van Puijenbroek E. Effectiveness of pharmacovigilance training of general practitioners: A

retrospective cohort study in the Netherlands comparing two methods. Drug Saf2011;34(9):755-62.

7. Kshirsagar N, Ferner R, Figueroa BA, Ghalib H, Lazdin J.Pharmacovigilance methods in public health programmes: The example of miltefosine and visceral leishmaniasis. Trans RSoc Trop Med Hyg2011;105(2):61-7.
8. LazarouJ, Pomeranz BH, CoreyPN. Incidence of adverse drug reactions in hospitalized patients: A meta-analysis of prospective studies. JAMA 1998;279(15):1200-5.
9. Danan G, Benichou C. Causality assessment of adverse reactions to drugs--I. A novel method based on the conclusions of international consensus meetings: Application to drug-induced liver injuries. J Clin Epidemiol1993;46(11):1323-30.
10. Agbabiaka TB, SavovicJ, Ernst E. Methods for causality assessment of adverse drug reactions: A systematic review. DrugSaf2008;31(1):21-37.
11. Macedo AF, Marques FB, Ribeiro CF, TexeiraF. Causality assessment of adverse drug reactions: Comparison of the results obtained from published decisional algorithms and from the evaluations of an expert panel. Pharmacoepidemiol Drug Saf2005;14(12):885-90.
12. Dangoumau J, Evreux JC, Jouglard J. Mehtod for determination of undesirable effects of drugs. Therapie1978;33(3):373-81.
13. KramerMS, Leventhal JM, Hutchinson TA, Feinstein AR. Analgorithm for the operational assessment of adverse drug reactions. I. Background, description, and instructions for use. JAMA1979;242(7):623-32.
14. Naranjo CA, Busto U, Sellers EM, Sandor P, Ruiz I, Roberts EA, *et al.* A method for estimating the probability of adverse drug reactions. Clin Pharmacol Ther1981;30(2):239-45.
15. Lagier G, VincensM, Castot A. Imputability in drug monitoring. Principles of the balanced drug reaction assessment method and principal errors to avoid. Therapie1983;38(3):303-18.
16. VenuletJ, Ciucci A, Berneker GC. Standardized assessment of drug-adverse reaction associations – Rationale and experience. Int J Clin Pharmacol Ther Toxicol 1980;18(9):381-8.
17. Loupi E, Ponchon AC, VentreJJ, Evreux JC. Imputability of a teratogenic effect. Therapie1986;41(3):207-10.
18. Mashford ML. The Australian method of drug-event assessment. Special workshop – regulatory. Drug Inf J1984;18(3-4):271-3.

19. Hutchinson TA. Computerized Bayesian ADE assessment. Drug Inf J 1991;25:235-41.
20. Hutchinson TA, Dawid AP, Spiegel halter DJ, Cowell RG, Roden S. Computerized aids for probabilistic assessment of drug safety: I. A spreadsheet program. Drug Inf J1991;25:29-39.
21. World Health Organization (WHO), Uppsala Monitoring Centre. The use of the WHO-UMC System for Standardized Case Causality Assessment. Available from: http://www.who-umc.org/graphics/4409.pdf.7

www.ingramcontent.com/pod-product-compliance
Ingram Content Group UK Ltd.
Pitfield, Milton Keynes, MK11 3LW, UK
UKHW052227270726
14060UKWH00004B/644

9 789391 910518